I0470857

Comparative Effectiveness Review
Number 82

Bariatric Surgery and Nonsurgical Therapy in Adults With Metabolic Conditions and a Body Mass Index of 30.0 to 34.9 kg/m²

Prepared for:
Agency for Healthcare Research and Quality
U.S. Department of Health and Human Services
540 Gaither Road
Rockville, MD 20850
www.ahrq.gov

Contract No. 290-2007-10062-I

Prepared by:
Southern California Evidence-based Practice Center
Santa Monica, CA

Investigators:
Margaret A. Maglione, M.P.P.
Melinda Maggard Gibbons, M.D.
Masha Livhits, M.D.
Brett Ewing, M.S.
Jianhui Hu, M.P.P.
Alicia Ruelaz Maher, M.D.
Zhaoping Li, M.D. Ph.D.
Tanja Perry, B.H.M.
Paul G. Shekelle, M.D., Ph.D.

AHRQ Publication No. 12(13)-EHC139-EF
June 2013

Addendum - Bariatric Surgery and Nonsurgical Therapy in Adults With Metabolic Conditions and a Body Mass Index of 30.0 to 34.9 kg/m²

As part of the preparation of a paper to appear in the Journal of the American Medical Association (JAMA), we added to our analysis two additional elements:

1. We updated our literature search through September 2012. This resulted in including eight additional surgical observational studies (1-8 below).
2. We attempted to compare the weight loss and glucose control outcomes of bariatric surgery with nonsurgical therapy in the two RCTs that directly compared these in patients with diabetes for only those patients with a body mass index (BMI) of 30.0 to 34.9 kg/m². The mean baseline BMI was 37.0 kg/m² in both RCTs. For the trial reported by Schauer and colleagues, we used the results of an analysis presented as supplemental material with their original publication. This analysis found no statistically significant evidence that the study outcomes differed in patients above and below the mean BMI of 37 kg/m². For the trial reported by Dixon and colleagues, we obtained patient-level data from the authors, and compared weight loss and glucose outcomes in the 13 patients included in that trial that had a BMI of less than 35 kg/m². There were statistically significantly better weight loss and glucose control outcomes in the patients treated with bariatric surgery compared to those treated nonsurgically.

These additions did not change our conclusions regarding the effectiveness and safety bariatric surgery in this population.

For further information, see:

Maggard-Gibbons M, Maglione M, Livhits M, et al. Bariatric surgery for weight loss and glycemic control in nonmorbidly obese adults with diabetes: a systematic review. JAMA. 2013 June 5;309(21):2250-2261. DOI 10.1001/jama.2013.4851.

References:

1. Abbatini F, Capoccia D, Casella G, Coccia F, Leonetti F, Basso N. Type 2 diabetes in obese patients with body mass index of 30-35 kg/m²: sleeve gastrectomy versus medical treatment. Surg Obes Relat Dis. 2012 Jan-Feb;8 (1):20-4. PMID 21924686.

2. Boza C, Munoz R, Salinas J, et al. Safety and efficacy of Roux-en-Y gastric bypass to treat type 2 diabetes mellitus in non-severely obese patients. Obes Surg. 2011 Sep;21 (9):1330-6. PMID 21744283.

3. Cohen RV, Pinheiro JC, Schiavon CA, Salles JE, Wajchenberg BL, Cummings DE. Effects of gastric bypass surgery in patients with type 2 diabetes and only mild obesity. Diabetes Care. 2012 Jul;35 (7):1420-8. PMID 22723580.

4. Gianos M, Abdemur A, Fendrich I, Gari V, Szomstein S, Rosenthal RJ. Outcomes of bariatric surgery in patients with body mass index <35 kg/m². Surg Obes Relat Dis. 2012 Jan-Feb;8 (1):25-30. PMID 22019140.

5. Kim MK, Lee HC, Lee SH, et al. The difference of glucostatic parameters according to the remission of diabetes after Roux-en-Y gastric bypass. Diabetes Metab Res Rev. 2012 Jul;28 (5):439-46. PMID 22407971.

6. Lee WJ, Hur KY, Lakadawala M, Kasama K, Wong SK, Lee YC. Gastrointestinal metabolic surgery for the treatment of diabetic patients: a multi-institutional international study. J Gastrointest Surg. 2012 Jan;16 (1):45-51; discussion -2. PMID 22042564.

7. Sun ZC, Yu WS, Na Y, et al. Modified Roux-en-Y gastric bypass for type 2 diabetes mellitus in China. Hepatogastroenterology. 2012 Jul 25;60 (121) PMID 22829557.

8. Zhu L, Mo Z, Yang X, et al. Effect of laparoscopic Roux-en-Y gastroenterostomy with BMI < 35 kg/m^2 in type 2 diabetes mellitus. Obes Surg. 2012 Oct;22 (10):1562-7. PMID 22692669.

This report is based on research conducted by the Southern California Evidence-based Practice Center (EPC) under contract to the Agency for Healthcare Research and Quality (AHRQ), Rockville, MD (Contract No. 290-2007-10062-I). The findings and conclusions in this document are those of the author(s), who are responsible for its contents; the findings and conclusions do not necessarily represent the views of AHRQ. Therefore, no statement in this report should be construed as an official position of AHRQ or of the U.S. Department of Health and Human Services.

The information in this report is intended to help health care decisionmakers—patients and clinicians, health system leaders, and policymakers, among others—make well-informed decisions and thereby improve the quality of health care services. This report is not intended to be a substitute for the application of clinical judgment. Anyone who makes decisions concerning the provision of clinical care should consider this report in the same way as any medical reference and in conjunction with all other pertinent information, i.e., in the context of available resources and circumstances presented by individual patients.

This report may be used, in whole or in part, as the basis for development of clinical practice guidelines and other quality enhancement tools, or as a basis for reimbursement and coverage policies. AHRQ or U.S. Department of Health and Human Services endorsement of such derivative products may not be stated or implied.

Persons using assistive technology may not be able to fully access information in this report. For assistance, contact EffectiveHealthCare@ahrq.hhs.gov.

None of the investigators have any affiliations or financial involvement that conflicts with the material presented in this report.

Suggested citation: Maglione MA, Maggard Gibbons M, Livhits M, Ewing B, Hu J, Ruelaz Maher A, Li Z, Perry T, Shekelle PG. Bariatric Surgery and Nonsurgical Therapy in Adults With Metabolic Conditions and a Body Mass Index of 30.0 to 34.9 kg/m². Comparative Effectiveness Review No. 82. (Prepared by the Southern California Evidence-based Practice Center under Contract No. 290-2007-10062-I.) AHRQ Publication No. 12(13)-EHC139-EF. Rockville, MD: Agency for Healthcare Research and Quality. June 2013. www.effectivehealthcare.ahrq.gov/reports/final.cfm.

Preface

The Agency for Healthcare Research and Quality (AHRQ), through its Evidence-based Practice Centers (EPCs), sponsors the development of systematic reviews to assist public- and private-sector organizations in their efforts to improve the quality of health care in the United States. These reviews provide comprehensive, science-based information on common, costly medical conditions, and new health care technologies and strategies.

Systematic reviews are the building blocks underlying evidence-based practice; they focus attention on the strength and limits of evidence from research studies about the effectiveness and safety of a clinical intervention. In the context of developing recommendations for practice, systematic reviews can help clarify whether assertions about the value of the intervention are based on strong evidence from clinical studies. For more information about AHRQ EPC systematic reviews, see www.effectivehealthcare.ahrq.gov/reference/purpose.cfm

AHRQ expects that these systematic reviews will be helpful to health plans, providers, purchasers, government programs, and the health care system as a whole. Transparency and stakeholder input are essential to the Effective Health Care Program. Please visit the Web site (www.effectivehealthcare.ahrq.gov) to see draft research questions and reports or to join an email list to learn about new program products and opportunities for input.

We welcome comments on this systematic review. They may be sent by mail to the Task Order Officer named below at: Agency for Healthcare Research and Quality, 540 Gaither Road, Rockville, MD 20850, or by email to epc@ahrq.hhs.gov.

Carolyn M. Clancy, M.D.
Director
Agency for Healthcare Research and Quality

Jean Slutsky, P.A., M.S.P.H.
Director, Center for Outcomes and Evidence
Agency for Healthcare Research and Quality

Stephanie Chang M.D., M.P.H.
Director, EPC Program
Center for Outcomes and Evidence
Agency for Healthcare Research and Quality

Mary Nix M.S., M.T.(A.S.C.P.), S.B.B., P.M.P.
Task Order Officer
Center for Outcomes and Evidence
Agency for Healthcare Research and Quality

Acknowledgments

The authors gratefully acknowledge Roberta Shanman, M.L.S., who was instrumental in supporting the EPC team's effort to find and obtain relevant literature. The authors also gratefully acknowledge the following individuals for their contributions to this project:

Key Informants

Caroline M. Apovian, M.D., FACP, FACN
Boston University School of Medicine
Boston, MA

Pam Davis, R.N., CBN, CCM
Centennial Center for the Treatment of
Obesity
Nashville, TN

Jim Fivecoat, M.B.A.
Member, Obesity Action Coalition
Taylors, SC

Jeff Haaga
Member, Obesity Action Coalition
West Jordan, UT

Monali Misra, M.D., FRCSC, FACS
Dr. Feiz and Associates
Beverly Hills, CA

John Morton, M.D., M.P.H., FACS
Stanford School of Medicine
Stanford, CA

Joe Nadglowski
President and CEO
Obesity Action Coalition
Tampa, FL

Jamshid Nazarian, M.D., FACS
Beverly Hills, CA

Chuck Stemple, M.D.
Humana
Cincinnati, OH

Technical Expert Panel

Caroline M. Apovian, M.D., FACP, FACN
Boston University School of Medicine
Boston, MA

George Bray, M.D.
Pennington Biomedical Research
Foundation
Baton Rouge, LA

John B Dixon, M.B.B.S., Ph.D., FRACGP
Monash University, Baker IDI Heart and
Diabetes Institute
Melbourne, Australia

David Heber, M.D.
Ronald Reagan UCLA Medical Center
Los Angeles, CA

Edward Harry Livingston, M.D., FACS, UT
Southwestern Medical Center
Dallas, TX

John Morton, M.D., M.P.H., FACS
Stanford School of Medicine
Stanford, CA

Christine J. Ren-Fielding, M.D.
NYU Langone Medical Center
New York, NY

Bruce Wolfe, M.D.
Oregon Health & Science University
Portland, OR

Peer Reviewers

David Arterburn, M.D., M.P.H.
University of Washington
Seattle, WA

Alison Avenell, Ph.D.
University of Aberdeen
Aberdeen, Scotland, U.K.

Scott A. Cunneen, M.D.
Cedars-Sinai Medical Center
Los Angeles, CA

Ken Fujioka, M.D.
Scripps Clinic Del Mar
San Diego, CA

James Hill, Ph.D.
University of Colorado
Denver, CO

Joe Nadglowski
President and CEO
Obesity Action Coalition
Tampa, FL

Bariatric Surgery and Nonsurgical Therapy in Adults With Metabolic Conditions and a Body Mass Index of 30.0 to 34.9 kg/m²

Structured Abstract

Objectives. To systematically review the scientific evidence on efficacy, safety, and comparative effectiveness of various types of bariatric surgery for treating adult patients with a body mass index (BMI) of 30.0 to 34.9 kg/m² and diabetes or impaired glucose tolerance (IGT) and to compare effectiveness of surgery versus nonsurgical interventions in this population.

Data sources. Systematic reviews, case series, cohort, case control studies and controlled trials, found through searching PubMed®, Embase, CINAHL, Cochrane Central Register of Controlled Trials (CENTRAL), Cochrane Database of Abstracts of Reviews of Effects (DARE), and Clinicaltrials.gov through March, 2012.

Review methods. To be included, studies had to report on laparoscopic adjustable gastric banding (LAGB), Roux-en-Y gastric bypass (RYGB), biliopancreatic diversion with duodenal switch (BPD), sleeve gastrectomy (SG), or nonsurgical treatment, and had to include patients with a BMI of at least 30 kg/m² but less than 35 kg/m² with diabetes or IGT. The following studies were excluded: (1) those with no outcomes of efficacy, effectiveness, or safety/adverse events; (2) nonsurgical studies with less than one year followup; (3) nonsurgical studies already included in previous systematic reviews; and (4) studies with a sample size of less than three. Two reviewers, each trained in the critical analysis of scientific literature, independently reviewed and abstracted each study.

Results. We found only 24 studies reporting bariatric surgery results in this specific target population. Two were trials comparing different procedures, three were trials of surgical versus nonsurgical interventions, and the rest were observational studies. Both weight and blood glucose improved significantly for surgery patients in the trials. In the observational studies, surgery patients showed much greater weight loss at 1 year than reported in systematic reviews and randomized controlled trials (RCTs) on diet, exercise, medication, and other behavioral interventions. While both behavioral interventions and medications lowered HbA1c (glycosylated hemoglobin) levels significantly, the decreases reported in surgery patients were much greater. Improvements in blood glucose measures were reported as early as one month postsurgery. Improvements in hypertension, low-density lipoprotein (LDL) cholesterol, and triglycerides were also reported in some studies. Short-term rates of adverse events associated with bariatric surgery were relatively low. One death, a case of sepsis at 20 months in an LAGB patient, was reported. Short-term complications were minor and tended not to require major intervention. Due to the dearth of long-term studies of bariatric surgery in this particular target population, few data exist about long-term adverse effects, and we found no evidence regarding major clinical endpoints such as all-cause mortality, cardiovascular mortality and morbidity, and peripheral arterial disease.

Conclusions. According to blood glucose outcomes, there is moderate strength evidence of efficacy for RYGB, LAGB, and SG as treatment for diabetes and IGT in patients with a BMI between 30 kg/m^2 and 35 kg/m^2 in the short term (up to 2 years). The strength of evidence for BPD is rated low because there are fewer studies, and these have smaller sample sizes. Evidence on comparative effectiveness of surgical procedures is insufficient. Short-term adverse events are relatively minor; strength of evidence is low due to small sample size with low power to detect rare events. Strength of evidence is insufficient regarding adverse events in the long-term (2 years or more postsurgery). Longitudinal studies of bariatric surgery patients are needed to assess overall safety and comparative effectiveness regarding diabetes-related morbidity such as kidney failure and blindness.

Contents

Appendixes

Executive Summary

Background

Bariatric surgery, also known as weight-loss surgery, refers to surgical procedures usually performed on people who are morbidly obese for the purpose of losing weight and to treat, as well as prevent, obesity-related comorbidities. Bariatric surgery has evolved since its introduction in the 1950s, with some procedures that were popular initially (like jejunoileal bypass) having been abandoned because of unacceptable complication rates. The types of bariatric surgery that are most commonly performed now include laparoscopic adjustable gastric banding (LAGB); Roux-en-Y gastric bypass (RYGB); biliopancreatic diversion with duodenal switch (BPD); and sleeve gastrectomy (SG), also referred to as gastric sleeve. Newer procedures—gastric sleeve with ileal interposition, duodenal-jejunal bypass, and duodenal-jejunal exclusion—are being studied outside of the United States (one study in the United States was conducted in 2008, but the results were not published). The mechanism of weight loss and metabolic impact are under investigation, but they are not regularly performed in the United States currently. Thus, they are beyond the scope of this report.

Studies show that these procedures cause significant weight loss in morbidly obese patients. In addition, bariatric surgeries such as LAGB and RYGB in morbidly obese patients have been found to be far more effective than conventional nonsurgical therapy at lowering blood sugar to improve diabetes in the short term. Improvement in diabetes has been demonstrated to start rapidly after bariatric surgery, especially for patients undergoing RYGB, before significant weight loss has occurred. The mechanism of postoperative metabolic improvements has not been fully elucidated and may in part be independent from weight loss, suggesting that bariatric surgery may improve metabolic comorbidities, even for patients who are not morbidly obese.

Bariatric surgery is an accepted practice for patients with a body mass index (BMI) of 40 kg/m² or greater, and for patients with a BMI of between 35 and 40 kg/m², who have significant obesity-related comorbidities such as diabetes, hypertension, cardiovascular disease, dyslipidemia, obstructive sleep apnea, and degenerative arthritis. The National Institutes of Health (NIH) criteria state that patients should undergo medically supervised weight loss attempts before bariatric surgery.

In the past few years, bariatric surgery has been suggested as an option for patients with a lower BMI (at least 30 kg/m², but less than 35 kg/m²) as a way to treat diabetes and other metabolic conditions. Given a lack of consensus regarding the minimum BMI requirement and uncertainties regarding the comparative effectiveness of different bariatric procedures, especially in the long term, a review of the relative risks and benefits of the various surgical and more conservative approaches to treatment of diabetes or impaired glucose tolerance (IGT) in patients whose BMI is between 30 and 35 kg/m² was suggested by a constituent group. The topic was refined by the Southern California Evidence-based Practice Center (EPC) in conjunction with Key Informants, including bariatric surgeons, researchers, consumers, and payers.

Objectives

This systematic review aims to address the following Key Questions (KQs).

KQ1. What does the evidence show regarding the comparative effectiveness of bariatric surgery for treating adult patients with a BMI of 30.0 to 34.9 kg/m² and metabolic conditions, including diabetes? Are certain surgical procedures more effective than others (LAGB, RYGB, or SG)?

KQ2. What does the evidence show regarding the comparative effectiveness of bariatric surgery versus conventional nonsurgical therapies for treating adult patients with a BMI of 30.0 to 34.9 kg/m² and metabolic conditions?

KQ3. What are the potential short-term adverse effects and/or complications associated with bariatric surgery for treating adult patients with a BMI of 30.0 to 34.9 kg/m² who have metabolic conditions?

KQ4. Does the evidence show racial and demographic disparities with regard to potential benefits and harms associated with bariatric surgery for treating adult patients with a BMI of 30.0 to 34.9 kg/m² and metabolic conditions? What other patient factors (social support, counseling, preoperative weight loss, compliance with recommended treatment) are related to successful outcomes?

KQ5. What does the evidence show regarding long-term benefits and harms of bariatric surgery for treating adult patients with a BMI of 30.0 to 34.9 kg/m² and who have metabolic conditions? How do the long-term benefits and harms of bariatric surgery compare to short-term outcomes (within 1 year after surgery)?

Analytic Framework

Figure A presents the analytic framework for this comparative effectiveness review (CER). Using data from controlled trials, cohort studies, and case series, we sought evidence of the benefits and harms of different types of bariatric surgeries and in treating targeted patients (those with diabetes or IGT and a BMI of ≥ 30 kg/m^2 and < 35 kg/m²). The evidence for both short- and long-term outcomes was assessed. Planned comparisons included (1) among different surgical procedures such as RYGB, LAGB, SG, and BPD to answer KQ1; and (2) surgical procedures to conventional nonsurgical therapies (e.g., diet, exercise, and pharmaceuticals) to answer KQ2. Documented short- and long-term benefits and harms of surgical procedures were compared to answer KQ3 and KQ5.

Benefits and harms for specific subpopulations (by gender, age, and race/ethnicity) and other patient factors (social support, counseling, preoperative weight loss, and compliance with recommended treatment) were examined and summarized to answer KQ4.

Figure A. Analytic framework for evaluating the effectiveness and safety of alternative approaches to treatment of metabolic conditions in the patient population with BMI ≥ 30 < 35

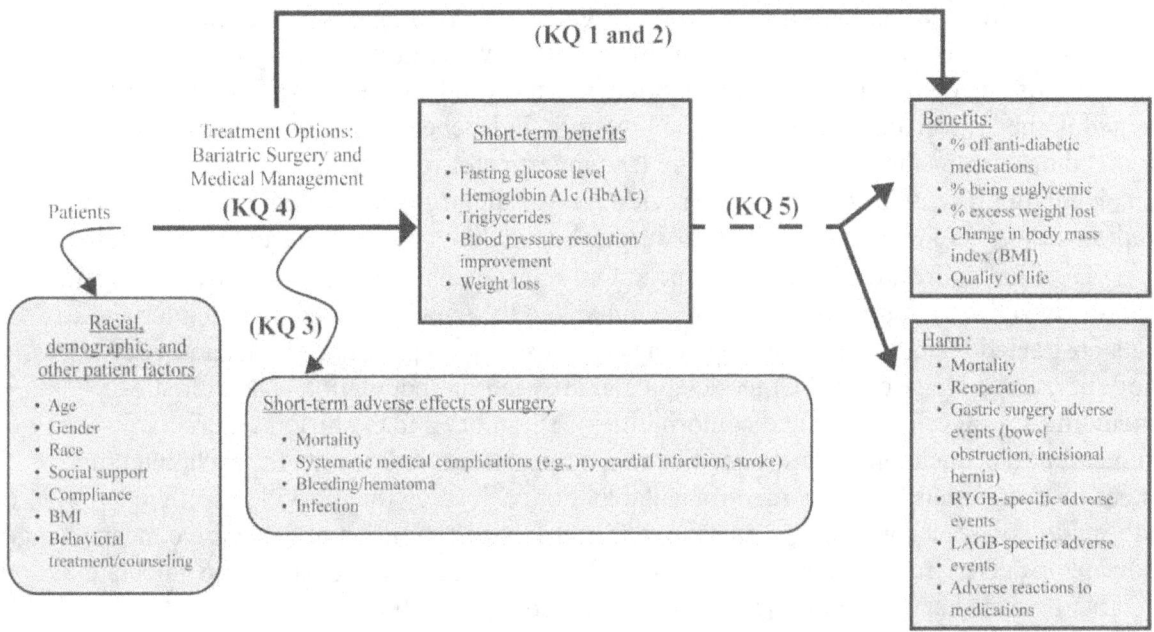

KQ = Key Question; LAGB = laparoscopic adjustable gastric banding LAGB; RYGB = Roux-en-Y gastric bypass

Methods

We searched the electronic databases PubMed®, Embase®, CINAHL (Cumulative Index to Nursing and Allied Health Literature), the Cochrane Database of Systematic Reviews, the Cochrane Central Register of Controlled Trials (CENTRAL), and the Cochrane Database of Abstracts of Reviews of Effects (DARE) for studies addressing our KQs. Other sources included Clinicaltrials.gov, references of included studies and relevant reviews, and personal files from projects with related topics. The original search was conducted in March 2010; electronic search updates were conducted monthly through March 2012. We used various search terms for each type of procedure and for nonsurgical interventions. Further details and surgery strategies are included in the full report. There were no limits on publication date or language.

We searched the literature for systematic reviews, case series, cohort, case control studies and controlled trials. To be included, studies had to report on one of the surgical procedures listed above or nonsurgical treatment, and had to include patients with a BMI of at least 30 kg/m² but less than 35 kg/m² with diabetes or IGT. The following studies were excluded: (1) studies that did not report any outcomes of efficacy, effectiveness, or safety/adverse events; (2) nonsurgical studies with less than 1 year followup; (3) nonsurgical studies already included in previous systematic reviews; and (4) studies with fewer than three subjects.

We note here that we are dealing with two concepts—weight and disorders of glucose metabolism—that are a continuum physiology, but in the KQs, are treated as dichotomous. In other words, we expect the risk of excess weight to be similar for a person with a BMI of 29.5 kg/m² and a person with a BMI of 31.5 kg/m², yet our KQs deal with the latter and not the former. Indeed, the published literature does not always conform to the same threshold specified in the KQs. We judged that studies that included substantial numbers of patients within the threshold of our KQs, but also some outside the range, were still informative and were included. Thus, if a study included patients with a BMI of 29 kg/m²–37 kg/m², we judged that it would be more relevant to the KQs to include rather than exclude, it. Similar decisions were made about the presence of IGT and the clinical diagnosis of diabetes.

We reviewed the studies retrieved from the various sources against our exclusion criteria. Items included specific surgical procedures or nonsurgical treatments, study design, sample size, and types of outcomes reported (i.e. metabolic, mortality, adverse events). Two reviewers, each trained in the critical analysis of scientific literature, independently reviewed each study and resolved disagreements by consensus. The lead investigator resolved any disagreements that remained after discussions between the reviewers. Results from controlled trials, case-control studies, cohort studies, and case series of surgical procedures were abstracted by researchers using Distiller® software (Evidence Partners, Ottawa, Canada). Because of study heterogeneity, meta-analysis was not possible; thus, we summarized the data by procedure and intervention. Data abstracted included metabolic outcomes (glucose, blood pressure, lipids) and weight loss, mortality, and adverse events. Other details included setting; population characteristics (including sex, age, ethnicity, and comorbidities); eligibility and exclusion criteria; any cointerventions, including allowed medication; comparisons; and results for each outcome. Intent-to-treat results were recorded if available. For each study that provided sufficient information, we calculated the mean change from baseline to followup. A negative mean change indicated a decrease in outcome measure (e.g. BMI). We used these estimates to calculate a weighted mean change within surgery type and outcome.

The overall strength of evidence for intervention efficacy was assessed by using guidance suggested by the Agency for Healthcare Research and Quality (AHRQ) for its Effective Health Care Program. This method is based loosely on one developed by the GRADE working group, and classifies the grade of evidence according to the following criteria:

High = High confidence that the evidence reflects the true effect. Further research is very unlikely to change our confidence on the estimate of effect.

Moderate = Moderate confidence that the evidence reflects the true effect. Further research may change our confidence in the estimate of effect and may change the estimate.

Low = Low confidence that the evidence reflects the true effect. Further research is likely to change our confidence in the estimate of effect and is likely to change the estimate.

Insufficient = Evidence is either unavailable or does not permit a conclusion.

The evidence grade is based on four primary (required) domains and four optional domains. The required domains are risk of bias, consistency, directness, and precision; the additional domains are dose-response, plausible confounders that would decrease the observed effect, strength of association, and publication bias. For this review, global implicit judgment about "confidence" was used in the result.

Results

Figure B displays the results of our literature search. We identified 7,088 titles through our electronic database searches, by reference mining, and by locating those suggested by our Technical Expert Panel. We also reviewed scientific information packets received from device manufacturers. Our researchers selected 2,376 for further review; almost half were rejected upon abstract review. Of the 1,220 studies that underwent full-text review, we retained 24 surgical studies, 12 systematic reviews, and 10 nonsurgical studies. The most common reasons for exclusion of surgical studies were focus on patients outside the BMI range (516 studies) or that the study did not include patients with diabetes or IGT (94 studies). The most common reasons for excluding nonsurgical studies were followup of less than 1 year or inclusion in previous systematic reviews.

Of the 24 studies reporting bariatric surgery results in patients with diabetes or IGT and a BMI of at least 30 but less than 35 kg/m², we found two head-to-head trials, one cohort study, and one case series comparing surgical procedures. We identified three controlled trials and two small cohort studies comparing surgery with nonsurgical intervention. (One of the trials contained two different surgical arms.) The remaining included studies were observational, with no comparison group. Six of the studies included only a portion of patients with diabetes or IGT; in the rest, all patients had one of these disorders.

Figure B. Study/literature flow diagram

```
┌─────────────────────┐   ┌─────────────────────┐   ┌─────────────────────┐
│ Literature searches │   │ Titles identified from│  │ Titles from external│
│     N=5,528         │   │  reference mining     │  │     sources         │
│                     │   │     N=1,511           │  │     N=49            │
└──────────┬──────────┘   └──────────┬───────────┘  └──────────┬──────────┘
           │                         │                         │
           └─────────────────────────┼─────────────────────────┘
                                      ▼
           ┌──────────────────────────────────────────────────┐
           │        Total number of titles identified          │
           │                   N=7,088                          │
           └──────────────────────┬───────────────────────────┘
                                   ▼
           ┌──────────────────────────────────────────────────┐
           │        Titles selected for abstract review         │
           │                   N=2,376                          │
           └──────────────────────┬───────────────────────────┘
                                   │        ┌─────────────────────┐
                                   ├───────▶│  Abstracts rejected │
                                   │        │     N=1,111         │
                                   ▼        └─────────────────────┘
           ┌──────────────────────────────────────────────────┐
           │   Abstracts accepted for short form review of      │
           │             article   N=1,265                      │
           └──────────────────────┬───────────────────────────┘
                                   │        ┌───────────────────────────┐
                                   ├───────▶│  45 articles not retrievable│
                                   ▼        └───────────────────────────┘
           ┌──────────────────────────────────────────────────┐
           │    Accepted and sent out for short form review     │
           │                   N=1,220                          │
           └──────────────────────┬───────────────────────────┘
```

Rejected based on short form review
N=1,177

Background:	19
Case report:	3
No diabetes or impaired glucose tolerance:	94
BMI > 35:	516
Non systematic review:	11
Non surgical treatment with follow-up < 1 year:	210
Published before 1990:	42
Treatment not of interest:	64
Non-surgical already included in systematic reviews:	210
N < 10, case control/case series:	4
Wrong population – cancer patients:	1
Other:	3

Accepted based on short form review
N=43
The total number of surgical and non-surgical studies exceeds the number accepted as some studies fall into both categories.

Surgical N=24	Non-surgical > 1 year published after systematic reviews N=10

RCTs: surgery vs. non-surgical N=3
Small cohort: surgery vs. non-surgical N=2
RCTs: surgery vs. surgery N=1
Cohort: surgery vs. surgery N=1
Case series: surgery vs. surgery N=1
Case control N=1
Case series N=8
Cohort N=7

Systematic reviews on either: N=12

BMI = body mass index; RCT = randomized controlled trial

Of the 24 surgery studies, there were 13 RYGB arms, 7 LAGB arms, 5 BPD arms, and 3 gastric sleeve arms. We also included 20 systematic reviews on diet, exercise, medication, or bariatric surgery in our target population. Table A presents a summary of our findings.

Short-Term Outcomes

Based primarily on glucose control outcomes, there is moderate strength evidence of efficacy of bariatric surgery in treating diabetes in patients with a BMI of at least 30 but less than 35 kg/m^2 in the short term. At 1 year, surgery patients show much greater weight loss than usually seen in studies of diet, exercise, or other behavioral interventions. With the exception of GLP-1T agonists, diabetes medications do not cause significant weight loss. While both behavioral interventions and various medications lower HbA1c (glycosyated hemoglobin) levels significantly, the decreases reported in bariatric surgery patients at one year are greater. Improvements in glucose control outcomes have been reported as early as 1 month post-surgery. Several studies report improvement in hypertension and cholesterol at 1 year. We rated the overall evidence as moderate due to sparseness of data—three randomized controlled trials (RCTs) directly compared surgical with nonsurgical interventions, and two came from the same group of researchers. Observational data, which start as low strength evidence, were upgraded due to consistency of results regarding BMI and blood sugar. Thus, the total body of evidence is considered moderate strength, based on moderate strength of evidence for BMI and glucose outcomes. Strength of evidence for cholesterol and blood pressure outcomes is low.

Long-Term Outcomes

There are few long-term data on patients with diabetes or IGT in this weight class who have undergone bariatric surgery. We identified only two studies with followup of more than 2 years. One, a case series of LAGB patients in Italy, reported followup at 5 years for 29 of the 210 initial patients, for a followup rate of only 13.8 percent. Another very small Italian study followed seven BPD patients for at least 5 years Thus, despite promising short-term outcomes reported, the evidence that bariatric surgery is an effective way to treat diabetes in patients with a BMI of at least 30 kg/m^2 but less than 35 kg/m^2 in the long term is insufficient. Strength of evidence is insufficient for all outcomes, including BMI, blood glucose, cholesterol, and hypertension. In contrast, behavior and medication interventions have been studied extensively for decades; several large, long-term RCTs have found improved HbA1c continues for 10 years. Several long-term trials and meta-analyses have reported clinically significant improvements in microvascular and macrovascular outcomes as a result of behavioral or medication interventions.

Specific Bariatric Procedures

We found two head-to-head trials comparing bariatric procedures (one also had a medication-only group). An average-size trial (N=60) conducted in Taiwan compared RYGB with SG; the RYGB group had better weight and diabetes outcomes at 1 year postsurgery. A recent U.S. trial comparing these same procedures found similar results.

We also found two observational studies that compared procedures. One conducted in the United States compared RYGB with LAGB. This study was fairly large (N=235), and had an adequate followup rate (61.9% for RYGB, 69.2% for LAGB) at 6 to 12 months. Some patients were followed for 2 years. Weight loss was similar among groups; diabetes outcomes were generally better for RYGB patients. The other study, conducted in Germany, compared results for 12 BPD patients with 4 RYGB patients. Both groups lost a significant amount of weight. At 1 year, decrease in HbA1c was significantly greater in the BPD group.

Observational studies of surgical procedures without a comparison arm reported clinically meaningful decreases in BMI with all types of bariatric surgery at less than 1 year. Clinically meaningful diabetes outcomes were also reported at less than 1 year for all surgery types. At a year or more, weight loss was maintained or improved in all groups; RYGB patients had the greatest decrease in BMI.

Taking into consideration the entire body of evidence, we rate the strength of evidence of efficacy as moderate for RYGB, LAGB, and SG in treating diabetes and IGT in patients with a BMI of between 30 kg/m^2 and 35 kg/m^2 in the short term (up to 2 years), based primarily on glucose control outcomes. For BPD, both the number of studies and their sample sizes are much lower; thus the strength of evidence of efficacy is rated low. Evidence on comparative effectiveness of surgical procedures is insufficient.

Table A. Summary of data on interventions and outcomes in patients with diabetes or impaired glucose tolerance

Outcome	Behavioral Changes (Data Almost Entirely From Systematic Reviews, RCTs)	Intervention Medications (Data Almost Entirely From Systematic Reviews, RCTs)	Bariatric Surgery (Data Primarily From Observational Studies)
Weight loss at 1 year	2.8 kg for diet, exercise, behavioral vs. usual care	Weight gain from 1 to 5 kg with some drugs. 2.8 kg weight loss with GLP-1R agonists; no weight change with metformin	BMI loss of 5 to 7 kg/m^2 (about 15 to 20 kg for someone 5 feet 6 inches tall)
Weight loss at 2 years	2.7 kg for diet, exercise, behavioral vs. usual care	Data unavailable	BMI loss of 4 to 8 kg/m^2 (about 11 to 23 kg for someone 5 feet 6 inches tall)
Long-term weight loss (5 years and more)	1.7 kg for diet, exercise, behavioral vs. usual care at 5 years	Few data; the U.S. Diabetes Prevention Program Outcomes Study (DPPOS) found no significant change with metformin at 10 years	BMI loss of 5.7 kg/m^2 at 5 years, in one study of 29 LAGB patients
HbA1C, percentage of total hemoglobin, at 1 year	Decrease of 0.3 to 2.2 percentage points	Decrease of 0.5 to 1.0 percentage points	Decrease of 2.6 to 3.7 percentage points
HbA1C at 2 years	No significant change	Data unavailable	Decrease of 1.8 to 3.1 percentage points
HbA1C at 5 years and more	Few data; the U.S. Diabetes Prevention Program Outcomes Study (DPPOS) found HbA1C concentrations lower in behavioral group at 10 years (vs. placebo)	Few data; the U.S. Diabetes Prevention Program Outcomes Study (DPPOS) found HbA1C concentrations lower in metformin group at 10 years (vs. placebo)	Data unavailable

Table A. Summary of data on interventions and outcomes in patients with diabetes or impaired glucose tolerance (continued)

Outcome	Behavioral Changes (Data Almost Entirely From Systematic Reviews, RCTs)	Intervention Medications (Data Almost Entirely From Systematic Reviews, RCTs)	Bariatric Surgery (Data Primarily From Observational Studies)
Other metabolic outcomes at 1 year	Diet improved fasting glucose (1.3%-36.6% reduction) and triglycerides (11.3%-58.9% reduction); the Spain PREDIMED study found Mediterranean diet reduced metabolic syndrome prevalence by 13.7% at 1 year; the Finnish Diabetes Prevention Study (DPS) found behavioral change reduced metabolic syndrome prevalence at 3.9 years (odds ratio: 0.62)	Most medications had minimal effects on systolic & diastolic blood pressure (< 5 mmHg change); metformin and second-generation sulfonylureas generally decreased LDL cholesterol levels	Mixed results, one RYGB and one BPD study reported slight increase in triglycerides at 1 year
Other metabolic outcomes at 5 years and more	Data unavailable	Data unavailable	Of 7 BPD patients followed, all had normal serum cholesterol and triglycerides
Microvascular outcomes (renal disease, neuropathy, retinopathy, etc.)	Data unavailable	U.K. Prospective Diabetes Study (UKPDS) found patients taking sulfonylurea, insulin, or metformin had 24% risk reduction for microvascular disease at 10 years	Data unavailable
Macrovascular outcomes (cardiovascular disease, stroke, heart attack)	Few data; the China Da Qing Diabetes Prevention Study (CDQDPS) found no significant difference in first CVD event, CVD mortality and all-cause mortality between intervention and control group	Meta-analysis of 5 trials with 33,040 participants found that on an average A1C reduction of 0.9% there was a 19% reduction in non-fatal myocardial infarction and a 15% reduction on coronary heart disease, and no statistically significant effect on stroke or all-cause mortality	Data unavailable
Prevention of diabetes	Hazard ratio 0.51 for behavioral interventions vs. standard advice at 1 to 5 years; the U.S. Diabetes Prevention Program (DPP) found diabetes incidence in 10 years reduced by 34% by behavioral change vs. placebo, and the China Da Qing Diabetes Prevention Study (CDQDPS) found it was 43% lower in behavioral group over 20 years	Hazard ratio 0.70 for oral medications vs. control at 1 to 5 years; the U.S. Diabetes Prevention Program (DPP) found diabetes incidence in 10 years reduced by 18% in the metformin group vs. placebo	Data unavailable

BMI = body mass index; BPD = biliopancreatic diversion with duodenal switch; CVD = cardiovascular disease; LAGB = laparoscopic adjustable gastric banding; LDL = low-density lipoproteins; RCT = randomized controlled trial; RYGB = Roux-en-Y gastric bypass

Adverse Events

The strength of evidence for short-term harms is low for all four surgical procedures. In the two RCTs comparing SG with RYGB, complications were minor, and rates were similar between groups. The surgical complications reported for RYGB and LAGB in observational studies were fairly consistent; they differ due to the nature of the procedures. Complications related to LABG include band slippage, tube problems, and band erosion, while those related to RYGB include stricture, ulcer, and on rare occasions, hemorrhage.

Studies were included in our mortality analyses only if they reported or mentioned either the number of deaths or lack of any deaths. Thus, 14 studies were included, which accounted for five LAGB arms, one gastric sleeve arm, nine RYGB arms, and one BPD arm. Only one death was reported—an LAGB patient with complications of a gastric perforation. Thus, the reported rate of mortality was 0.48 percent for LAGB and 0.0 percent for gastric sleeve, RYGB, and BPD.

The low strength of evidence reflects several limitations in the data. The majority of the adverse events data were submitted by surgeons, and thus subject to possible publication bias. Few studies were clear exactly when adverse events took place, and patients who were lost to followup had no adverse events data. In addition, definitions of complications varied from study to study.

We found no data on long-term adverse events of bariatric surgery in diabetes or IGT patients in our specific BMI range. Thus, strength of evidence for long-term adverse events is rated insufficient.

Discussion

The literature on bariatric surgery for diabetes or IGT patients with BMI of at least 30 kg/m² and less than 35 kg/m² has many limitations. Most important, very few studies of this target population have long-term followup. Only two studies followed patients for more than 2 years; one has a followup rate of only 13.8 percent and the other includes only seven patients. Thus, we have almost no data on long-term efficacy and safety. No evidence was found on major clinical endpoints such as all-cause mortality, cardiovascular mortality or morbidity, or peripheral arterial disease. The studies of bariatric surgery in this population have measured only intermediate or surrogate endpoints regarding glucose control. While control of glucose is certainly important, the available evidence from the diabetes literature indicates it may be premature to assume that controlling glucose to normal or near normal levels completely mitigates the risk of microvascular and macrovascular events. Thus, claims of a "cure" for diabetes based on glucose control within 1 or 2 years require longer term data before they can be substantiated.

Randomized controlled trials are considered the highest level of medical evidence. We found three RCTs of surgery versus nonsurgical treatment (one of these also compared two procedures) and another RCT comparing surgical procedures. This was expected given the difficulty in conducting RCTs of surgery. Still, we identified only two observational studies comparing surgical procedures and two small cohort studies comparing surgery with nonsurgical approaches. The rest of our data came from studies with no comparison group and with data submitted primarily by the practicing surgeons. The sample sizes, regardless of methodological design, are far smaller than those of most trials of diet, exercise, and medications.

Applicability of this research to the larger treatment population of diabetes and IGT patients with BMI between 30.0 kg/m^2 and 34.9 kg/m^2 is important in interpreting the results. The participation rate, population characteristics, representativeness of the setting, and representativeness of the individuals are used to assess applicability. One RCT comparing surgery with nonsurgery was performed in the United States and included two of the more commonly performed procedures—RYGB and SG. However, it was of modest size and was conducted in an academic setting in a select group of patients with uncontrolled type II diabetes at baseline. Two RCTs of LAGB versus nonsurgical interventions conducted in Australia comprised primarily Caucasian patients. However, the RCT comparing LAGB with SG was conducted in Taiwan, where diets and lifestyle may differ considerably from those of the West. One of the cohort studies comparing procedures was conducted in the United States, but only three of the remaining observational studies were conducted here. The others were conducted in Western Europe, South America, India, Asia, and Australia. Diet, behavior, and culture in many of these locations may differ dramatically from that in the United States. In addition, there may be biological or genetic differences. Thus, the results seen in studies in other countries may not be directly applicable to patients in the United States.

Data reported on adverse events also have several limitations. Most studies were not primarily designed to assess these outcomes and reflect surgeon or surgery team-reported events. There were only 20 instances in which 100 or more patients contributed data to a particular adverse event category; thus, the rate estimate for most adverse events is imprecise. Additionally, in 76 percent of instances, only a single study contributed data to a particular adverse event rate calculation, meaning the generalizability of the estimate is questionable. Followup times and rates were variable, and many studies did not state exactly when adverse events occurred, other than "within a year postsurgery." As such, the rates of adverse events may be biased and lower than actual. Comparisons between procedure types are limited for the same reasons. Again, we found almost no long-term adverse events data for our target population.

Finally, although our literature-search procedures were extensive and included canvassing experts for studies we may have missed, the possibility of publication bias still exists. For all surgical procedures, there is the concern that published studies usually come from academic medical centers with high-performing surgical teams and careful patient selection. Outcomes for such patients may not reflect the outcomes achieved in the wider community. (The difference between complication rates seen in the major clinical trials of carotid endarterectomy and those observed in the general Medicare population is one well-known example of this phenomenon.) For bariatric surgery, there are media reports (Los Angeles Times) on several deaths following LAGB surgery. Whether there is any causal relationship between the surgery and the deaths has not yet been assessed in a peer-reviewed publication, so no conclusions can be drawn. Still, it illustrates the potential for there to exist adverse events and/or beneficial outcomes in as-yet-undescribed populations.

Future Research

Future research should focus on long-term outcomes of bariatric surgery in U.S. patients with diabetes or IGT and a BMI of 30 kg/m^2 to 34.9 kg/m^2. In this population, there is no evidence that bariatric surgery is effective in preventing the clinical consequences of diabetes—microvascular and macrovascular endpoints such as diabetic retinopathy, kidney failure, and myocardial infarction. Studies with followup of 5 to 10 years are needed.

We found one trial and one cohort study comparing procedures performed in the United States. The cohort study used the BOLD (Bariatric Outcomes Longitudinal Database), a resource created by the Surgical Review Corporation to monitor outcomes from the Bariatric Surgery Center of Excellence (BSCOE) program. As of June 2009, 235 patients with diabetes within our BMI range were in the BOLD database. The study we identified reported outcomes at 6 to 12 months. Outcomes at 12 to 24 months were reported for only a small number of patients (6.8 percent) presumably because that followup time had not expired for most of the patients. Continued followup of these patients and publication of findings will shed light on which, if any, bariatric procedures mitigate long-term sequelae of diabetes.

In addition, according to the U.S. clinical trials database (Clinicaltrials.gov), several bariatric surgery trials are being conducted in the target population. In addition to monitoring weight loss, these studies will frequently collect important metabolic data, including measures of blood sugar, cholesterol, triglycerides, and blood pressure. Long-term followup of the research subjects, if funded, could add to our knowledge base on the effects of bariatric surgery and cardiovascular morbidity and mortality. Collection and reporting of psychological and quality of life outcomes will also help inform prospective patients and providers.

Glossary

Bariatric surgery: Surgery on the stomach and/or intestines to help a person lose weight. Biliopancreatic diversion with duodenal switch (BPD): Surgery that involves removing 70 percent of the stomach, along with bypassing a significant proportion of small intestine.

Body mass index (BMI): An individual's weight, in kilograms, divided by his or her height, in meters squared. It is used to define normal weight, overweight, obesity, and morbid obesity.

GLP-1 agonists: Glucagon-like peptide-1 agonists, a class of diabetes drugs targeting the incretin system.

HbA1c: Glycosylated hemoglobin.

Impaired glucose tolerance (IGT): Prediabetic state of high blood sugar associated with insulin resistance.

Laparoscopic adjustable gastric banding (LAGB): A surgical weight-loss procedure that involves the placement of an adjustable belt around the upper portion of the stomach, restricting the size of the stomach and the amount of food it can hold.

LDL (low-density lipoprotein) cholesterol: Cholesterol that may collect in the walls of blood vessels, causing blockage.

Metabolic condition: A constellation of syndromes including impaired fasting glucose (prediabetes) and diabetes mellitus that increase the risk of cardiovascular disease.

Roux-en-Y gastric bypass (RYGB): A surgical weight-loss procedure that involves the creation of a small stomach pouch to restrict food intake and construction of bypasses of the duodenum and other segments of the small intestine to cause malabsorption (decreased ability to absorb nutrients from food). Often referred to as gastric bypass.

Sleeve gastrectomy (SG): A surgical weight-loss procedure in which the stomach is reduced to about 15 percent of its original size by surgical removal of a large portion of the stomach. There are variations on the sleeve gastrectomy that involve the addition of intestinal bypasses.

References

Please refer to the reference list in the full report for documentation of statements contained in the Executive Summary.

Introduction

In 2010, diabetes affected 25.8 million people in the United States, or 8.3 percent of the population. About 1.9 million people aged 20 years or older were newly diagnosed with diabetes in 2010. In 2005-2008, based on fasting glucose or hemoglobin A1c levels, 35 percent of U.S. adults (79 million people) aged 20 years or older had prediabetes (50 percent of adults aged 65 years or older).[1] Among adults with diabetes, the prevalence of individuals considered as overweight or higher (body mass index [BMI] $\geq$ 25 kg/m²) was 80.3 percent; and the prevalence of obesity or higher (BMI >= 30 kg/m²) was 49.1 percent.[1]

Diabetes is considered a chronic, progressive disease. Traditional medical therapy focuses on glycemic control and control of long-term complications such as retinopathy, renal failure, and cardiovascular disease. Management may involve injecting insulin daily or using oral medications for a life time.

Studies show that bariatric surgeries such as laparoscopic adjustable gastric banding (LAGB), Roux-en-Y gastric bypass (RYGB), and biliopancreatic diversion with duodenal switch (BPD) in morbidly obese patients have been found to be far more effective than conventional nonsurgical therapy at improving diabetes in the short term.[2] A recent randomized controlled study (RCT) studying a population with BMI >35 kg/m² found that no patients in the medical treatment alone group had resolution of diabetes (defined as HgA1c<6.5 percent and fasting blood glucose<100 mg/dL) compared with 75 percent resolution in RYGB and 95 percent in BPD.[3]

Improvement in diabetes has been demonstrated to start rapidly after bariatric surgery, especially for patients undergoing RYGB, before significant weight loss has occurred. Additionally, the degree of weight loss achieved may not predict the improvement in hyperglycemia.[3] The mechanism of postoperative metabolic improvements has not been fully elucidated and may in part be independent from weight loss, suggesting that bariatric surgery may improve metabolic comorbidities even for patients who are not morbidly obese.

Bariatric surgery is an accepted practice for patients with a BMI of 40 kg/m² or greater, and for patients with a BMI of between 35-40kg/m² who have significant obesity-related comorbidities such as diabetes, hypertension, cardiovascular diseases, dyslipidemia, obstructive sleep apnea, and degenerative arthritis.

In the past few years bariatric surgery has been suggested as an option for lower BMI (at least 30 kg/m² but less than 35 kg/m²) patients as a way to treat diabetes and other metabolic conditions. Given a lack of consensus regarding the minimum BMI requirement and uncertainties regarding the comparative effectiveness of different bariatric procedures, especially in the long term, a review of the relative risks and benefits of the various surgical and conservative approaches to treatment of diabetes or impaired glucose tolerance (IGT) in patients whose BMI is at least 30 kg/m² and less than 35 kg/m² was suggested by a constituent group; the topic was refined by the Southern California Evidence-based Practice Center in conjunction with Key Informants, including bariatric surgeons, researchers, consumers, and payers.

Conventional Therapy for Obesity and Diabetes

Conventional nonsurgical therapy for overweight patients with diabetes or IGT includes diet, exercise, and medications (summarized below). Most interventions combine multiple modalities such as diet and exercise and must be sustained long-term to prevent weight regain.

Diet

A variety of diets have been proposed to assist obese patients in losing weight. Low calorie diets are typically high in carbohydrates (55 percent – 60 percent of total daily energy intake), low in fat (< 30 percent of energy intake), and produce a negative energy balance. Other strategies focus on decreasing the proportion of carbohydrates or fats. Low carbohydrate, high fat/protein diets (e.g. Atkins) induce weight loss primarily through decreased calorie intake but can have mixed effects on lipid profiles. Very-low-calorie diets (VLCDs) – typically 800 kcal per day – can be effective to induce rapid weight loss, especially when used as a short-term adjunct prior to bariatric surgery. More recently, the Mediterranean diet, which emphasizes eating fruit, vegetables, and whole grains has become popular. Finally, the low glycemic index diet, originally designed for diabetes patients, ranks carbohydrate foods from 1 to 100 according to glucose level, with 100 as the reference for pure glucose.

Exercise

Aerobic exercise can induce weight loss as well as decrease blood sugar levels for those with impaired glucose tolerance, though it is often difficult for morbidly obese patients due to comorbidities such as osteoarthritis. There is some debate regarding the optimal level of physical activity necessary to induce weight loss. The National Heart, Lung and Blood Institute (NHLBI) Obesity Education Initiative Expert and the United States (U.S.) Preventive Services Task Force guidelines suggest that at least 30 minutes of aerobic activity daily (amounting to an energy expenditure of 2,500 to 3,500 kcal per week) is necessary to promote weight loss and reduce comorbidities.[4]

Behavior Modification

These interventions include individual counseling and community-based programs to provide detailed strategies to assist with weight loss. Recommendations may include those regarding diet and exercise, as well as counseling regarding the deleterious effects of obesity and associated comorbidities. Cognitive behavioral therapy, targets specific psychological processes that may interfere with weight loss or maintenance, can be included in a behavior modification program.

Medications

Anti-obesity medications rely on increasing metabolism, decreasing appetite or altering food absorption. Commonly used drugs have included orlistat, which inhibits pancreatic lipases and prevents fat absorption, and sibutramine, a serotonin-norepinephrine reuptake inhibitor that decreases appetite. The latter was recently withdrawn from the United States and other markets due to increased risks of myocardial infarction and stroke.[5] Phentermine, approved for short-term weight loss, is another popular appetite suppressant. Conventional pharmaceutical therapy for weight loss has not been very effective at producing significant and sustained weight loss in obese patients.[6,7] The combination of diet and weight loss medications like orlistat results in a mean weight loss of only 3-4 kg at one year.[6] Such medications can improve glycemic control and dyslipidemia in obese patients with type 2 diabetes, but this improvement is modest.[8]

Conventional therapy for diabetes also includes specific medications meant to lower plasma glucose levels. Pharmacotherapy for obese patients with diabetes includes insulin or oral hypoglycemic agents, which work through a variety of mechanisms (e.g. sulfonylureas, which increase insulin secretion; biguanides, which reduce hepatic glucose production; and thiazolidinediones or glitazones, which reduce insulin resistance mainly in the periphery). Medications used for obese patients with diabetes, such as insulin or sulfonylureas (e.g. glyburide), do not produce significant weight loss and can even cause weight gain, exacerbating insulin resistance and glucose intolerance.[9] Recently developed GLP-1 receptor agonists such a liraglutide and exenatide treat diabetes by reducing meal-related hyperglycemia by increasing insulin secretion and delaying gastric emptying. These drugs have been shown to cause weight loss in clinical trials.[10,11] Cardiovascular risk reduction medications (statins, aspirin, angiotensin converting enzyme inhibitors, etc.) are also mainstays of diabetes management.

Bariatric Surgery

Bariatric surgery was first introduced in the 1950s and has evolved significantly since that time, leading to some procedures that were initially performed being abandoned due to unacceptably complication rates secondary to malabsorption that led to reduced nutrient intake (e.g. jejunoileal bypass) or poor long-term benefit (i.e., vertical banded gastroplasty). The most common procedures currently performed are RYGB, laparoscopic adjustable gastric banding, and gastric sleeve. These procedures result in weight loss via different mechanisms and most likely involve a combination. Pre-surgery assessments of weight history, food preferences, psychological issues and medical history impact decisions regarding which surgery is most appropriate.

Researchers are still learning about all the specifics of how weight loss is achieved. Two general components employed, alone or in combination, include (1) restricting the size of the stomach to limits the quantity of food a patient can consume at a single meal, and (2) inducing malabsorption which decreases the proportion of nutrients that are absorbed from a meal. These procedures can also produce behavior changes, such as aversions to high carbohydrate foods. As the gastrointestinal tract communicates with the central nervous system, these procedures also appear to lead to hunger control and satiety, the details of which are still being studied. Descriptions of selected bariatric procedures (those performed currently) are provided below.

Gastric Bypass (RYGB)

The most common bariatric procedure, Roux-en-Y gastric bypass, often referred to as "gastric bypass," achieves weight loss through complex mechanisms. The surgery involves creating a small gastric pouch (and outlet) along with a proximal intestinal bypass. This small pouch (30 cc) is connected to a segment of the jejunum (which is downstream), thus bypassing the duodenum and very proximal small intestine. Although the procedure generates minimal malabsorption, significant changes in hormones and neural signals to the gastrointestinal tract lead to hunger control and satiety. In addition, following ingestion of high-density carbohydrates, some patients may experience the resultant "dumping" syndrome, whose unpleasant symptoms include flushing, palpitations, abdominal pain, cramping, and diarrhea. As a result, these patients develop an aversion to high-carbohydrate foods that leads to behavior changes in diet and eating habits. RYGB for weight loss has been performed regularly since the early 1980s. It was first performed laparoscopically in the early 1990s and is now one of the most common types of weight loss procedures.

Laparoscopic Adjustable Gastric Band (LAGB)

Gastric banding achieves weight loss predominately by gastric restriction. The uppermost portion of the stomach is encircled by a band to create a gastric pouch with a capacity of approximately 15 to 30 cubic centimeters (cc). The band consists of an inflatable doughnut-shaped balloon whose diameter can be adjusted in the clinic by adding or removing saline via a reservoir port positioned beneath the skin. The bands are adjustable to allow the size of the gastric outlet to be modified as needed, depending on clinical symptoms and eating behaviors. A full understanding of how weight loss is achieved is still being investigated, but likely includes components of behavioral diet and eating changes as well as inducing satiety through neuropeptide changes. Currently, banding procedures are performed laparoscopically (laparoscopic adjustable gastric banding). While this procedure is technically reversible (e.g., removal of the band for failed weight loss), doing so exposes the patient to potential risks associated with a second operation and, of course, will necessitate identifying an alternative method for weight loss.

Sleeve Gastrectomy

Also known as gastric sleeve, vertical sleeve gastrectomy, is a relatively new restrictive type of procedure. Approximately 60 to 80 percent of the stomach is removed laparoscopically, leaving a small tube (or "sleeve") which remains connected to the original stomach outlet. The cutaway part of the stomach is removed, making this procedure irreversible, and no foreign objects are implanted in the body.

The mechanism by which gastric sleeve induces weight loss is not clear. At least one study has demonstrated increased or rapid gastric emptying following gastric sleeve resection, leading to a possible mechanism of neural-hormonal phenomena similar to RYGB. This procedure may also lower plasma ghrelin, a natural hormone, which produces hunger. Originally gastric sleeve surgery was the first stage of two-stage procedure, biliopancreatic diversion with duodenal switch in high risk patients. (discussed below). However, many patients lost sufficient weight after the gastric sleeve such that the second stage surgery was not needed, and it has been gaining popularity as a stand-alone procedure since the early 2000s. In South America, the procedure has been paired with ileal interposition, with very good results reported. However, as that process is considered experimental and rarely performed in the United States, it is beyond the scope of this report.

Biliopancreatic Diversion/Duodenal Switch (BPD)

BPD involves removing 70 percent of the stomach along with bypassing a significant proportion of small intestine. By reducing the size of the stomach, less acid is produced, but the remaining capacity is generous compared with that achieved with RYGB. As such, patients eat relatively normal-sized meals and do not need to restrict intake severely. Malabsorption is a component of how weight loss is generated, but it has not been clearly established as the main cause. Malabsorption is generated by (1) the diversion of food downstream, decreasing the opportunity for nutrient absorption and (2) reduction in the quantities of enzymes and bile in the bypassed segment, which decreases absorption. Patients develop steatorrhea from the decrease in fat absorption.

Although this procedure is not as commonly performed as either banding procedures or RYGB, the approach is favored by some bariatric surgery specialists. The partial biliopancreatic diversion with duodenal switch is a variant of the BPD procedure that, until recently, was performed mostly in Italy and only rarely performed in the United States. Recently, a number of centers in the United States and Canada have begun to perform this procedure, which involves resection of the greater curvature of the stomach, preservation of the pyloric sphincter, and transection of the duodenum above the ampulla of Vater with a duodeno-ileal anastomosis and a lower ileo-ileal anastomosis.

Newer procedures, gastric sleeve with ileal interposition, duodenal-jejunal bypass, and duodenal-jejunal exclusion, are being studied outside in the United States (one study in the United States in 2008 was conducted but the results were not published). The mechanism of weight loss and metabolic impact are under investigation and they are not standardly performed in the United States currently. Thus, they are beyond the scope of this report.

Bariatric Surgery in Lower Weight Patients

Currently the standard criteria for bariatric surgery candidates include having a BMI ≥ 40 kg/m² or ≥ 35 kg/m² with significant obesity-related comorbidities. This is based on National Institutes of Health (NIH) guidelines[12] and has been endorsed by the Center for Medicare & Medicaid Services (CMS), which covers a variety of bariatric procedures for patients with BMI ≥ 35 kg/m² and comorbidities.[13] Bariatric surgery has been shown to improve or resolve metabolic conditions such as diabetes in the short term, at least in part due to the associated weight loss.[14] However, there may be other mechanisms involved (particularly for RYGB) as metabolic improvements are often seen rapidly after surgery, before significant weight loss has occurred. Bariatric surgery has therefore been advocated as a treatment for metabolic conditions even for the non-morbidly obese patients. Though experts have suggested that the minimum BMI requirement for bariatric candidates with type 2 diabetes be lowered below 35 kg/m², CMS in 2006 denied coverage for lower BMI patients with diabetes, specifically for open and laparoscopic RYGB, LAGB, and open and laparoscopic BPD/DS.[15] In 2011, the International Diabetes Federation recommended that diabetic patients with BMI of at least 30 kg/m² to 35 kg/m² be eligible for bariatric surgery if they have a HbA1c level of $> 7.5\%$.[16] More recently, the Food and Drug Administration (FDA) expanded the indications for a specific brand of laparoscopic adjustable gastric banding to include patients with a BMI between 30 kg/m² and 34.9 kg/m² and at least one obesity-related comorbidity.[17]

Methods

Original Proposed Key Questions (KQs)

KQ1. What does the evidence show regarding the comparative effectiveness of bariatric surgery for treating adult patients with a BMI of 30.0 to 34.9 kg/m² and metabolic conditions, including diabetes? Are certain surgical procedures more effective than others (LAGB, RYGB, or SG)?

KQ2. What does the evidence show regarding the comparative effectiveness of bariatric surgery versus conventional nonsurgical therapies for treating adult patients with a BMI of 30.0 to 34.9 kg/m² and metabolic conditions?

KQ3. What are the potential short-term adverse effects and/or complications associated with bariatric surgery for treating adult patients with a BMI of 30.0 to 34.9 kg/m² who have metabolic conditions?

KQ4. Does the evidence show racial and demographic disparities with regard to potential benefits and harms associated with bariatric surgery for treating adult patients with a BMI of 30.0 to 34.9 kg/m² and metabolic conditions? What other patient factors (social support, counseling, preoperative weight loss, compliance with recommended treatment) are related to successful outcomes?

KQ5. What does the evidence show regarding long-term benefits and harms of bariatric surgery for treating adult patients with a BMI of 30.0 to 34.9 kg/m² and who have metabolic conditions? How do the long-term benefits and harms of bariatric surgery compare to short-term outcomes (within 1 year after surgery)?

Technical Expert Panel

For each Agency for Healthcare Research and Quality (AHRQ) evidence report, a Technical Expert Panel (TEP) is assembled to provide clinical expertise and context. We invited a distinguished group of scientists and clinicians, including individuals with expertise in obesity, surgery, and metabolic conditions such as diabetes, to participate in the TEP for this report. A list of members is included in the front matter of this report. A TEP conference call was held on October 4, 2010. On the call, staff presented the KQs as well as the preliminary literature search results and asked experts to help define the scope of the review (e.g. types of metabolic conditions and bariatric procedures to include). Panel members reviewed a draft version of this report and provided feedback.

Analytic Framework

Figure 1 presents the analytic framework for this comparative effectiveness review (CER). Using data from controlled trials, cohort studies, and case series, we documented evidence of the benefits and harms of different types of bariatric surgeries and conventional nonsurgical therapies in treating targeted patients (those with diabetes or impaired glucose tolerance [IGT] and a body mass index [BMI] of 30 to 34.9 kg/m²). The evidence for both short- and long-term outcomes was assessed. Comparisons included: (1) among different surgical procedures such as Roux-en-Y gastric bypass (RYGB), laparoscopic adjustable gastric banding (LAGB), sleeve gastrectomy (SG), and biliopancreatic diversion with duodenal switch (BPD) to answer KQ1, and (2) of surgical procedures to conventional nonsurgical therapies (e.g., diet, exercise, and pharmaceuticals) to answer KQ2. Documented short- and long-term benefits and harms of surgical procedures were compared to answer KQ3 and KQ5.

Benefits and harms for specific subpopulations (by gender, age, and race/ethnicity) and other patient factors (social support, counseling, preoperative weight loss, compliance with recommended treatment) were examined, where available, to answer KQ4.

Figure 1. Analytic framework for evaluationg the effectiveness and safety of alternative approaches to treatment of metabolic conditions in the patient population with BMI ≥ 30 < 35

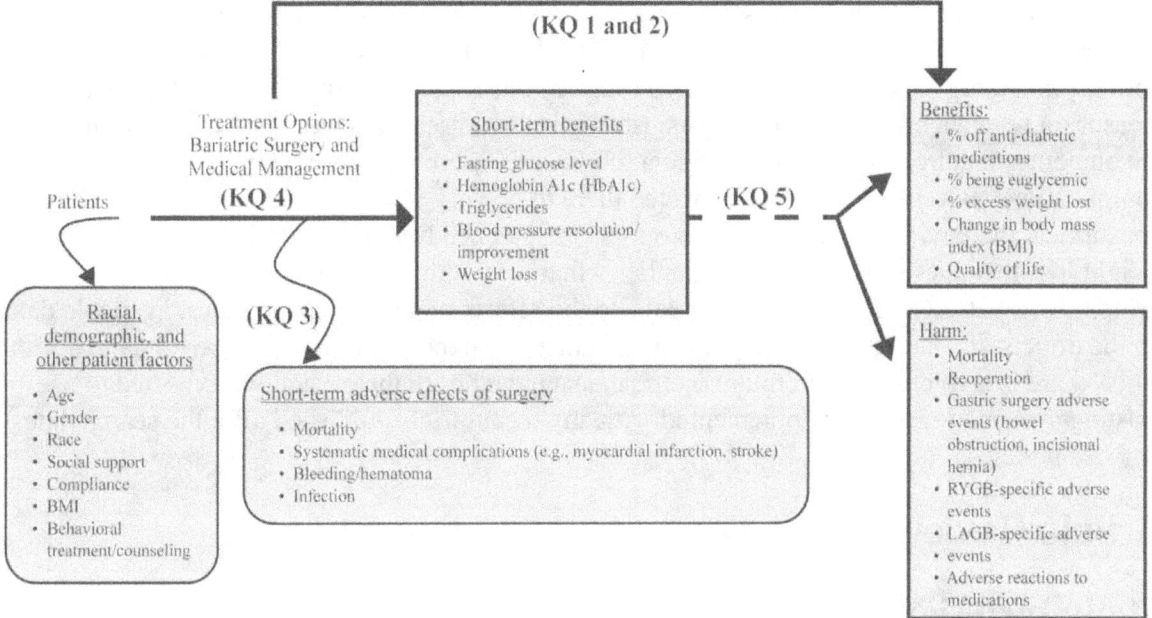

KQ = Key Question; LAGB = laparoscopic adjustable gastric banding LAGB; RYGB = Roux-en-Y gastric bypass

A protocol for this review was available for public comment on the AHRQ Effective Healthcare Web site http://effectivehealthcare.ahrq.gov/index.cfm/search-for-guides-reviews-and-reports/?productid=595&pageaction=displayproduct.

Literature Search

Our search for studies began in April 2009, with an electronic search of PubMed® and Embase® for reports on bariatric surgery and patients with diabetes or IGT. We also searched the CINAHL (Cumulative Index to Nursing and Allied Health Literature), Cochrane library of systematic reviews, Cochrane Central Register of Controlled Trials (CENTRAL) and the Cochrane Database of Abstracts of Reviews of Effects (DARE). (The Cochrane Collaboration is an international organization that helps people make well-informed decisions about health care by preparing, maintaining, and promoting the accessibility of systematic reviews on the effects of heath care interventions.) Other sources included Clinicaltrials.gov, references of included studies, and relevant reviews, and personal files from projects with related topics. Reviewers performed additional reference mining by scanning titles listed in the reference section of each selected study to identify additional potential articles. The literature search was updated in March 2010, and October 2010 after the TEP call, and search updates were conducted monthly through March 2012. Appendix A shows our specific search terms. We also searched for studies of nonsurgical treatments (diet, exercise, education, medications, and other interventions). The following bariatric procedures: laparoscopic adjustable gastric banding (LAGB), sleeve gastrectomy (SG), Roux-en-Y gastric bypass (RYGB), and biliopancreatic diversion (BPD) were included in our searches. Jejunoileal bypass, one of the earliest procedures performed for weight loss, was not included, as this procedure was abandoned about 25 years ago due to a high rate of complications. We used various search terms for each type of procedure. For example, for Roux-en-Y gastric bypass, we also used gastric bypass, RYGB, laparoscopic gastric bypass, and open gastric bypass. We ordered all articles on metabolic conditions and weight loss interventions, regardless of language or publication date.

The strongest evidence to assess the relative benefits and harms of bariatric surgery with nonsurgical therapy would come from randomized controlled trials comparing the treatment options, including only patients in the BMI range of our KQs (30 kg/m^2 – 34.9 kg/m^2) and measuring relevant outcomes such as glucose control and use of diabetic medications, but also the outcomes that treating diabetes is meant to prevent: microvascular and macrovascular complications. Because a priori we expected there to be very few RCTs comparing surgical with nonsurgical therapy, we expected – as in our prior Evidence Report on surgical and nonsurgical weight loss therapies in more obese patients[18] – that we would need to make indirect comparisons between the best available data on the effects of surgery and the best available data on the effects of nonsurgical therapy. For the former, we expected to use case series data. For the latter, there is a voluminous literature on the management of diabetes, and we expected to use existing systematic reviews supplemented with any recent trials published after the search dates of these reviews.

Article Review

Study Inclusion

We searched the literature for systematic reviews, case series, cohort, case control and controlled trials. Editorials, historical pieces, and descriptive articles without data were excluded. The studies included in this report are of one of the following types.

Review articles identified by the search were classified as either systematic (including meta-analyses) or nonsystematic. *Systematic reviews* were identified by reading the methods section of the article to determine whether an acceptable method was employed to identify evidence (such as a description of the name of the computerized database searched and the full set of search terms used, as well as details about the method for accepting and rejecting identified articles).

Randomized controlled trials (RCTs) are studies where the participants are definitely assigned prospectively to one of two (or more) alternative forms of intervention, using a process of random allocation (e.g., random number generation, coin flips).

Controlled clinical trials (CCTs) are studies where participants (or other units) are either

    (a) definitely assigned prospectively to one of two (or more) alternative forms of health care using a quasi-random allocation method (e.g., alternation, date of birth, patient identifier) OR

    (b) possibly assigned prospectively to one of two (or more) alternative forms of health care using a process of random or quasi-random allocation.

Observational studies (such as cohort and cases series) are those where the investigators do not control who gets the interventions.

To be included, studies had to report on one of the surgical procedures or conservative nonsurgical treatments described in the introduction, and had to include patients with BMI 30.0

to 34.9 kg/m² with diabetes or IGT. Systematic reviews of interventions both surgical and nonsurgical were the exception to this rule, since they often synthesized data over a number of studies with varying BMI patient population. The following studies were excluded: (1) studies that did not report any outcomes of efficacy, effectiveness, or safety/adverse events; (2) nonsurgical studies with less than one year followup; (3) nonsurgical studies already included in previous systematic reviews; (4) background articles; and (5) studies with less than three subjects. We note here that we are dealing with two concepts, weight and disorders of glucose metabolism, that are a continuum physiology, but in the KQs are treated as dichotomous. In other words, we expect the risk of weight to be similar for a person with a BMI of 29.5 kg/m² and a person with a BMI of 31.5 kg/m², yet our key questions deal with the latter and not the former. Indeed, the published literature does not always conform to the same threshold specified in the KQs. We judged that studies that included substantial number of patients within the threshold of our KQs, but perhaps also some outside the range, were still informative, and were included. Thus, if a study included patients with a BMI of 29 kg/m²–37 kg/m² we judged that it would be more informative to the KQs to include rather than exclude it. Similar decisions were made about the presence of impaired glucose tolerance and the clinical diagnosis of diabetes.

Screening

Using a single-page "screening form" (included in Appendix B), we reviewed the studies retrieved from the various sources against our exclusion criteria. Items included specific surgical procedure or nonsurgical treatment, study design, sample size, and type of outcomes reported (i.e. metabolic conditions, mortality, adverse events). Two reviewers, each trained in the critical analysis of scientific literature, independently reviewed each study and resolved disagreements by consensus. The lead investigator resolved any disagreements that remained after discussions between the reviewers.

Data Abstraction and Synthesis of Results

Results from controlled trials, case-control studies, cohort studies, and cases series were abstracted by researchers using Distiller® software. Because of study heterogeneity, meta-analysis was not possible; thus, we summarize the data both quantitatively and qualitatively. Data abstracted included metabolic outcomes (glucose, blood pressure, lipids) and weight loss, mortality, and other adverse events. Other details included trial name (if applicable), setting, population characteristics (including sex, age, ethnicity, and diagnosis), eligibility and exclusion criteria, any co-interventions, other allowed medication, comparisons, and results for each outcome. Intent-to-treat results were recorded if available. For each study that provided sufficient information, we calculated the mean change from baseline to followup, where a negative mean change indicates decrease in outcome measure (e.g. BMI). We used the estimates to calculate a weighted mean change within surgery type and outcome.

Assessment of Methodological Quality

To arrive at a quantitative measure for controlled trials, the Jadad scale was used, which was originally developed for drug trials.[19] This method measures quality on a scale that ranges from 0–5, assigning points for randomization and blinding and accounting for withdrawals and dropouts. (Across a broad array of meta-analyses, an evaluation of the scale found that trials scoring from 0–2 report exaggerated results when compared with trials scoring from 3–5.[20] The latter scores indicate studies of "good" quality and the former indicate those of "poor" quality.) For any disagreement that arose during the quality assessment, issues were discussed in the project meeting, and group decisions were made by the research team.

To assess the quality of included systematic reviews and meta-analyses, we used AMSTAR—a measurement tool for the assessment of multiple systematic reviews.[21] This tool contains eleven yes/ no items, such as whether the literature search was comprehensive, if dual abstraction was used, and if individual study characteristics are displayed. The tool has strong face and content validity, inter-rater reliability, and construct validity.[22] A copy is included in Appendix B.

Grading the Evidence for Each KQ

The overall strength of evidence for intervention effectiveness was assessed by using guidance suggested by AHRQ for its Effective Health Care Program.[23,24] This method is based loosely on one developed by the GRADE working group,[25] and classifies the grade of evidence according to the following criteria:

High = High confidence that the evidence reflects the true effect. Further research is very unlikely to change our confidence on the estimate of effect.

Moderate = Moderate confidence that the evidence reflects the true effect. Further research may change our confidence in the estimate of effect and may change the estimate.

Low = Low confidence that the evidence reflects the true effect. Further research is likely to change our confidence in the estimate of effect and is likely to change the estimate.

Insufficient = Evidence either is unavailable or does not permit a conclusion.

The evidence grade is based on four primary (required) domains and four optional domains. The required domains are risk of bias, consistency, directness, and precision; the additional domains are dose-response, plausible confounders that would decrease the observed effect, strength of association, and publication bias. Information on the required domains is presented in Table 1 below.

Table 1. Grading the strength of a body of evidence: required domains and their definitions

Domain	Definition and Elements	Score and Application
Risk of Bias	Risk of bias is the degree to which the included studies for a given outcome or comparison have a high likelihood of adequate protection against bias (i.e., good internal validity), assessed through two main elements: • Study design (e.g., RCTs or observational studies) • Aggregate quality of the studies under consideration. Information for this determination comes from the rating of quality (good/fair/poor) done for individual studies.	Use one of three levels of aggregate risk of bias: • Low risk of bias • Medium risk of bias • High risk of bias
Consistency	The principal definition of consistency is the degree to which reported effect sizes from included studies appear to have the same direction of effect. This can be assessed through two main elements: • Effect sizes have the same sign (that is, are on the same side of "no effect") • The range of effect sizes is narrow.	Use one of three levels of consistency: • Consistent (i.e., no inconsistency) • Inconsistent • Unknown or not applicable (e.g., single study) As noted in the text, single-study evidence bases (even megatrials) cannot be judged with respect to consistency. In that instance, use "Consistency unknown (single study)."
Directness	The rating of directness relates to whether the evidence links the interventions directly to health outcomes. For a comparison of two treatments, directness implies that head-to-head trials measure the most important health or ultimate outcomes. Two types of directness, which can coexist, may be of concern: Evidence is indirect if: • It uses intermediate or surrogate outcomes instead of health outcomes. In this case, one body of evidence links the intervention to intermediate outcomes and another body of evidence links the intermediate to most important (health or ultimate) outcomes. • It uses two or more bodies of evidence to compare interventions A and B – that is, studies of A versus placebo and B versus placebo, or studies of A versus C and B versus C but not A versus B. Indirectness always implies that more than one body of evidence is required to link interventions to the most important health outcomes. Directness may be contingent on the outcomes of interest. EPC authors are expected to make clear the outcomes involved when assessing this domain.	Score dichotomously as one of two levels directness • Direct • Indirect If indirect, specify which of the two types of indirectness account for the rating (or both, if that is the case)—namely, use of intermediate/ surrogate outcomes rather than health outcomes, and use of indirect comparisons. Comment on the potential weaknesses caused by, or inherent in, the indirect analysis. The EPC should note if both direct and indirect evidence was available, particularly when indirect evidence supports a small body of direct evidence.
Precision	Precision is the degree of certainty surrounding an effect estimate with respect to a given outcome (i.e., for each outcome separately). If a meta-analysis was performed, this will be the confidence interval around the summary effect size.	Score dichotomously as one of two levels of precision: • Precise • Imprecise A precise estimate is an estimate that would allow a clinically useful conclusion. An imprecise estimate is one for which the confidence interval is wide enough to include clinically distinct conclusions. For example, results may be statistically compatible with both clinically important superiority and inferiority (i.e., the direction of effect is unknown), a circumstance that will preclude a valid conclusion.

EPC = Evidence-based Practice Center; RCT = randomized controlled trial

11

For this systematic review, we focused on the inherent risk of bias in study design (e.g., in general, randomized controlled trials have less bias than observational studies) and within study design, certain aspects of execution and reporting (e.g. proportion lost to followup, baseline differences between the comparison groups). Regarding consistency, we judged the evidence as consistent if, *all other factors being equal*, a super majority of the studies reported results in the same direction. For directness, we judged the evidence to be direct if, *all other factors being equal*, studies reported relevant health outcomes such as weight loss, micro or macrovascular complications of diabetes, stroke myocardial infarction, etc. rather than indirect outcomes such as fasting blood sugar or HbA1c. We consider weight loss per se to be a health outcome since it is something patients can feel, although it is also an intermediate towards improvement in comorbid conditions. For precision, we defined the evidence as precise if, all other factors being equal, the data were sufficiently within its 95% confidence interval to support a decision, i.e. if the evidence is on one side of a decision threshold. The most important additional domain was publication bias, because surgeons submitting case series for publication may be unrepresentative of the community as a whole.

Peer Review and Public Commentary

A draft of this report was prepared in September 2011. The AHRQ Effective Healthcare Program Scientific Resource Center located at Oregon Health Sciences University coordinated peer review by experts and stakeholders. The report was also posted on AHRQ's Web site for a month for public comment. Resulting comments were considered by the EPC in preparation of the final report. Synthesis of the scientific literature presented here does not necessarily represent the views of individual reviewers, and service as a peer reviewer or member of the TEP cannot be construed as endorsement of the report's findings.

Results

Figure 2 displays the results of our literature search. We identified 7,088 titles through our electronic database searches, reference mining, scientific information packets received from manufacturers, and expert panel suggestions. Our researchers selected 2,376 for further review; almost half were rejected upon abstract review. Of the 1,220 studies that underwent full-text review, we included 24 studies that included a surgical arm, 12 systematic reviews, and ten large studies of nonsurgical interventions published after those reviews. The most common reasons for exclusion of surgical studies were wrong body mass index (BMI) range (516 studies) or the study did not include patients with diabetes or impaired glucose tolerance (IGT) (94 studies). The most common reasons for excluding nonsurgical studies were followup of less than one year or inclusion in previous systematic reviews.

Figure 2. Study/Literature flow diagram

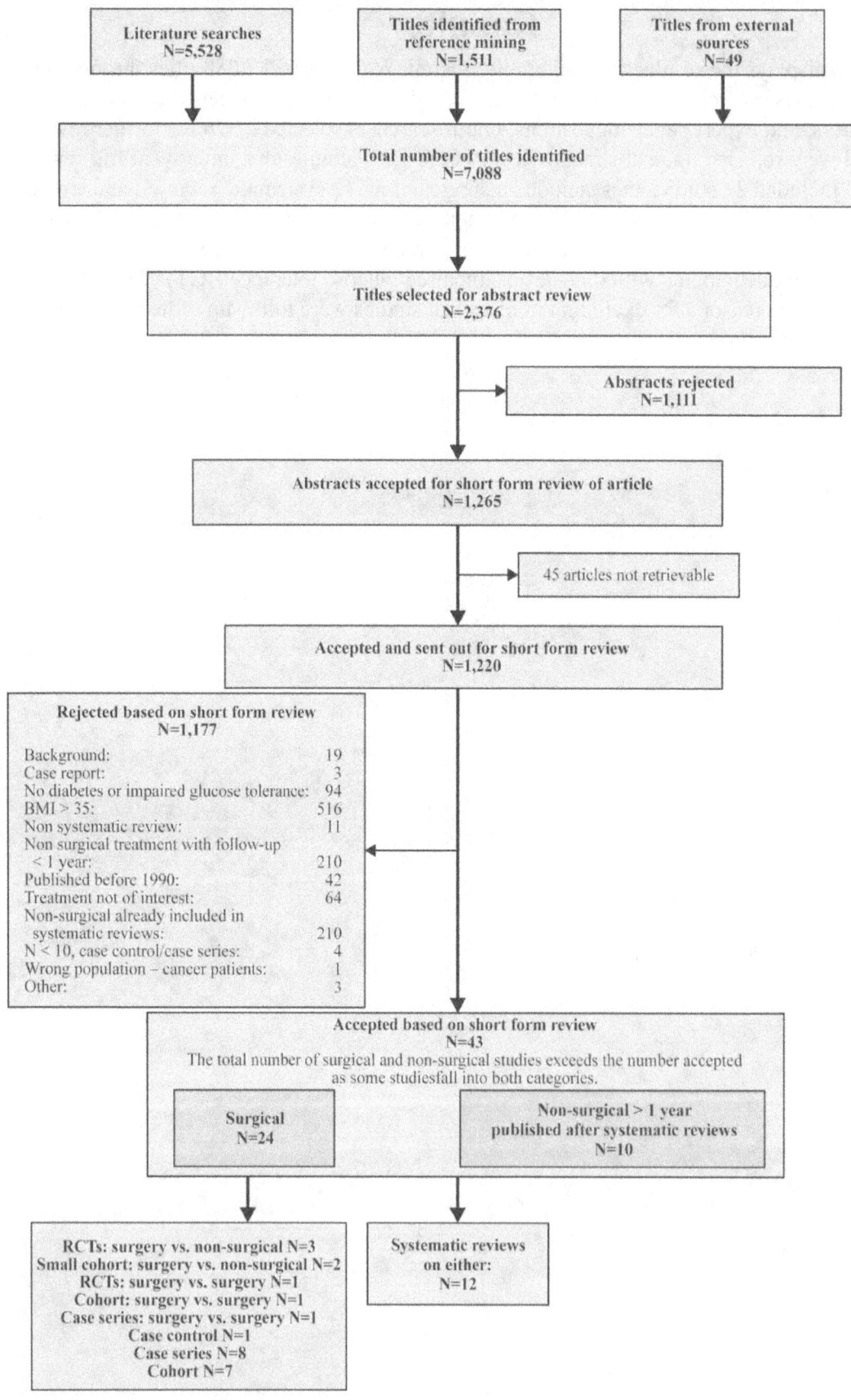

BMI = body mass index; RCT = randomized controlled trial

Key Question (KQ)1: What does the evidence show regarding the comparative effectiveness of bariatric surgery for treating adult patients with BMI of 30 to 34.9 and metabolic conditions, including diabetes? Are certain surgical procedures more effective than others (laparoscopic adjustable gastric banding, gastric bypass, or sleeve gastrectomy)?

KQ2: What does the evidence show regarding the comparative effectiveness of bariatric surgery versus conventional nonsurgical therapies for treating adult patients with BMI of 30 to 34.9 and metabolic conditions?

Of the 24 studies reporting bariatric surgery results in patients with diabetes or IGT and a BMI of $\geq 30 < 35$ kg/m^2, we found two head to head, one cohort study, and one case series comparing surgical procedures. We also identified three controlled trials with a nonsurgical comparison arm (one of which also compared two surgical procedures) and two small cohorts with a nonsurgical arm. The rest of the studies were observational with no comparison group. Six studies included only a portion of patients with diabetes or IGT; in the rest, all patients had these disorders. The majority of the surgical studies came represented single institutions. Of these, three studies reported that only one surgeon performed the cases, three others reported that two surgeons performed the cases, and one study reported procedures were performed by three surgeons. It is unknown how many surgeons performed the cases in the remaining studies.

There were thirteen Roux-en-Y gastric bypass (RYBG) arms, seven laparoscopic adjustable gastric banding (LAGB) arms, five biliopancreatic diversion with duodenal switch (BPD) arms, and three sleeve gastrectomy (SG) arms. Table 2 displays the followup times for each study, along with whether BMI, HbA1c, and/or fasting glucose were measured at each point. Many studies measured additional metabolic outcomes; however, no studies reported on diabetes sequelae such as nephropathy or retinopathy. The vast majority of the studies included followup between 10 and 12 months postsurgery. Unfortunately, few studies followed patients more than two years. It is important to note that when assessing outcomes across time points (for example, 4–6 month data and 10–12 month data) the patients contributing data at 4–6 months may not be the same patients contributing data at 10–12 months, either within study across studies.

Table 2. Bariatric outcomes by followup time

Study	Surgery	0-3 mths	4-6 mths	7-9 mths	10-12 mths	13-24 mths	>24 mths
Cohen, 2006[26]	RYGB					§	
Lee, 2008[27]	RYGB				† § #		
DeMaria, 2010[28]	RYGB	†	†		†	†	
Shah, 2010[29]	RYGB	§ #	§ #	† § #			
Boza, 2011[30]	RYGB				#		
de Sa, 2011[31]	RYGB					† § #	
Frenken, 2011[32]	RYGB				† #		
Huang, 2011[33]	RYGB		† § #		† § #		
Lee, 2011[34]	RYGB	† #	† #		† #		
Lee,2011[35]	RYGB	† § #	† § #		† § #	† § #	
Ramos, 2011[36]	RYGB					#	
Schauer, 2012[37]	RYGB	† § #	† § #	† § #	† § #		
Serrot,2011[a38]	RYGB				† #		
Angrisani, 2004[39]	LABG		†		†	†	†
O'Brien, 2006[40]	LABG		†		†	† §	
Parikh, 2006[41]	LABG				†	†	†
Dixon, 2008[42]	LABG					† #§	
Sultan, 2009[43]	LABG		†		†	†	
Choi, 2010[b44]	LABG						
DeMaria, 2010[28]	LABG	†	†		†	†	
Lee, 2011[34]	Sleeve	† #	† #		† #		
Lembach,2011, T2DM[45]	Sleeve				† § #		
Lembach,2011,IR[c45]	Sleeve				† §		
Schauer, 2012[37]	Sleeve	† § #	† § #	† § #	† § #		
Noya, 1998[46]	BPD			†			
Scopinaro, 2007[47]	BPD				† §	† §	
Chiellini, 2009[48]	BPD				† #	† #	
Frenken, 2011[d32]	BPD				† #		
Scopinaro, 2011, OB[e49]	BPD	† § #	† § #	† § #	† § #	† § #	
Scopinaro, 2011, OW[f49]	BPD	† § #	† § #	† § #	† § #	† § #	

BMI = body mass index;BPD= biliopancreatic diversion; BPD/DS = biliopancreatic diversion with duodenal switch; IR = insulin resistant patients; LABG = laparoscopic adjustable gastric banding; mths = months; OB = obese; OW = overweight; RYGB = Roux-en-Y gastric bypass; Sleeve = sleeve gastrectomy; T2DM = type 2 diabetes mellitus
†BMI.
#HbA1c.
§ Glucose.
[a] Only reported Median, used in outcome table.
[b] Only usable outcome is % diabetes remission: defined as "% improved/resolved" not otherwise specified.
[c] IR=insulin resistant patients.
[d] BPD-DS & BPD treated as 1 group.
[e] Obese (BMI 30-35).
[f] Overweight (BMI 25-30).

Head-to-Head Trials of Bariatric Surgery Versus Nonsurgical Interventions

We identified three randomized controlled trials (RCTs) comparing bariatric surgery with a nonsurgical intervention. One study by Schauer[37] compared medical treatment alone with medical treatment following laparoscopic RYGB or gastric sleeve in diabetic patients. Approximately one third of subjects had a baseline BMI in the target range (38%, 28%, and 36% respectively). Outcomes were assessed at 12 months. Two RCTs from an Australian research group assessed weight loss and diabetes outcomes for LAGB compared with nonsurgical interventions in our target population. O'Brien[40] focused on patients with BMI 30 kg/m^2–35 kg/m^2 and Dixon[42] included patients with somewhat higher BMI (range 30 kg/m^2–40 kg/m^2). The comparison arms included medical care and usual diabetes care. Patients were followed up to 24 months. Information on these studies is displayed in Table 3.

Schauer[37] conducted a recent RCT in 150 patients with uncontrolled type 2 diabetes (HbA1c >7.0%) and BMI of 27–43 kg/m^2 comparing intensive medical treatment alone with medical treatment following either RYGB or gastric sleeve. Study inclusion/exclusion criteria and randomization protocol were described in detail. Ninety-three percent of patients completed the 12 month follow-up. Eight patients withdrew from the study (seven in the medical therapy only group did not attend follow-up appointment and one subject in the SG group decided against surgery). Two additional patients in the medical therapy only group did not complete their nine month or 12 month follow-up—leaving 41 patients in the medical therapy alone group, 50 patients in the RYGB group and 49 in the SG group at 12 month followup.

The medical therapy alone group lost less weight at 12 months (–5.4 kg+/–8 kg) than medical therapy with RYGB (–29.4+/–9 kg,) or SG (–25.2+/–8.5 kg, p<.0001 for both comparisons). More patients in the surgical arms achieved glycemic control of HbA1c <6.0 percent: 12 percent in medical group, 42 percent in RYGB (p=0.002), and 37 percent in SG (p=0.008). Mean HbA1c at one year was lower following surgery: 7.5+/–1.8 percent for medical group, 6.4+/–0.9 percent for RYGB (p<0.001), and 6.6+/–1.0 percent for SG (p=0.003). The surgical groups reduced the mean number of both cholesterol medication and hypertension medications significantly compared with the surgical group. (p<.0001).

O'Brien[40] performed an RCT comparing LAGB (n=40) and medical management (n=40) which included low calorie diet, pharmacotherapy, and behavioral change. Patients had a mean baseline BMI of 33 kg/m^2 and were well-matched for baseline characteristics; the randomization process was well-described, as were dropouts. No patients were excluded from the analysis. One patient randomized to the surgical arm dropped out preoperatively; seven patients in the medical management did not attend followup at 24 months.

Both groups lost a similar amount of weight at six months (13.8 percent of initial weight in both arms). The surgical arm continued to lose weight out to 24 months (21.6 percent of initial weight), but the medical arm regained much of the weight they initially lost. At that followup, the surgical arm (n=39) had a mean BMI of 26.4 kg/m^2 and the medical arm (n=33) mean BMI was 31.5 kg/m^2. The surgical group experienced significantly greater weight loss (p<0.001). The majority of other outcomes were improved to a statistically significant degree in the surgical arm as compared with the medical arm, including diastolic blood pressure and lipid levels. Fasting blood glucose was lower in the surgical patients at 24 months as compared with the medical group (which did not experience a decrease). Metabolic syndrome was present in 37.5 percent of patients in both groups at baseline and decreased to 2.7 percent in the surgical patients (p<0.001) and 24 percent in the medical patients (p=0.22) at followup. A greater proportion of patients in the surgical group improved metabolic syndrome than in the medical group (p=.0006). Other laboratory values, such as HbA1c or use of diabetes medications, were not reported. Of note, quality of life (by short form 36) scores improved to a statistically significant degree in 5 of the 8 domains in the surgical group (8 of 8 subscores) as compared with the medical group (3 of 8).

Dixon et al[42] performed a similar study but included patients of somewhat higher BMI (mean baseline 37 kg/m^2). Sixty patients were randomized to LAGB or diabetes care as usual. Usual care focused on weight loss via conventional methods including counseling on diet and exercise. Authors described the randomization process and dropouts; patient baseline characteristics were similar following randomization.

At two years, 55 of 60 patients completed the followup. Surgical patients lost a mean of 21.1 kg initial weight compared with 1.5 kg in the conventional treatment arm (p<0.001 between groups). BMI decreased to 29.6 kg/m^2 in the surgery patients and 36.7 kg/m^2 in the conventional therapy group (p<.001 between groups). Fasting blood glucose (105.2 versus 139.6) was significantly lower in the surgery patients at two years as compared with the medical group (mean difference -32.8 [95% confidence interval (CI) -53.1, -12.3]). HbA1c was also improved to a greater degree in the surgical patients at two years as compared with the convention therapy group (6.00 versus 7.21; mean difference -1.43 [95% CI -2.1, -0.80]). Remission of type 2 diabetes was seen in 73 percent of the surgical group and 13 percent of the usual care group; relative risk of remission was 5.5 (95% CI 2.2, 14.0). Remission of diabetes was defined as fasting plasma glucose levels less than 126 mg/dL and HbA1c less than 6.2 percent without the use of oral hypoglycemic or insulin. Eighty percent of surgery patients had HbA1c <6.2 percent at 24 months compared with 20 percent of conventional therapy group (p<0.001). Resolution of type 2 diabetes was related to weight loss and lower baseline HbA1c levels.

Table 3. RCTs with comparison nonsurgical arms

Author/ Study Type	Procedure/ # Patients	Weight Outcomes at 12 Months		Diabetes and Metabolic Syndrome Outcomes at 12 Months				
		Weight Change, kg (SD)	BMI at 12 mo	Fasting Blood Glucose Change, mg/dL (SD)	HbA1c, % (SD)	HbA1c <6.0% at 12 mo	Average # Diabetes Meds, at 12 mo,	Diabetes Remission*, % at 12 mo [Change]
Schauer [37] RCT	Medical therapy +RYGB (n=50)	-29.4 (9.0)	26.5	99	6.4 (0.9)	42%	0.3	
	Medical therapy + GS (n =50)	-25. (8.5)	27.2	97	6.6 (1.0)	37%	0.9	
	Medical therapy alone (n=50)	-5.4 (8.0)	34.4	120	7.5 (1.8)	12%	3.0	
		p<0.0001†	p<0.001†	p<=0.002†	p<=0.003†	p<=0.002†	p<0.001†	

Author/ Study Type	Procedure/ # Patients	Weight Outcomes at 24 mo		Diabetes and Metabolic Syndrome Outcomes at 24 mo				
		Weight Change, kg (SD)	BMI at 24 mo [95% CI]	Fasting Blood Glucose change, mg/dL (SD)	HbA1c, % (SD)	HbA1c <6.0% at 12 mo	Average # Diabetes Meds, at 12 mo,	Metabolic Syndrome, % at 24 mo, [change]
O'Brien [40] RCT	LAGB (n=40)	-20.5, (6.4)	26.4 [25.6, 27.2]	-7.3 (15.2)	---	---	---	2.7, [-35]
	Medical Care (n=40)	-6.1, (8.5)	31.5, [30.6, 32.4]	0.35 (8.3)				24, [-12]
	Betw grp comparison Baseline BMI = 33.5 (SD =1.4)	95% CI [-18.9, -11.6]	p<0.001	95% CI [-13, -0.7]				p=.0006

Author/ Study Type	Procedure/ # Patients	Weight Change, kg (SD)	BMI at 24 mo [Change]	Fasting Blood Glucose Change, mg/dL (SD)	HbA1c, % Change, (SD)	HbA1c <6.2% at 24 mo	Taking DM Meds, % at 24 mo, [Change]	Diabetes Remission, % at 24 mo* [Change]
Dixon [42] RCT	LAGB (n=30)	-21.1 (10.5)	29.6, [-7.4]	-51.2, (37.2)	-1.81, (1.24)	80%	13.3, [-79.7]	73 [-73]
	Conventional (n=30)	-1.5 (5.4)	36.7, [-0.5]	-18.4, (41.2)	-0.38, (1.26)	20%	73.3, [-13.4]	13 [-13]
	Betw grp comparison Baseline BMI = 37.0 (SD = 2.7)	-19.6 [23.8,15.2] p<0.001	p<0.001	-32.8 [-53.1, -12.3] p=0.002	-1.43 [-2.1, -0.80] p<0.001	p<0.001	p<0.001	p<0.001

betw = between; BMI = body mass index; CI = confidence interval; DM = diabetes mellitus; grp = group; LAGB = laparoscopic adjustable gastric banding; meds = medications; mo = months; RCT = randomized controlled trial; RYGB = Roux-en-Y gastric bypass; SD = standard deviation

*Diabetes remission defined as fasting blood glucose <126mg/dL, HbA1c <6.2% without the use of insulin or oral hypoglycemics.

†Medical treatment compared with each surgical group.

Note: n=33 in the Medical Care Group.

Head-to-Head Trials of Surgical Procedures

We identified two RCTs comparing surgical procedures in our target population (Table 4). Lee[34] randomized 60 diabetic patients in Taiwan to RYGB or SG. Baseline demographics and clinical characteristics (mean BMI=30.3 kg/m^2) were similar between the groups. At 12 months followup the RYGB group had lost more weight: BMI was 22.8 kg/m^2 for RYGB, compared with 24.4 kg/m^2 for SG (p=0.009). Diabetes outcomes were also better in the RYGB group with 93 percent remission compared with 47 percent in SG group (p=0.02). Diabetes type 2 remission was defined as fasting plasma glucose levels less than 126 mg/dL and HbA1c values less than 6.5 percent without the use of oral hypoglycemics or insulin. HbA1c decreased by 4.2 percentage points in the RYGB versus 3.0 percentage points in the SG patients (p<0.05). Fasting glucose was lower in the RYGB patients compared with SG (99.3 versus 140.1; p<0.001). Total cholesterol level, triglycerides, low-density lipoprotein (LDL) cholesterol, and high-density lipoprotein (HDL) cholesterol improved in both groups but to a greater degree in the RYGB patients. A composite measure of diabetes improvement (HbA1c<7 percent, LDL<100 mg/dL, and triglycerides<150 mg/dL) revealed greater improvement in the RYGB group (57 percent versus 0 percent; p<0.001). Complication rates were similar between groups and were minor. Operative time and hospital stay were no different.

Schauer randomized 150 U.S. patients to either RYGB, SG, or intensive medical therapy alone (discussed earlier). The surgical groups also received the same intensive medical therapy. Patients' baseline characteristics were similar. Mean BMI was 37.0 ± 3.3 for the RYGB group, compared with 36.2 ± 3.9 for the gastric sleeve group. At 12 month followup, the bypass group had lost significantly more weight (p=.02) and had a slightly lower mean BMI (26.8 vs. 27.2). Changes in blood glucose were similar; however, all patients in the bypass group who achieved a pre-determined target glycated hemoglobin level (6 percent) did so without medications, while 28 percent in the sleeve group required medications to reach this level.

Changes in blood pressure and cholesterol did not differ significantly by surgical group.

Table 4. RCT with comparison surgical arms – Outcomes at one year

Author/ Study Type	Procedure/ # Patients	Weight Change (%)	BMI, kg/m² (SD)	Fasting Blood Glucose Mean, mg/dL (SD)	HbA1c %, Mean (SD)	Metabolic Syndrome No (%)	Successful Treatment Diabetes,[†] No (%)	Diabetes Remission,[‡] No (%)
Lee[34] RCT	Roux–en-Y gastric bypass (n=30)	-23.3	22.8 (2.2)	99.3 (19.4)	5.7 (0.5)	2 (6.6)	17 (57)	28 (93)
	Sleeve gastrectomy (n=30)	-19.9	24.4 (2.4)	140.1 (53.0)	7.2 (1.5)	18 (60.0)	0 (0)	14 (47)
	Betw grp comparison*	p=0.02	p=0.009	p<0.001	p<0.001	p<0.001	p<0.001	p=0.02
Schauer[37] RCT	Roux-en-Y gastric bypass (n=50)	-27.6	26.8	99.0	6.4 (0.9)	N/A	21 (42)	21 (42)
	Sleeve gastrectomy (n=49)	-25.0	27.2	97.0	6.6 (1.0)	N/A	18 (37)	13 (27)
	Betw grp comparison*	p=.02[§]	p=.03[§]	p=.86	p=.23	N/A	p=.59	p=.10

BMI = body mass index; btw = between; grp = group; LDL-C = low-density lipoprotein cholesterol; N/A = not applicable; No = number; RCT = randomized clinical trial; SD = standard deviation

*Between group comparisons are mean difference and 95% CI.

[†]Successful treatment of diabetes mellitus (HbA1c <7%, LDL-C <100 mg/dL, and triglycerides <150 mg/dL in Lee; HbA1c ≤ 6 percent in Schauer).

[‡]Remission defined as fasting plasma glucose levels less than 126 mg/dL and HbA1c values less than 6.5% without the use of oral hypoglycemics or insulin in Lee; HbA1c values ≤ 6 percent without use of oral hypoglycemic or insulin in Schauer.

[§] p for mean change from baseline.

Observational Studies With Surgical Procedure Comparisons

One cohort study compared RYGB with LAGB. Demaria[28] accessed a large retrospective database of patients operated on in the United States from 2005 to 2007 (n=66,264) and identified 235 who met the lower weight criteria (BMI ≥30 and <35 kg/m²). 109 patients underwent RYGB, the same number had had laparoscopic adjustable gastric band. (The remaining 17 underwent other procedures.) The study methods did not comment on the rationale of procedure choice for patients, but groups did not differ by baseline weight (33.7 kg/m² versus 33.9 kg/m²), gender, race, or age. Followup was 61.9 percent and 69.2 percent at 6-12 months for RYGB and laparoscopic adjustable gastric band patients, respectively. At 6-12 months, RYGB patients lost more weight than those undergoing laparoscopic adjustable gastric band (6-12 months: BMI 27.1 kg/m² and 30.9 kg/m²; p=0.0002). RYGB achieved better diabetes control for all time intervals as the number of patients off diabetes medications (at 6-12 months: 55.2 percent versus 27.2 percent; p=.0199), with the exception of the latest followup at 12-24 months (but only 4 RYGB and 11 LAGB patients were followed up at that time interval). For patients with diabetes controlled with oral medications, 60.9 percent and 38.5 percent, for RYGB and laparoscopic adjustable gastric band, respectively, were able to stop their diabetes medications within 3-6 months. For patients on insulin and oral medications, 50 percent and 11.1 percent, respectively, were able to stop their medications. Complications, while minor, occurred more commonly in the RYGB group (18 percent versus three percent, p<0.05).

One small study conducted in Germany compared results for twelve BPD patients with the results for four RYGB patients.[32] Both groups lost a significant amount of weight. At one year, decrease in HbA1c in the RYGB group was significantly greater than in the BPD group.

Small Cohorts: Surgery Versus Nonsurgical Interventions

We found two small cohort studies matching data from surgical patients with data from similar patients who did not have bariatric surgery. One small study by Chiellini[48] compared patients undergoing BPD (n=5) with those managed by diet (n=7). The study did not specify what variables the patients were matched on and only one month followup was reported. In this very short-term followup, HbA1c and weight were significantly lower in both groups. The BPD group did see a significant decrease in the blood glucose (at 2 hr) during an oral glucose tolerance test, whereas the diet arm did not.

Serrot[38] retrospectively compared data for 17 diabetic patients who underwent RYGB with 17 matched patients on routine medical management for diabetes / weight control. The nonsurgical group received counseling regarding diet, physical activity, and weight management. At one year, BMI did not change significantly in the routine management group, but decreased significantly from 34.6 kg/m^2 to 25.8 kg/m^2 in the RYGB group. HbA1c decreased significantly from a mean 8.2 percent at baseline to 6.1 percent at one year in the RYGB group, but did not change significantly in the comparison group. Systolic blood pressure and LDL cholesterol did not change significantly in either group; however, 41% of the RYGB group ceased use of antihypertension medications and 35% ceased use of antihyperlipidemia medications despite lack of clinically meaningful improvement on these outcomes.

Observational Studies—Diabetes Outcomes

Tables 5 and 6 display data from the observational studies. Table 5 presents data for the studies where all patients entering had type 2 diabetes or IGT; Table 6 displays the remaining handful of studies where only a portion of patients had these metabolic conditions. The tables are organized by outcome, surgery type, and followup time. Each table displays BMI, HbA1c, fasting glucose, percentage of patients off diabetes medication, and percentage of diabetes patients in remission, at three post-surgery intervals: 0 to 3 months, 6 to 11 months, and 12 months or more. Unlike RCTs, which try to measure outcomes at exact followup times, in these observational studies patient outcomes are measured at a wide range of times, depending on availability / convenience. Thus, we also include a column displaying the exact range of followup points included.

BMI

At up to three months followup, mean decrease in BMI ranged from 2.3 kg/m^2 in one study of LABG to 4.4 kg/m^2 in three studies of RYGB. Between six and 11 months followup, BMI decrease continued. Decreases were similar for BPD (5.2 kg/m^2), sleeve (5.3 kg/m^2) and RYGB (5.4 kg/m^2). The one LABG study that reported BMI during this time showed a decrease of 6.8 kg/m^2 (in contrast, this study reported a mean decrease of 4.0 kg/m^2 from baseline to 12 months.) At 12 to 24 months, mean BMI decrease was 5.6 kg/m^2 for BPD, 6.4 kg/m^2 for SG, and 7.9 kg/m^2 for RYGB.

Blood Glucose

Metabolic improvements after surgery were reported various ways including changes in HbA1c and plasma glucose, percentage of patients who no longer required diabetes medication, and remission or resolution of diabetes. There were six surgery arms reporting change in HbA1c at six to 11 months. Baseline HbA1c values were quite high ranging from 9.3 percent for BPD to 10.0 percent for SG. Considerable decreases were reported after surgery, with a mean drop of 2.9 percentage points for BPD, 2.6 percentage points for sleeve and 3.7 percentage points for RYGB. Unfortunately, none of the observational studies of LAGB reported HbA1c outcomes. Studies that reported HbA1c at one year or more also reported clinically significant improvement. RYGB patients had a mean decrease of 2.4 percentage points, compared with 3.1 percentage points for SG and 3.1 percent points for BPD patients.

Studies also reported clinically significant improvements in plasma glucose levels. Many patients were hyperglycemic preoperatively. In studies reporting results at six to 11 months, baseline levels ranged from 203.3 mg/dL for RYGB patients to 220.0 mg/dL for sleeve. These studies reported decreases in plasma glucose of 68.0 mg/dL for BPD to 102.0 mg/dL in the one sleeve study. Studies with followup of at least one year reported decreases in plasma glucose ranging from 62.6 mg/dL in one sleeve study to 92.4 mg/dL for BPD. At this time point, most surgical patients were euglycemic.

Medication Needs

A few studies reported the percentage of patients who no longer required diabetes medication after surgery. The majority of these studies regularly measured and reported corresponding data on HbA1c, fasting glucose, C-Peptite, etc. One LAGB study (Parikh, 2006[41] reported only the data regarding medication use, making it impossible to confirm whether discontinuation was appropriate; all eight diabetic patients discontinued medication.[41] At three months or less, two RYGB studies reported that 46.6 percent of their patients no longer needed diabetes medication, compared with 21.1 percent of patients in one LABG study. Two RYGB studies reported that 70.5 percent of patients no longer required medication at six to 11 months after surgery compared with 27.5 percent in an LABG study and 30.0 percent in a BPD study. At 12 months, the LABG study reported 36.4 percent of patients discontinued medications. At 24 months, a BPD study of seven patients reported that all had discontinued medications. Three RYBG studies reported a mean 87.2 percent of patients had discontinued diabetes medications between 12 to 20 months. At 12 to 24 months followup, discontinuation rate was 87.2 percent in three RYGB studies.

Remission/Resolution

Eight studies reported at 12 months or more. Definitions of remission and resolution varied; however, all these studies monitored metabolic data regularly. 87.2 percent of RYGB patients in six studies had resolved their diabetes, along with half of SG patients in one study and 83.5 percent of BPD patients in one study.

Table 5. Bariatric surgery results—by surgery type, studies of only diabetes or IGT patients

Outcome	F-Up	F-Up Range	# Studies	Surg Type	BL (N)	BL Mean (%)	BL (SE)	F-Up (N)	F-Up Mean (%)	F-Up (SE)	Mean Chg
BMI	0-3m	0-3m*	3	RYGB	201	32.1	1.2	163	27.7	2.3	-4.4
BMI	0-3m	0-3m*	1	LABG	109	33.9		90	31.6		-2.3
BMI	0-3m	3m	1	Sleeve	30	30.3		30	26.0		-4.3
BMI	0-3m	1m	1‡	BPD	30	30.6	2.5	30	26.7	2.4	-3.9
HbA1c	0-3m	3m	3	RYGB	107	9.8	0.1	90	6.3	0.4	-3.5
HbA1c	0-3m			LABG							
HbA1c	0-3m	3m	1	Sleeve	30	10.0		30	7.8		-2.2
HbA1c	0-3m	1m	1‡	BPD	30	9.3	0.2	30	7.3	0.0	-2.0
Glucose	0-3m	3m	2	RYGB	77	203.0	14.7	60	115.5	1.9	-89.6
Glucose	0-3m			LABG							
Glucose	0-3m			Sleeve							
Glucose	0-3m	1m	1‡	BPD	30	220.0	14.0	30	165.0	11.0	-55.0
% on Diabetes Meds	0-3m	0-3m*	2	RYGB	124	100.0	0.0	103	53.4	22.0	-46.6
% on Diabetes Meds	0-3m	0-3m*	1	LABG	109	100.0		90	78.9		-21.1
% on Diabetes Meds	0-3m			Sleeve							
% on Diabetes Meds	0-3m			BPD							
Diabetes Remission/Resolution	0-3m			RYGB							
Diabetes Remission/Resolution	0-3m			LABG							
Diabetes Remission/Resolution	0-3m			Sleeve							
Diabetes Remission/Resolution	0-3m			BPD							
BMI	6-11m	6-<12m*	5	RYGB	124	31.8	0.9	44	25.5	1.4	-5.4
BMI	6-11m	6-<12m*	1	LABG	109	33.9		40	27.1		-6.8
BMI	6-11m	6	1	Sleeve	30	30.3		30	25.0		-5.3
BMI	6-11m	8m	2‡	BPD	40	31.3	1.7	40	26.1	1.0	-5.2
HbA1c	6-11m	6-9m	4	RYGB	129	9.7	0.1	107	5.9	0.1	-3.7

Table 5. Bariatric surgery results—by surgery type, studies of only diabetes or IGT patients (continued)

Outcome	F-Up	F-Up Range	# Studies	Surg Type	BL (N)	BL Mean (%)	BL (SE)	F-Up (N)	F-Up Mean (%)	F-Up (SE)	Mean Chg
HbA1c	6-11m		0	LABG							
HbA1c	6-11m	6m	1	Sleeve	30	10.0		30	7.4		-2.6
HbA1c	6-11m	6m	1‡	BPD	30	9.3	0.2	30	6.4	0.5	-2.9
Glucose	6-11m	6-9m	3	RYGB	99	203.3	9.2	77	103.4	5.9	-102.0
Glucose	6-11m		0	LABG							
Glucose	6-11m			Sleeve							
Glucose	6-11m	8m	1‡	BPD	30	220.0	14.0	30	152.0	19.0	-68.0
% on Diabetes Meds	6-11m	6-<12m*	2	RYGB	124	100.0	0.0	44	29.5	21.2	-70.5
% on Diabetes Meds	6-11m	6-<12m*	1	LABG	109	100.0		40	72.5		-27.5
% on Diabetes Meds	6-11m			Sleeve							
% on Diabetes Meds	6-11m	8m	1	BPD	10	40.0		10	10.0		-30.0
Diabetes Remission/Resolution	6-11m	6m	1	RYGB				37	97.3		
Diabetes Remission/Resolution	6-11m		0	LABG							
Diabetes Remission/Resolution	6-11m		1	Sleeve							
Diabetes Remission/Resolution	6-11m		0	BPD							
BMI†	12-24m	12-24m	8	RYGB	315	32.2	0.6	168	23.9	0.5	-7.9
BMI	12-24m	>12m*	1	LABG	109	33.9		11	29.9		-4.0
BMI	12-24m	12-13m	2	Sleeve	42	31.9	2.5	42	25.5	1.7	-6.4
BMI	12-24m	12-24m	4‡	BPD	54	31.3	1.1	54	25.7	0.6	-5.6
HbA1c†	12-24m	12-24m	9	RYGB	433	8.6	0.3	275	5.9	0.1	-2.4
HbA1c	12-24m		0	LABG							
HbA1c	12-24m	12-13m	2	Sleeve	42	9.2	1.3	42	6.3	1.4	-2.9
HbA1c	12-24m	12-24m	3‡	BPD	47	9.1	0.2	47	6.0	0.4	-3.1
Glucose	12-24m	12-24m	5	RYGB	192	178.2	10.0	150	94.0	3.6	-79.3
Glucose	12-24m		0	LABG							
Glucose	12-24m	12-13m	1	Sleeve	12	150.6		12	88.0		-62.6
Glucose	12-24m	24m	2‡	BPD	37	226.2	12.8	37	133.9	16.1	-92.4

Table 5. Bariatric surgery results—by surgery type, studies of only diabetes or IGT patients (continued)

Outcome	F-Up	F-Up Range	# Studies	Surg Type	BL (N)	BL Mean (%)	BL (SE)	F-Up (N)	F-Up Mean (%)	F-Up (SE)	Mean Chg
% on Diabetes Meds	12-24m	12-20m	3	RYGB	293	100.0	0.0	188	12.8	4.6	-87.2
% on Diabetes Meds	12-24m	12m*	1	LABG	109	100.0		11	63.6		-36.4
% on Diabetes Meds	12-24m		0	Sleeve							
% on Diabetes Meds	12-24m	24m	1	BPD	7	71.4		7	0.0		-71.4
Diabetes Remission/Resolution	12-24m	12-20m	6	RYGB				323	77.7	5.3	
Diabetes Remission/Resolution	12-24m		0	LABG							
Diabetes Remission/Resolution	12-24m	12m	1	Sleeve				30	46.7		
Diabetes Remission/Resolution	12-24m	12m	1‡	BPD				30	83.5	16.5	

BL= baseline; BMI = body mass index; BPD = biliopancreatic diversion; chg = change; F-up = followup; IGT = impaired glucose tolerance; IQR = inter-quartile range; LAGB = laparoscopic adjustable gastric banding; m = month; meds = medications; N = sample size; RYGB = Roux-en-Y gastric bypass; SE = standard error ; Sleeve = sleeve gastrectomy

*DeMaria et al. 2010[28] reported results as 0-3m, 3-6m, 6-12m,12-24m. The range 6-12m was reported in the 6-11m category, 12-24m was reported in the >=12mth category.

†Serrot, 2011 (6027) only reported median and IQR. Median value used instead of mean for summary calculations.

‡Scopinaro et al. 2001[49] reports data for obese and overweight patients separately, both subgroups contribute to this analysis but it is only counted as 1 study/article.

26

Table 6. Bariatric surgery results—by surgery type, studies with less than 100% diabetes or IGT patients

Outcome	F-Up	F-Up Range	# Studies	Surg Type	BL (N)	BL Mean (%)	BL (SE)	F-Up (N)	F-Up Mean (%)	F-Up (SE)	Mean Chg
BMI	6-11m		0	RYGB							
BMI	6-11m	6m	2	LABG	263	33.74	0.32	244	30.68	1.04	-3.11
BMI	6-11m		0	Sleeve							
BMI	6-11m		0	BPD							
HbA1c	6-11m		0	RYGB							
HbA1c	6-11m		0	LABG							
HbA1c	6-11m		0	Sleeve							
HbA1c	6-11m		0	BPD							
Glucose	6-11m		0	RYGB							
Glucose	6-11m		0	LABG							
Glucose	6-11m		0	Sleeve							
Glucose	6-11m		0	BPD							
% on Diabetes Meds	6-11m		0	RYGB							
% on Diabetes Meds	6-11m		0	LABG							
% on Diabetes Meds	6-11m		0	Sleeve							
% on Diabetes Meds	6-11m		0	BPD							
Diabetes Remission/Resolution	6-11m		0	RYGB							
Diabetes Remission/Resolution	6-11m	6m	1	LABG				210	100.00		
Diabetes Remission/Resolution	6-11m		0	Sleeve							
Diabetes Remission/Resolution	6-11m		0	BPD							

27

Table 6. Bariatric surgery results—by surgery type, studies with less than 100% diabetes or IGT patients (continued)

Outcome	F-Up	F-Up Range	# Studies	Surg Type	BL (N)	BL Mean (%)	BL (SE)	F-Up (N)	F-Up Mean (%)	F-Up (SE)	Mean Chg
BMI	12-24m		0	RYGB							
BMI	12-24m	24m	3	LABG	356	33.47	0.38	302	28.09	0.68	-5.47
BMI	12-24m	12m	1	Sleeve	9	33.60		9	23.40		-10.20
BMI	12-24m		0	BPD							
HbA1c	12-24m		0	RYGB							
HbA1c	12-24m		0	LABG							
HbA1c	12-24m		0	Sleeve							
HbA1c	12-24m		0	BPD							
Glucose	12-24m		0	RYGB							
Glucose	12-24m		0	LABG							
Glucose	12-24m	12m	1	Sleeve	9	99.20		9	76.00		-23.20
Glucose	12-24m		0	BPD							
% on Diabetes Meds	12-24m		0	RYGB							
% on Diabetes Meds	12-24m		0	LABG							
% on Diabetes Meds	12-24m		0	Sleeve							
% on Diabetes Meds	12-24m		0	BPD							
Diabetes Remission/Resolution	12-24m		0	RYGB							
Diabetes Remission/Resolution	12-24m	12m	1	LABG				66	33.33		
Diabetes Remission/Resolution	12-24m		0	Sleeve							
Diabetes Remission/Resolution	12-24m		0	BPD							

28

Table 6. Bariatric surgery results—by surgery type, studies with less than 100% diabetes or IGT patients (continued)

Outcome	F-Up	F-Up Range	# Studies	Surg Type	BL (N)	BL Mean (%)	BL (SE)	F-Up (N)	F-Up Mean (%)	F-Up (SE)	Mean Chg
BMI*	36m		2	LABG	303	33.53	0.55	277	26.85	0.26	-6.76
BMI*	48m		1	LABG	210	33.90		210	27.90		-6.00
BMI*	60m		1	LABG	210	33.90		210	28.20		-5.70
% on Diabetes Meds*	36m		1	LABG	93	8.60		67	0		-8.60

BL= baseline; BMI = body mass index; BPD = biliopancreatic diversion with duodenal switch; chg = change; F-up = followup; IGT = impaired glucose tolerance; LAGB = laparoscopic adjustable gastric banding; m = month; meds = medications; N = sample size; RYGB = Roux-en-Y gastric bypass; SE = standard error ; Sleeve = sleeve gastrectomy

*Angrisani et al. 2004[39] has BMI data for 36m-60m, Parikh et al. 2006[41] has BMI data at 36m and % off diabetes meds at 36m.

Observational Studies – Other Health Outcomes

Blood Pressure

Eight surgery studies reported blood pressure outcomes; measures reported included percent of patients with hypertension, percent able to discontinue blood pressure medication, and mean systolic and diastolic blood pressure. One study (primarily of non-diabetics) followed patients for 12 months after undergoing LAGB and found that the percentage of patients with hypertension decreased from 4.3 percent to 0.5 percent.[39] Another reported that hypertension improved or resolved in 28.6 percent of patients, 18 months after receiving LAGB.[44] Two LAGB studies reported the number who no longer required antihypertensive medications; one found that 75 percent were able to discontinue 24 months after surgery, while another found that 46 percent were able to 36 months post-op.[41,43] Unfortunately, these two studies did not report corresponding systolic or diastolic blood pressure data. Four RYGB studies reported blood pressure outcomes. One reported that 41 percent of patients were off hypertension medications at one year; however, they did not report baseline percentage taking the medications. Mean systolic blood pressure in this RYGB group actually increased from 126.0 at baseline to 132.0 at one year.[38] Another RYGB study[30] reported hypertension resolved in 46.7 percent of patients at one year; however diastolic and systolic blood pressure data were not reported. Another RYGB study[29] reported a mean 11 point drop in systolic blood pressure at six months. One study[50] reported a mean decrease of 9 mmHg in diastolic and 11 mmHg in systolic blood pressure at six months.

Cholesterol and Triglycerides

Cholesterol and triglyceride outcomes were reported inconsistently. One small BPD study followed seven patients at one, two, three, and five years[47] and reported that none had hypercholesterolemia or high triglycerides at any followup. Baseline mean triglycerides were 311.6 mg/dL in this study. Another study of 10 BPD patients reported a mean decrease of 106.3 mg/dL in total cholesterol at followup of two to 18 months. One LAGB study[43] reported that 33.3% of patients no longer needed cholesterol medications at two years but gave no other details on this outcome. Lemback[45] reported SG results separately for patients with diabetes versus impaired glucose tolerance (IGT) at one year post-surgery. Triglycerides decreased 69 mg/dL and 76 mg/dL respectively.

Five RYGB studies[26,27,29,37,38] reported on cholesterol. Decreases in LDL ranged from only 3 mg/dL to 53.8 mg/dL at one year. Two studies reported change in total cholesterol. Shah[29] reported a decrease of 40 mg/dL at nine months, while Cohen[26] reported a decrease of 80 mg/dL at 20 months.

GERD and Sleep Apnea

A few studies reported on gastroesophageal reflux disease (GERD) and obstructive sleep apnea (OSA); these studies included a small subset of patients who had preoperative GERD or OSA who underwent LAGB. In one study that included five patients with preoperative GERD, all had complete resolution at one year after surgery.[39] In a slightly larger study that included 22 patients with preoperative GERD, only 31.3 percent experienced improvement or resolution at one year after LAGB.[44] Neither study detailed the exact methods of diagnosing resolution of GERD. Of the three studies that reported on OSA, one study found that half of the 19 patients had complete resolution (defined as discontinuation of continuous positive airway pressure

[CPAP] mask use) at two years after LAGB and an additional 30 percent had improvement (decreased CPAP use).[43] In another study that included seven patients with preoperative OSA, six had OSA resolution (did not require CPAP use) by three years after LAGB.[41] In a third study, only three of nine patients with OSA had improvement or resolution at one year (definition of improvement or resolution not specified).[44]

Systematic Reviews on Behavioral Interventions

The effects of interventions such as exercise, diet, and health education on weight loss and diabetes outcomes have been studied for decades. Thus, the primary literature on these topics is extensive. In such cases we attempt to find existing reviews.[51] We identified six fair to excellent quality systematic reviews; four focused on adults with pre-existing diabetes while the other two focused on diabetes prevention in adults with impaired glucose tolerance. Details on the reviews are displayed in Table 7.

Pooling 22 RCTs with a total of 4,659 participants and a followup interval of 1 to 5 years, Norris and colleagues[52] assessed the effectiveness of lifestyle and behavioral interventions on weight loss or weight control among adults with type 2 diabetes (mean BMI = 33.2kg/m², mean duration of diabetes = 6.5 years). Interventions examined included physical activity, low calorie diet, and behavioral interventions such as self-monitoring blood glucose and spousal involvement in education. Comparisons of three groups of studies were conducted: any intervention versus usual care, very low-calorie diet versus low-calorie diet, and physical activity versus no or less intensive physical activity. The pooled weight loss for intervention group (any intervention) in comparison with usual care was 1.7 kg at 1 and 2 years of followup, and the pooled weight loss for very low-calorie diets in comparison with low-calorie diets was 3.0 kg at 72 and 104 weeks of followup. Among those who received identical dietary and behavioral interventions, the pooled weight loss for intensive physical activity in comparison with no or less physical activity was 3.9 kg. Of the six intervention types (including usual care and different combinations of interventions), all interventions were associated with significant weight loss, but a very low-calorie diet combined with physical activity and behavioral therapy produced the largest weight loss effect. However, changes in glycated hemoglobin level were not significant.

Kirk and colleagues (2008) evaluated 13 studies (including nine RCTs) that examined effects of carbohydrate-restricted diets in type 2 diabetes patients (mean weight = 77 to 132 kg, mean HbA1c = 6.9 – 9.8) in North America.[53] Seven outcomes were reported: weight, fasting glucose, HbA1c, total cholesterol, HDL cholesterol, LDL cholesterol, and triglycerides. At 3 to 26 weeks followup, weight loss after carbohydrate-restricted diets ranged from 0.5 to 8.7 kg, representing 0.5 percent to 7.5 percent changes from baseline; decrease in HbA1c ranged from 0.2 to 2.2, representing 2.9 percent to 22.4 percent changes from baseline; and reduction in fasting glucose ranged from 1.8 to 83.0, representing 1.3 percent to 36.6 percent changes from baseline. They also found a greater mean reduction in fasting glucose and HbA1c in the lower-carbohydrate diet phase compared with the higher-carbohydrate diet phase. While triglyceride reductions were observed in both lower- and higher-carbohydrate phases, an especially strong relationship was found in the lower-carbohydrate phase. No significant relationships were found for the three cholesterol outcomes.

Dyson, 2008[54] reviewed 6 studies (including one RCT) that examined short-term effect and associated risks of low and reduced carbohydrate diets in type 2 diabetes patients (mean BMI = 28.5 to 42.2kg/m², mean HbA1c = 7.3 to 9.7). Meta-analysis was not conducted due to heterogeneity of the studies. Sample size ranged from 10 to 206; only two studies had sample size over 100). Short-term effects (followup duration n= 14 days – 22 months but only two

31

studies with data beyond six months) were reported and carbohydrate levels ranged from <20g/day to 95g/day. All studies reported reductions in body weight and glycated hemoglobin: reductions in body weight ranged from 1.2 to 11.4 kg, reductions in BMI ranged from 0.4 to 4.1 kg/m², and reductions in HbA1c ranged from 0.5 to 1.7 points. A few studies also recorded either reduction or discontinuation of glucose-lowering medications such as metformin and thiazoladinediones.

Kodama and colleagues[55] conducted a meta-analysis to assess the influence of fat and carbohydrate proportions on glucose and lipid parameters in type 2 diabetes patients. Pooling 22 trials with a total of 306 participants (mean BMI = 22.7 to 33.1kg/m², diabetes duration = 5 to 8 years) and an intervention period of 1.4 to 12 weeks, the study compared the effects of a low-fat high-carbohydrate (LFHC) diet with a high-fat low-carbohydrate (HFLC) diet. While no significant differences in the reduction in HbA1c, total cholesterol, and LDL cholesterol were found between the LFHC and HFLC diets, LFHC diet led to significant increases in fasting insulin (8.4 percent, with marked elevations observed when the carbohydrate/fat ratio >=3) and triglycerides levels (13.4 percent), and a significant reduction in HDL cholesterol (6 percent). They also found significant positive relationships among the change in fasting plasma glucose, fasting insulin, and triglycerides. They concluded that replacing fat with carbohydrate have negative implications for diabetes patients.

Norris and colleagues[56] examined the effects of weight-loss interventions in 9 RCTs consisting a total of 5,168 overweight or obese participants (mean BMI = 25.8 to 34.0 kg/m², mean glycated hemoglobin (GHb) = 5.7 to 5.9) with pre-diabetes (impaired fasting glucose or impaired glucose tolerance). Most of the studies reported long-term data, with followup durations ranging from 1 to 10 years. Weight-loss strategies included diet, physical activity, and behavioral interventions, while comparison group interventions consisted of usual care or general information and counseling. Compared with usual care, these weight-loss interventions led to 2.8 kg weight loss at one year (representing 3.3 percent of baseline body weight) and 2.7 kg at two years; reduction in BMI was 1.4 kg/m² at 1 year. The most notable mean weight change was observed in the lifestyle intervention of the DPP (Diabetes Prevention Program) study, which had the largest study population. It reported a mean weight loss of 5.5 kg at an average followup of 2.8 years. A few studies reported small decreases in systolic and diastolic blood pressure, minor improvements in lipids, and 0.0 to 0.2 decreases in GHb. Three large trials also demonstrated a significant lower cumulative incidence of diabetes in the intervention versus control groups, at three to six years followup.

Gillies and colleagues[57] also reviewed studies that evaluated interventions to delay or prevent type 2 diabetes among patients with impaired glucose tolerance. Behavioral interventions included diet and exercise; pharmacological/herbal interventions included acarbose, flumamine, glipizide, metformin, phenformin, orlistat, and herbal iangtang busheng. They identified 21 RCTs and conducted a meta-analysis using 17 RCTs with a total of 8,084 participants (mean BMI = 23.8 to 37.3 kg/m², baseline risk of type 2 diabetes = 2.6 to 30.0 cases per 100 person years). They found high strength of evidence in favor of interventions compared with controls, the pooled effects (in terms of hazard ratios) were 0.51 for overall behavioral interventions (corresponding to a relative 49 percent reduction in risk of developing diabetes), 0.67 for diet, 0.49 for exercise, 0.49 for diet and exercise combined, 0.70 for oral diabetes drugs, 0.44 for orlistat, and 0.32 for the herbal Jiangtang busheng recipe. All except for the herbal Jiangtang busheng recipe were statistically significant. The authors concluded that behavioral interventions were at least as effective as pharmacological interventions.

In sum, compared with surgical options, the effects of nonsurgical weight loss or weight control strategies among type 2 diabetes patients have been widely investigated. Evidence has shown that exercise, diet, lifestyle, and behavioral interventions are associated with significant weight loss and improved blood sugar outcomes (e.g., decreasing HbA1c or fasting glucose) among adult patients with pre-existing type 2 diabetes. Evidence is stronger for the weight loss effect, compared with the diabetes improvement effect, and more intensive and sustained interventions seem more effective. These findings were consistent with those found in non-diabetic but high-risk population with impaired glucose tolerance or impaired fasting glucose. Among those patients, nonsurgical interventions were associated with reduced risk of developing diabetes in the long run. However, studies also pointed out that the magnitude of effects of nonsurgical interventions in reducing weight and improving blood sugar outcomes are often small, although statistically significant. Most of these systematic reviews reported that studies were very heterogeneous with respect to the interventions; thus the effects should be interpreted cautiously.

Table 7. Systematic reviews on nonsurgical interventions

Author / Year	Intervention	Patients	Search Through	# of Included Studies	AMSTAR	Findings
Norris, 2004[52]	Exercise, diet, behavioral	Type 2 DM mean BMI = 33 range 23-38 mean HbA1C* = 10 range 7–13 Mean age = 55	August 2003	22 RCTs duration 1 year– 5 years (16/22 ≤ 1.5 yr)	10	1.7 kg weight loss for all interventions pooled, vs. usual care, at 1–5 years. Physical activity + very low cal diet lost 3.0 kg more than physical activity + low cal diet (N = 126). Identical diets + more intense physical activity lost 3.9 kg more. Differences in glycated hemoglobin and fasting glucose not significant.
Kirk, 2008[53]	Low carbohydrate diets	Type 2 DM Mean weight = 77 – 132 kg Mean HbA1c* = 6.9 – 9.8 North America only	April 2006	13 studies (9 RCTs) duration 3 weeks–26 weeks	6	No pooling conducted. Weight loss ranged from 0.5 to 8.7 kg from baseline at 3 to 26 weeks Decrease in HbA1c ranged from 0.3 to 2.2 points.
Dyson, 2008[54]	Low carbohydrate diets	Type 2 DM Mean weight = 76 – 131 kg Mean BMI = 28 – 42 Mean age = 51 – 66	March 2007	6 trials (1 RCT) duration 14 days – 22 months	6	No pooling conducted. Weight loss ranged from 1.2 to 11.4 kg from baseline . Decrease in HbA1c* ranged from 0.5 to 1.4. Decrease in BMI ranged from 0.4 to 4.1 points.
Kodama, 2009[55]	Low carbohydrate diets vs. low fat diets	Type 2 DM Mean BMI = 23 – 33 Mean age = 48 – 66 Mean % on diabetes meds = 52	2007	19 RCTs duration < 1 year	9	Low carb high cholesterol diet led to significant increases in fasting insulin and triglycerides from base, and decreases in HDL. Changes in HbA1c* were not significant.

Table 7. Systematic reviews on nonsurgical interventions (continued)

Author / Year	Intervention	Patients	Search Through	# of Included Studies	AMSTAR	Findings
Norris, 2005[56]	Weight loss Interventions (diet, physical activity, behavioral)	Adults with IGT, BMI range 26-34 Mean BMI 28.7 Mean age 51.2 Mean GHb 5.8	August 2003	9 RCTs f/u 1 to 10 years 7 of the RCTs were diet vs. usual care/ counseling	10	Pooled results 2.8 kg weight loss at 1 year compared with usual care & decrease in BMI of 1.4; at 2 years, 2.7 kg weight loss. No pooling for GHb. Decrease in GHb ranged from 0.0 to 0.2 percentage points. 3 studies reported diabetes incidence; one reported decrease of 31% at 2.8 years.
Gillies, 2007[57]	Treatment to delay or prevent DM (pharma, diet, exercise)	Adults with IGT Mean age ranged 38.7 to 56.7 Mean BMI ranged 23.8 to 37.3	July 2006	12 RCTs of behavioral interventions 12 RCTs of herbal/ pharmacological 4 other studies	9	Hazard ratios for progression to diabetes: 0.51 for lifestyle vs. standard advice 0.70 for oral diabetes meds vs. control 0.44 for orlistat vs. control 0.32 for herbal jiang tang bushen vs. advice

AMSTAR = measurement tool to assess the methodological quality of systematic reviews; BMI = body mass index;
DM = diabetes mellitus; GHb = glycated hemoglobin IGT = impaired glucose tolerance; RCTs = randomized controlled trials
*HbA1C measured as a percentage of total hemoglobin.

Systematic Reviews of Diabetes Medications

Four high quality systematic reviews focused on the efficacy and safety of diabetes medications in patients with type 2 diabetes. Two of the reviews[11,58] examined incretin-based agents (exenatide, liraglutide, vildagliptin, and sitagliptin), another[59] examined oral agents (second-generation sulfonylureas, biguanides, thiazolidinediones, meglitinides, and α-glucosidase inhibitors), and one[60] examined newer agents available for blood glucose control (exenatide, sitagliptin and vildagliptin, glargine and detemir, and thiazolidinediones). These reviews provide evidence that most blood glucose control medications are effective in glycemic control; some of them also lead to weight loss. However, clinical data such as effects on all-cause and cardiovascular mortality are limited. Results are summarized in Table 8.

Fakhoury and colleagues[58] conducted a systematic review and a meta-analysis to compare incretin-based agents with placebo. They identified 38 RCTs directly comparing either exenatide and liraglutide, which are GLP-1R agonists, or the dipeptidyl / peptidase-4 (DPP-4) inhibitors, vildagliptin and sitagliptin with placebo. Mean baseline HbA1c of participants included in the study ranged from 6.7 to 9.4 percent, mean duration of diabetes from 1.7 to 9.0 years, and mean baseline weight from 61.5 to 104.0 kg. Duration of trials ranged from 4 to 52 weeks. While all incretin-based agents significantly reduced HbA1c level in comparison with placebo (weighted mean difference [WMD]= -0.79 percentage points, -0.75, and -0.67 percentage points for sitagliptin, exenatide, and vildagliptin, respectively), liraglutide was found to produce the greatest reduction (WMD= - 1.03 percentage points) although this value was not statistically different from the other incretin-based drugs. A statistically significant weight gain was found in vildagliptin and sitagliptin groups, while a statistically significant weight reduction was found in the exenatide and liraglutide groups, especially in the exenatide group. Participants in sitagliptin and exenatide groups were more likely to experience some hypoglycemia compared with participants in the placebo group. The authors concluded that incretin-based agents produced beneficial effect on glycemic control, and that exenatide and liraglutide also led to weight loss. A new meta-analysis on these two GLP-1R agonists was published recently.[11] RCTs comparing exenatide or liraglutide with placebo, oral antidiabetic medication, or insulin were included. The authors found that patients taking these GLP-1R agonists lost a mean 2.90 kg (95% CI 2.22 kg to 3.59kg) more than patients in the control groups. Decrease in systolic blood pressure averaged 3.57 mmHg (95% CI 5.49 to 7.66) more than in the control groups, while decrease in diastolic blood pressure was also significantly greater (1.38 mmHg, 95% CI 0.73 to 2.22). Reduction in HbA1c (0.63 percentage points, 95% CI 0.80 to 0.46) was also superior in the GLP-1R agonistic groups. Gastro-intestinal adverse events including nausea, vomiting, and diarrhea were more common in the groups taking these medications.

Bolen and colleagues[59] reviewed the benefits and harms of oral agents in treating type 2 diabetes patients in the United States Two hundred and sixteen controlled trials and cohort studies were included. No evidence was found to support the effectiveness of oral agents on major clinical end points such as all-cause mortality, cardiovascular mortality or morbidity, peripheral arterial disease, neuropathy, retinopathy, or nephropathy. However, most oral agents showed a beneficial effect on intermediate outcomes such as glycemic control: thiazolidinediones, metformin, and repaglinide decreased HbA1c level by about one percentage point; nateglinide and α-glucosidase inhibitors produced weaker reductions in HbA1c by about 0.5 percentage point. Most oral agents other than metformin were associated with one to five kg of weight gain. Different agents were associated with different adverse events: sulfonylureas and repaglinide were associated with greater risk for hypoglycemia, thiazolidinediones with greater risk for heart failure, and metformin with greater risk for gastrointestinal problems. The authors concluded that older agents such as second-generation sulfonylurea and metformin were at least as effective as other oral agents on intermediate outcomes such as glycemic control.

A group of UK researchers reviewed newer pharmacological agents[60] for blood glucose control in type 2 diabetes patients from four classes: the glucagon-like peptide-1 (GLP-1) analogue exenatide; dipeptidyl peptidase-4 (DPP-4) inhibitors sitagliptin and vildagliptin; the long-acting insulin analogues, glargine and detemir; and thiazolidinediones. While focused on cost-effectiveness and comparing newer agents with neutral protamine Hagedorn (NPH), the study found that exenatide and DPP-4 inhibitors were all clinically effective in glycemic control: in patients with inadequate control on dual oral combination therapy, adding exenatide produced a one percentage point reduction in HbA1c level; when combined with metformin, the DPP-4 inhibitors reduced HbA1c level by about 0.8 percentage point. Exenatide was found to be associated with an added benefit of weight loss. Hypoglycemia, weight gain, heart failures, fractures, and cardiovascular events were among the side effects associated with the agents.

Table 8. Systematic reviews of medications

Author / Year	Intervention	Patients	Search Through	# of Included Studies	AMSTAR	Findings
Fakhoury, 2010[58]	Incretin-based medications: exenatide, liraglutide, vildagliptin, and sitagliptin	Type 2 DM mean weight = 61.5 - 104.0 kg mean HbA1C* = 6.7 - 9.4 Mean age = 50.9 - 62.9	July 2009	38 RCTs Duration 4 - 52 weeks	7	All agents significantly reduced HbA1c* level in comparison with placebo (pooled results of weighted mean differences: -1.03, -0.79, -0.75, -0.67 percentage points for liraglutide, sitagliptin, exenatide, and vildaglitin, respectively); weight loss associated with exenatide (WMD= -1.10).
Waugh, 2010[60]	Exenatide, sitagliptin and vildagliptin, glargine and detemir, and thiazolidinediones	Type 2 DM mean weight/BMI/HbA1c* separately reported for each arm	April 2008	Hard to count # of included studies since reported separately for individual arms; but > 24 RCTs and 10 Systematic reviews Duration >=12 weeks	9	Exenatide and DPP-4 inhibitors were effective in glycemic control: adding exenatide produced a 1 percentage point point reduction in HbA1c* in patients with inadequate control on dual oral combination therapy; DPP-4 inhibitors + metformin reduced HbA1c by 0.8 percentage points; pioglitazone + insulin reduced HbA1c by 0.54 percentage points.
Bolen, 2007[59]	Oral medications: second-generation sulfonylureas, biguanides, thiazolidinediones, meglitinides, and α-glucosidase inhibitors	Type 2 DM	January 2006	216 Controlled trials and cohort studies 2 Systematic reviews Duration >= 3 mo	10	Pooled result: thiazolidinediones, metformin, and repaglinide decreased HbA1c* by one percentage point; No pooling for nateglinide and α-glucosidase inhibitors: reduced HbA1c by 0.5 percentage point; No effectiveness evidence on all-cause mortality, cardiovascular mortality or morbidity, peripheral arterial disease, neuropathy, retinopathy, or nephropathy.
Visboll, 2012[11]	GLP-1R agents: Exenatide, Liraglutide	Overweight or obese patients with or without Type 2 DM	May 2011	25 RCTs Duration ≥ 20 weeks	9	Patients with diabetes lost a mean 2.8kg on the drugs; weight loss was greater with higher doses. Control groups included placebo, insulin, and oral diabetic medication groups. GLP-1R agonist groups had significantly greater decreases in blood pressure, cholesterol, and HbA1c than control groups. Gastro-intestinal adverse events including nausea, vomiting, and diarrhea were common in the GLP-1R agonist groups.

AMSTAR = measurement tool to assess the methodological quality of systematic reviews; BMI = body mass index; DM = diabetes mellitus;DPP-4 = dipeptidyl peptidase-4; GLP-1R = GLP-1 Agonists: Glucagon-like peptide-1 agonists, a class of diabetes drugs targeting the incretin system; RCTs = randomized controlled trials, WMD = weighted mean difference
*HbA1C measured as percentage of total hemoglobin.

Major Trials Published After the Systematic Reviews

Since the systematic reviews discussed above were published, several long-term followups of included studies have been published. These studies assessed the long-term effects of nonsurgical interventions in China[61] (behavioral intervention), Finland[62] (behavioral), United States[63] (behavioral and medications), and the United Kingdom[64] (medications). Weight loss effects that were observed during active intervention period did not always persist in the long run, while the reductions in diabetes incidence and diabetes-related end points persisted. This effect was consistent across locations. However, behavioral interventions did not lead to any significant reduction in some major clinical end points such as mortality. Pharmacological interventions reduced mortality in the long run only in the U.K. study[64]. More long-term data are needed to investigate morbidity reduction effects of nonsurgical interventions.

In China, Li and colleagues[61] conducted a 20-year followup study of the China Da Qing Diabetes Prevention Study (CDQDPS), which compared behavioral interventions (diet, exercise, and diet plus exercise) with a control group among adults with impaired glucose tolerance. Long-term effect on the risk of diabetes, diabetes-related macrovascular and microvascular complications, and mortality were reported. Although changes in body weight during the entire 20-year followup period did not differ significantly by intervention and control groups, participants in the intervention group had a 43 percent lower incidence of diabetes over the 20-year period, compared with those in control group. The average annual incidence of diabetes and 20-year cumulative incidence of diabetes were lower in the intervention group (7 percent annual incidence and 80 percent cumulative incidence) than those in the control group (11 percent annual incidence and 93 percent cumulative incidence). Diabetes onset was delayed an average of 3.6 years in the intervention group. However, no significant difference was observed in the rate of first cardiovascular disease (CVD) event, CVD mortality, and all-cause mortality between intervention group and control group. The authors concluded that behavioral interventions produced a long-lasting reduction in the incidence of type 2 diabetes.

Ilanne-Parikka and colleagues[62] reported on the Finnish Diabetes Prevention Study and assessed effects of behavioral intervention on metabolic syndrome and its components. Mean BMI at baseline was 31.2, with a standard deviation of 4.6 kg/m^2. At mean followup of 3.9 years, they found that intensive behavioral intervention produced a significant reduction in the prevalence of metabolic syndrome (from 74.0 percent to 58.0 percent), compared with the standard care provided to the control group (from 74.0 percent to 67.7 percent). A reduction in the prevalence of abdominal obesity in the long term was also observed in intervention group (odds ratio = 0.48).

In the United States, Knowler and colleagues[63] conducted a 10-year followup study of the DPP and investigated the persistence of the diabetes incidence and weight loss effects of behavioral and medication interventions that were observed during the intervention period. The effect of an intensive behavioral intervention and metformin on diabetes incidence, weight loss, and cardiovascular disease risk were compared with that of placebo. During the 10-year followup period, the behavioral group lost the most weight initially, and then gradually regained weight (but still weighed less than they did at baseline), while the metformin group maintained a modest weight loss. Cumulative incidence of diabetes in the 10 years was reduced by 34 percent in the behavioral group and 18 percent in the metformin group. It remained lower in the behavioral and metformin groups than in the placebo group, although diabetes incidence during the 10-year followup did not differ significantly between groups. Diabetes onset was delayed in behavioral group and metformin group by four years and two years, respectively, compared with placebo group. The authors concluded that both behavioral and metformin interventions reduced cumulative incidence of diabetes; this effect persisted for at least 10 years.

Holman and colleagues[64] performed a 10-year followup study of the United Kingdom Prospective Diabetes Study (UKPDS), which compared effects of an intensive glucose therapy (sulfonylurea or insulin or, in overweight patients, metformin) with conventional dietary therapy. No significant difference in mean body weight had been found between groups. After one year, between-group differences in mean glycated hemoglobin levels were lost: participants in both groups had similar improvements. However, the sulfonylurea/insulin group maintained significant reductions in relative risk for any diabetes-related end point (risk reduction 9 percent) and microvascular disease (risk reduction 24 percent) observed during the active intervention period. Overtime, the sulfonylurea/insulin intervention reduced risks for diabetes-related mortality, myocardial infarction, and all-cause mortality by 17 percent, 15 percent, and 13 percent, respectively, compared with the conventional dietary therapy. Among overweight patients, over 10 years, metformin reduced risks for any diabetes-related end point, diabetes-related mortality, myocardial infarction, and all-cause mortality by 21 percent, 30 percent, 33 percent, and 27 percent, respectively.

Three large RCTs recently published initial findings that were not included in the systematic reviews. The studies assessed nonsurgical interventions in India,[65] Spain,[66] and the U.K. Findings suggest that interventions can be effective across different ethnic populations, despite different BMI and other clinical and diabetes related characteristics.

In India, Ramachandran and colleagues[65] conducted a RCT in urban Asian Indians (mean BMI 25.8, SD 3.5 kg/m^2) with persistent IGT that evaluated the effects of behavioral modifications and metformin on the development of type 2 diabetes. With a median followup duration of 30 months, they found that compared with the control group, both behavioral modification and metformin significantly reduced the cumulative incidence of diabetes at year 3 (39.3 percent, 40.5 percent, and 55.0 percent in behavioral modification, metformin, and control group, respectively), while no added benefit was observed to combine lifestyle modification and metformin (39.5 percent). This represented a relative risk reduction of 28.5 percent, 26.4 percent, and 28.2 percent with behavioral modification, metformin, and the combination, in comparison with control, respectively.

In Spain, Salas-Salvado and colleagues[66] reported one year data from the PREDIMED trial, which evaluated the effect of two diet interventions (Mediterranean diet plus virgin olive oil and Mediterranean diet plus nuts) on metabolic syndrome status compared with a control (low-fat diet advice) among older participants at high risk for CVD. Mean BMI at baseline was 29.3 kg/m^2. They found a significant reduction of overall prevalence of metabolic syndrome in the Mediterranean diet plus nuts group (prevalence reduced by 13.7 percent), compared with that in control group (prevalence reduced by 2.0 percent). Although no significant difference in the incidence rates of metabolic syndrome was observed among groups, the effect of Mediterranean diet plus nuts seemed more a consequence of higher rates of reversion among those who had the metabolic syndrome at the baseline. Mediterranean diet plus virgin olive oil showed a nonsignificant reduction in metabolic syndrome prevalence. The authors concluded that a beneficial effect on metabolic syndrome could be achieved by diet alone.

Finally, a 12-month RCT[67] was carried out in 13 sites in primary care in the UK to evaluate the effectiveness of a structured group education program focused on behavior change among newly diagnosed type 2 diabetes patients (mean BMI= 32.3 kg/m^2; mean HbA1c=8.1). In addition to weight loss and blood glucose outcomes, this study also reported behavioral outcomes (smoking status and physical activity), psychosocial outcomes (illness belief and depression), and quality of life at 4, 8, and 12 months. Compared with usual care, the education intervention was found to be associated with significant weight loss (2.98 kg in education intervention group vs. 1.86 kg in usual care group), a significant reduction in triglyceride levels at eight months, a significant reduction in smoking status at all time points, and a significantly greater increase in physical activity at 4 months. The education intervention group also showed significantly greater understanding of their illness and its seriousness, and had a lower depression score. However, changes in HbA1c level and quality of life scores were not significantly different between groups at any time point.

Summary

Table 9 displays a summary of data on interventions and outcomes in patients with diabetes or IGT. While direct comparisons of these interventions in many cases have not been assessed in randomized trials, it is nonetheless useful to present the data in a side-by-side format. We discuss the limitations of such comparisons in detail in the discussion section; readers should keep in mind that patients enrolled in the nonsurgical trials of medication and behavioral interventions differ in important ways from those participating in the surgical studies.

Short-Term Outcomes

Based on glucose outcomes, there is moderate strength evidence of efficacy of bariatric surgery in treating diabetes in patients with BMI of at least 30 but less than 35 kg/m^2 in the short term. At one year, surgery patients show much greater weight loss than usually seen in studies of diet, exercise, or other behavioral interventions. With the exception of GLP-1T agonists, diabetes medications do not cause significant weight loss. While both behavioral interventions and various medications have been shown to lower HbA1c levels significantly, the decreases reported in bariatric surgery patients at one year are greater. Improvements in glucose control outcomes have been reported as early as one month post-surgery.[68] Improvements in hypertension, and cholesterol have been reported at one year in some studies. We judged this evidence as moderate due to sparseness of data - only three RCTs directly compared surgery with nonsurgical interventions; two came from the same group of researchers. Observational data, which start as "low" strength evidence, were upgraded due to consistency of results regarding BMI and blood sugar. Thus, the total body of evidence is considered moderate strength.

Long-Term Outcomes

There are few long-term data on patients in this weight class with diabetes or IGT who have undergone bariatric surgery. We identified only two studies, both observational, with followup of three or more years. One, a case series of LAGB patients in Italy, reported followup at five years for 29 of the 210 initial patients, for a followup rate of only 13.8 percent. Another small Italian study followed BPD patients for over 10 years; there were only seven patients total. Thus, the evidence that bariatric surgery is an effective way to treat diabetes or IGT in patients with BMI of at least 30 kg/m^2 but less than 35 kg/m^2 in the long term is insufficient, due to the small number of patients followed. In contrast, behavior and medication interventions have been studied extensively for decades; several large long-term RCTs have found improved HbA1c levels continue for ten years. Some long-term trials and meta-analyses have reported clinically significant improvements in microvascular and macrovascular outcomes as a result of behavioral or medication interventions.

Specific Bariatric Procedures

Taking into consideration the entire body of evidence, we rate the strength of evidence as moderate for RYGB, LAGB and gastric sleeve for treating diabetes and IGT in patients with a BMI of between 30 kg/m^2 and 35 kg/m^2, in the short term (up to two years). Each of these procedures have shown efficacy in two randomized trials, in addition to numerous observational studies. In contrast, BPD has not been studied in randomized trials in this particular population, although five observational studies have been published. Thus, the strength of evidence for BPD is rated low.

In two RCTs, RYGB patients lost significantly more weight than gastric sleeve patients. Both RCTs reported better blood glucose outcomes for RYGB; the difference was statistically significant in one. Observational data echo these findings, and also support that RYGB patients have greater changes in weight and blood glucose in the short term than those undergoing LABG. These results must be balanced with the different adverse event profiles of the procedures, discussed in the results for KQ 3.

Table 9. Summary of data on interventions and outcomes in patients with diabetes or impaired glucose tolerance

Outcome	Behavioral Changes (Data Almost Entirely From Systematic Reviews, RCTs)	Intervention Medications (Data Almost Entirely From Systematic Reviews, RCTs)	Bariatric Surgery (Data Primarily From Observational Studies)
Weight loss at one year:	2.8 kg for diet, exercise, behavioral vs. usual care.	Weight gain from 1 to 5 kg with some drugs. 2.8 kg weight loss with GLP-1R agonists. No weight change with metformin.	BMI loss of 5 to 7 kg/m^2 (about 15 to 20 kg for someone 5 foot 6 inches tall)
Weight loss at two years:	2.7 kg for diet, exercise, behavioral vs. usual care.	Data unavailable.	BMI loss of 4 to 8 kg/m^2 (about 11 to 23 kg for someone 5 foot 6 inches tall)
Long term weight loss (five years and more):	1.7 kg for diet, exercise, behavioral vs. usual care at 5 years.	Few data; the U.S. Diabetes Prevention Program Outcomes Study (DPPOS) found no significant change with metformin at 10 years.	BMI loss of 5.7 kg/m^2 at 5 years, in one study of 29 LAGB patients
HbA1C, percentage of total hemoglobin, at one year:	Decrease of 0.3 to 2.2 percentage points.	Decrease of 0.5 to 1.0 percentage points.	Decrease of 2.6 to 3.7 percentage points.
HbA1C at two years:	No significant change.	Few data; the UKPDS study found no significant difference in HbA1c for sulfonylurea-insulin or metformin at 2 year time-point.	Decrease of 1.8 to 3.1 percentage points.
HbA1C at five years and more:	Few data; the U.S. Diabetes Prevention Program Outcomes Study (DPPOS) found HbA1C concentrations lower in behavioral group at 10 years (vs. placebo).	Few data; the U.S. Diabetes Prevention Program Outcomes Study (DPPOS) found HbA1C concentrations lower in metformin group at 10 years (vs. placebo).	Data unavailable.
Other metabolic outcomes at one year:	Diet improved fasting glucose (1.3%-36.6% reduction) and triglycerides (11.3% - 58.9% reduction); the Spain PREDIMED study found Mediterranean diet reduced metabolic syndrome prevalence by 13.7% at 1 year; the Finnish Diabetes Prevention Study (DPS) found behavioral change reduced metabolic syndrome prevalence at 3.9 years (odds ratio: 0.62).	Most medications had minimal effects on systolic & diastolic blood pressure (< 5 mmHg change). Metformin and second generation sulfonylureas generally decreased LDL cholesterol levels.	Mixed results, one RYGB and one BPD study reported slight increase in triglycerides at one year.

Table 9. Summary of data on interventions and outcomes in patients with diabetes or impaired glucose tolerance (continued)

Outcome	Behavioral Changes (Data Almost Entirely From Systematic Reviews, RCTs)	Intervention Medications (Data Almost Entirely From Systematic Reviews, RCTs)	Bariatric Surgery (Data Primarily From Observational Studies)
Other metabolic outcomes at five years and more:	Data unavailable.	Data unavailable.	Of 7 BPD patients followed, all had normal serum cholesterol and triglycerides.
Microvascular outcomes: (Renal disease, neuropathy, retinopathy, etc)	Data unavailable.	UK Prospective Diabetes Study (UKPDS) found patients taking sulfonylurea, insulin, or metformin had 24% risk reduction for microvascular disease at 10 years.	Data unavailable.
Macrovascular outcomes: (Cardiovascular disease, stroke, heart attack)	Few data; the China Da Qing Diabetes Prevention Study (CDQDPS) found no significant difference in first CVD event, CVD mortality and all-cause mortality between intervention and control group.	Meta-analysis of 5 trials with 33,040 participants found that on an average A1C reduction of 0.9% there was a 19% reduction in non-fatal myocardial infarction and a 15% reduction on coronary heart disease, and no statistically significant effect on stroke or all cause mortality.	Data unavailable.
Prevention of diabetes:	Hazard ratio 0.51 for behavioral interventions vs. standard advice at 1 to 5 years; the U.S. Diabetes Prevention Program (DPP) found diabetes incidence in 10 years reduced by 34% by behavioral change vs. placebo, and the China Da Qing Diabetes Prevention Study (CDQDPS) found it was 43% lower in behavioral group over 20 years.	Hazard ratio 0.70 for oral medications vs. control at 1 to 5 years; the U.S. Diabetes Prevention Program (DPP) found diabetes incidence in 10 years reduced by 18% in the metformin group vs. placebo.	Data unavailable.

HbA1C = Glycosylated hemoglobin; BPD = biliopancreatic diversion; BMI = body mass index; CVD = cardiovascular disease; GLP-1R = GLP-1 Agonists: Glucagon-like peptide-1 agonists, a class of diabetes drugs targeting the incretin system; LAGB = laparoscopic adjustable gastric banding; LDL = low-density lipoprotein cholesterol; RCT = randomized controlled trial; RYGB = Roux-en-Y gastric bypass

KQ3: What are the potential short-term adverse effects (AEs) and/or complications involved with bariatric surgery for treating adult patients with BMI of 30 to 34.9 who have metabolic conditions?

The incidence of adverse events following bariatric surgery is displayed in Table 10 for all studies, including case series, cohorts and controlled trials. Adverse events for the few nonsurgical arms of these studies are also displayed. Followup times varied widely from the day of surgery to 2 years; the exception are two studies that reported events up to 3 and 5 years post-surgery. Few studies were clear exactly when the adverse events took place, and patients who were lost to followup had missing adverse events data. Adverse events were often identified and self-reported by the surgical team, with definitions of some complications varying from study to study. Little administrative data were available to diminish these biases. In addition, there were

41

few studies that compared adverse events between different surgical procedures, making direct comparisons difficult.

Studies were included in our mortality analyses only if they reported/mentioned either the number of deaths or lack of any deaths. Thus, 14 studies were included, which accounted for five LAGB arms, one gastric sleeve arm, nine RYGB arms, and one BPD arm. Only one death was reported—an LAGB patient with complications of a gastric perforation. Thus, the reported rate of mortality was 0.48 percent for LAGB and 0.0 percent for gastric sleeve, RYGB and BPD.

Medical complications (cardiovascular, respiratory, gastrointestinal) were reported in several studies. Four studies reported cardiovascular or respiratory complications. A BPD study reported that one of ten patients had a pulmonary embolism, while an RYGB study reported one case of arrthyhmia and three cases of pneumonia. (It is not clear whether these cases were mutually exclusive or in separate patients.) Another study reported two cases of pneumonia in RYGB patients, one case in a gastric sleeve patient and none in the nonsurgical arm. This same study noted two patients with arrhythmias in the nonsurgical arm, one case in a gastric sleeve patient, and none in the RYGB arm. One study of LAGB versus nonsurgical treatment reported one transient ischemia attack (TIA) among 30 patients in the nonsurgical arm.

Metabolic issues were also reported. Self-reported hypoglycemia was common in one RCT of diabetes patients who were receiving aggressive medical treatment in both surgical and nonsurgical: 28 of 50 (56.0 percent) RYGB patients, 39 of 49 (79.6 percent) SG patients, and 35 of 43 (81.4 percent) nonsurgical patients. The same study reported ketoacidosis in one of the RYGB patients and none of the SG or nonsurgical patients. In another study, hypoglycemia was reported by one of 30 LABG patients and did not occur in the non-surgery arm. Vitamin deficiency was reported in one of 109 patients in an RYGB study, and one study each of RYGB and LAGB mentioned that no patients suffered from malnutrition. Anemia was reported in an RCT by 12.0 percent of RYBG, 12.2 percent of SG, and almost 7 percent of nonsurgical patients.

Gastrointestinal (GI) complications were reported at a relatively low rate. Feeding difficulties were reported by 3.6 percent of LAGB patients, 0.9 percent of RYGB patients, and 4.3 percent of nonsurgical patients. There were no reports of feeding difficulties among BPD or gastric sleeve patients. Similarly, hiatal hernia or reflux was reported in four of 146 LAGB patients (2.7 percent), but in no studies of the other procedures. In one RCT, dehydration was reported in 22.0 percent of RYGB patients, 9.3 percent of SG patients, and 8.16 percent of nonsurgical patients. Gastroplegia was reported in one study of 30 BPD patients; the rate was 13.33 percent.

Wound infections were reported in three RYGB studies; the rate was 4.3 percent. A study of 30 LAGB patients also reported one wound infection. Incisional hernias were reported in two RYGB studies; rate was 4.5 percent.

Anastomotic and pouch complications were reported in gastric sleeve and RYGB patients. Five percent of RYGB patients experienced stricture. One RYGB patient and one sleeve patient experienced an anastomotic leak. Ulcer was reported in nine percent of RYGB patients. One RYBG study reported an anastomotic hemorrhage in one of 22 patients. Likewise, one RYGB study reported an intra-abdominal hemorrhage in one of 109 patients.

Several complications specific to LAGB were reported. Band slippage was reported in 2.3 percent of patients, port or tube problems in about two percent, and 3.3 percent of LAGB patients had the band removed. Five of 40 patients in one study had unspecified surgical complications. 5.42 percent of LAGB patients had pouch dilation post-surgery.

Two gastric sleeve patients, six RYGB patients, and another BPD patient required re-operation for unspecified reasons. In addition, one BPD patient required a revision due to chronic diarrhea.

Summary

In the two RCTs comparing SG with RYGB complications were minor and rates were similar between groups. The surgical complications reported for RYGB and LAGB in observational studies were fairly consistent; they differ due to the nature of the procedures. Complications related to LABG include band slippage, tube problems, and band erosion, while those related to RYGB include stricture, ulcer, and on rare occasions, hemorrhage. We rate the strength of evidence for overall short term harms as low for all four procedure types.

The low strength of evidence reflects several limitations in the data. The majority of the adverse events data were submitted by surgeons, and thus subject to possible publication bias. There were only 20 instances where 100 or more patients contributed data to a particular adverse event category; thus, the rate estimate for most adverse events is imprecise. Additionally, in 76 percent of instances, only a single study contributed data to a particular adverse event rate calculation, meaning the generalizability of the estimate is questionable. Few studies were clear exactly when adverse events took place, and patients who were lost followup had no adverse events data. In addition, definitions of complications varied from study to study.

Table 10. Incidence of adverse events - surgical weight loss treatments

Adverse Event*	Subcategory	Nonsurgical Arms				LAGB				Gastric Sleeve				RYGB				BPD			
		# Arms	# With Event	N	%**	# Arms	# With Event	N	%**	# Arms	# With Event	N	%**	# Arms	# With Event	N	%**	# Arms	# With Event	N	%**
Cardiovascular/ Respiratory	Pulmonary embolism																	1	1	10	10.00
	TIA	1	1	30	3.33																
	Arrhythmia	1	2	43	4.65					1	1	49	2.04	2	1	159	0.63				
	Pneumonia	1	0	43	0.00					1	1	49	2.04	3	5	268	1.87				
Constitutional	Cellulitis (nonwound related)	1	1	43	2.33	1	1	30	3.33	1	0	49	0.00	1	0	50	0.00				
	Not specified	1	1	30	3.33																
	Anorexia or excessive weight loss	1	0	43	0.00					1	0	49	0.00	3	0	69	0.00				
	Cholecystitis/Other biliary	2	4	83	4.82	1	1	40	2.50	1	0	49	0.00	2	2	159	1.26				
	Dehydration	1	4	43	9.30					1	4	49	8.16	1	11	50	22.00				
	Excessive weight gain	1	3	43	6.98					1	0	49	0.00	1	0	50	0.00				
Gastro-intestinal	Feeding difficulties	2	3	70	4.29	2	3	83	3.61					1	1	109	0.92				
	Reflux/Hiatal hernia					2	4	146	2.74					1	0	37	0.00				
	Diarrhea	1	1	30	3.33									1	1	22	4.55				
	Gastroplegia																	1	4	30	13.33
	Ileus					1	1	109	0.92												
	Vomiting and/or nausea					1	1	109	0.92					1	4	109	3.67				
	Not specified	2	10	70	14.29	1	1	30	3.33												
Metabolic	Ketoacidosis	1	0	43	0.00					1	0	49	0.00	1	1	50	2.00				
	Anemia	1	3	43	6.98					1	6	49	12.24	1	6	50	12.00				
	Hypoglycemia†	2	36	73	49.32	1	1	30	3.33	1	39	49	79.59	2	28	67	41.79				
	Hypokalemia	1	1	43	2.33					1	2	49	4.08	1	2	50	4.00				
	Vitamin deficiency													1	1	109	0.92				
Renal	Kidney stone	1	1	43	2.33					1	0	49	0.00	1	0	50	0.00				
	Renal insufficiency	1	0	43	0.00					1	0	49	0.00	1	1	50	2.00				

Table 10. Incidence of adverse events - surgical weight loss treatments (continued)

SURGICAL

Adverse Event*	Subcategory	Nonsurgical Arms				LAGB				Gastric Sleeve				RYGB				BPD			
		# Arms	# With Event	N	%**	# Arms	# With Event	N	%**	# Arms	# With Event	N	%**	# Arms	# With Event	N	%**	# Arms	# With Event	N	%**
Band Related	Band erosion					1	1	66	1.52												
	Band removal					1	7	210	3.33												
	Port or tubing complication					5	9	462	1.95												
	Band slippage					6	13	571	2.28												
	Pouch dilation					2	13	240	5.42												
Bleeding/Hematoma	Anastomotic hemorrhage													1	1	22	4.55				
	Intraabdominal hemorrhage													1	1	109	0.92	1	1	30	3.33
	Transfusion NOS									1	1	49	2.04	1	1	50	2.00				
	Incisional hernia									1	0	49	0.00	2	3	67	4.48				
Minor Surgical	Wound infection/seroma	1	0	43	0.00	1	1	30	3.33	1	0	49	0.00	3	8	186	4.30				
	Not specified									1	3	30	10.00	1	3	30	10.00				
Pouch/Anastomosis	Leak									1	1	49	2.04	3	1	239	0.42				
	Fistula													1	1	147	0.68				
	Stricture													4	18	363	4.96				
	Ulcer									1	0	49	0.00	2	6	67	8.96				
Reoperation	Not specified									2	2	98	2.04	3	6	180	3.33	1	1	10	10.00
Revision	Revision secondary to diarrhea																	1	1	30	3.33
Other	Morbidity major - unspecified													1	2	44	4.55				
	Other adverse event - unspecified													1	1	109	0.92				
	Readmission									1	1	30	3.33	1	1	30	3.33				
	Internal hernia													1	1	109	0.92				
	Surgical NOS					1	5	40	12.50	1	0	30	0.00	3	0	72	0.00	1	0	30	0.00

BPD = biliopancreatic diversion with duodenal switch; gastric sleeve = sleeve gastrectomy; LAGB = laparoscopic adjustable gastric banding; N = number; NOS = not otherwise specified; RYGB = Roux-en-Y gastric bypass; TIA = transient ischemia attack

*Studies may have reported on >1 adverse event category and the majority reported on >1 surgical weight loss treatment. Some patients had >1 adverse event. The total number of adverse events was counted for each category.

**% = number of patients with adverse event/total number of patients.

†Schauer et al. 2012[37] hypoglycemia was self-reported.

KQ4: Does the evidence show racial and demographic disparities with regard to potential benefits and harms associated with bariatric surgery for treating adult patients with BMI of 30 to 34.9 and metabolic conditions? What other patient factors (social support, counseling, pre-operative weight loss, compliance) are related to successful outcomes?

There were insufficient data in the included surgery studies to assess whether racial and demographic disparities exist in terms of weight loss and metabolic outcomes. However, previous research shows that some patient-level factors are associated with successful weight loss after bariatric surgery. Regardless of procedure type, patients who lose more weight tend to be younger, have a lower preoperative BMI, and be non-diabetic.[69-71]

One recent systematic literature review identified a number of psychosocial patient factors that may be associated with weight loss after bariatric surgery.[72,73] This review was based on observational studies that included all bariatric patients, including those with baseline BMI> 35 kg/m^2 and those without diabetes. Data specific to patients with a BMI less than 35 kg/m^2 and diabetes are not available. Preoperative factors include baseline BMI, with heavier patients losing less weight than their lighter counterparts in 37 out of 62 studies. Meta-analysis revealed a decrease of 10.1 percent more EWL (excess weight loss) for super obese versus non-super obese patients (95% CI 3.7 percent – 16.5 percent). Some programs request that bariatric candidates lose a modest degree of weight (generally 10-20 pounds) in the weeks immediately prior to surgery. This mandatory preoperative weight loss was associated with successful outcomes after bariatric surgery in many studies. In a meta-analysis on the association between preoperative weight loss versus no weight loss and postoperative weight loss, the preoperative weight loss group lost a mean of 5.0 percent greater EWL (95% CI 2.7 to 7.3 percent).[74]

Social support is believed to be an important component of successful weight loss, and support group attendance in particularly is associated with improved weight loss outcomes after surgery. For example, one study of RYGB patients found that when controlling for time elapsed since surgery, the number of support group meetings attended explained some variance in weight loss (R2 = .09, P<0.05).[75] Another study of patients who underwent LAGB reported that patients who attended support groups had greater weight loss starting at 6 months after surgery, and continuing at 12 months (9.7 vs. 8.1 BMI points decrease at 12 months, P<0.05).[76,77]

Support groups can help to provide continuing postoperative education regarding behavior modification, as well as identify any problems early on. Increased postoperative physical activity was also associated with greater postoperative weight loss in the majority of studies (11 out of 13 studies). A meta-analysis assessing the association of exercise versus no exercise and postoperative weight loss at 12 months showed that the exercise group lost a mean of 4.2 percent greater total BMI (95% CI 0.3 to 8.1 percent).[72] Other factors that may be predictive of postoperative weight loss include specific eating habits or disorders, such as hunger and emotional eating. The emotional and physical stresses of such dramatic weight loss can trigger maladaptive responses in patients with preexisting eating disorders. The impact of other eating disorders and psychiatric disorders such as depression is not clear. This is in part due to variability in how eating and psychiatric disorders are defined from study to study, which survey instruments are used, and the followup time.

Summary

There was insufficient evidence in the studies of patients with diabetes or IGT and BMI 30 to 34.9 kg/m^2 on demographic disparities regarding benefits and harms of bariatric surgery. The same is true for patient factors related to successful outcomes. A recent systematic review on patients with higher BMI found that mandatory pre-operative weight loss, social support, and increased physical activity were associated with better outcomes.

KQ5: What does the evidence show regarding long-term benefits and harms of bariatric surgery for treating adult patients with BMI of 30 to 34.9 and who have metabolic conditions? How do they compare to short-term outcomes (within 1 year from surgery)?

Few long-term data exist on patients with diabetes or IGT in this weight class who have undergone bariatric surgery. Fifteen surgical studies reported outcomes at 13 to 24 months; however, only a handful included followup of more than two years. This section focuses on those studies.

A case series of 210 LAGB patients in Italy with baseline BMI of 30 to 34.9 kg/m^2 included only four patients with diabetes. The authors reported that diabetes had resolved in all four at one year, but resolution was not defined and metabolic evidence was not presented. Authors attempted to followup on the entire group at two, three, four, and five years. Five-year data were reported for only 29 of the 210 initial patients, for a followup rate of only 13.8 percent.[39] No other diabetes related outcomes were reported. Another study of 93 LAGB patients of one surgeon in Australia[41] reported on followup at one, two, and three years. Response rate was good, ranging from 79 to 89 percent per year. Only eight patients had diabetes at baseline; none needed diabetes medications at three years. Again, no other metabolic evidence was presented. For the entire group, mean BMI decreased from 32.7 kg/m^2 at baseline to 27.0 kg/m^2 at one year, and this BMI was maintained at two and three years. Finally, one author followed seven BPD patients with diabetes and BMI < 35 kg/m^2 for over five years in Italy.[47] Serum glucose was normalized at one, two, and three years in all patients. At five years, serum glucose had increased to above 125 mg/dL in five patients. Diabetes had "resolved" in the other two patients. At each follow-up, all patients had normal cholesterol and triglyceride levels. None of these studies reported long-term (over two years) adverse events, although the Italian LAGB study reported a death at 20 months post-surgery from sepsis due to perforation of a dilated gastric pouch.

For comparison, one RCT of surgery versus nonsurgical treatment in our target population[40] reported BMI at six, 12, 18 and 24 months. Both LAGB and medical management groups lost 13.8 percent of excess weight at six months. However, the medical management group gained weight at each subsequent followup while the LAGB group continued to lose weight. Mean BMI decreased from 33.7 kg/m^2 at baseline to 28.9 kg/m^2 at six months, 27.0 kg/m^2 at 12 months, 26.7 kg/m^2 at 18 months, and 26.4 kg/m^2 at two years. (Detailed results for LAGB versus usual care in this study are discussed in the section on KQs 1 and 2.) Metabolic outcomes were not reported at these intervals.

Though not within the parameters of this systematic review, we note the results of a recent European study on long-term outcomes of laparoscopic adjustable gastric band[78] because it reports the longest followup we identified in the bariatric literature published to date. Of 151 consecutive patients from a single institution operated on from 1994-1997, the mean preoperative BMI was 41.57 kg/m^2 (range, 35-57). Of these patients, 82 (54.3 percent) were available for long-term followup at 13 years. The number of patients varied somewhat for each outcome depending on preoperative data availability. For example, complete weight loss data were available for 70 of 151 patients. Overall, 43 percent maintained a loss of excess weight, nearly 60 percent required reoperation, and obesity-related comorbidities such diabetes, hypertension, and sleep apnea persisted. Of 78 patients, 20 (25.6 percent) were treated for hypertension before band insertion and 23 (29.5 percent) were treated for hypertension 12 years after their laparoscopic adjustable gastric band (p=.72). Of 78 patients, 5 (6.4 percent) had type 2 diabetes before band insertion and 11 had diabetes 12 years after surgery. Of the 78 patients, two (2.6 percent) needed continuous positive pressure for sleep apnea before surgery and 6 (7.7 percent) after surgery. Nearly one-third of patients experienced band erosion, while 17 percent were converted to a RYGB. Intent to treat excess weight loss was 33.92 percent (range 24 percent – 143 percent). 36 patients (51.4 percent) still had the band in place and their mean excess weight loss was 48 percent (range 38 percent – 58 percent).

This study on long-term outcomes included patients with preoperative weight higher than that of our target population. It is not clear how these results translate to a lower weight group. Additionally, the study was limited in its ability to draw conclusions as almost 50 percent of patients were not available for followup, which may contribute to significant bias. Still, the study described above draws attention to the importance of having long-term outcomes following bariatric surgery as some obesity-related comorbidities were not resolved at 12 years and there was a high rate of significant band-related complications.

Summary

Due to the dearth of data available, the strength of evidence that bariatric surgery is an effective way to treat diabetes or IGT in patients with BMI of at least 30 kg/m² but less than 35 kg/m² in the long term is insufficient. There are very few long-term (over two years) studies, each includes only a handful of patients in our target population, and none includes a comparison group. We identified no long-term reports of surgery-related adverse events in our target population; thus strength of evidence for harms is also insufficient.

Summary and Discussion

We conducted an extensive literature search, data abstraction, and quantitative analysis where possible, to assess the comparative effectiveness of bariatric surgery in patients with diabetes or impaired glucose tolerance (IGT) and a body mass index (BMI) of at least 30 but less than 35. Here we describe the limitations of our systematic review then present our conclusions. We also discuss the implications of our findings for future research.

Limitations

The research on bariatric surgery in patients with BMI of at least 30 kg/m^2 and less than 35 kg/m^2 and diabetes or IGT has many limitations. Most importantly, very few studies have long term followup (more than two years). Two report data at five years or more; one has a followup rate of only 13.8 percent, while the other includes only seven patients. Thus, we have almost no data on long-term efficacy and safety. No evidence was found on major clinical end points such as all-cause mortality, cardiovascular mortality or morbidity, or peripheral arterial disease. Some evidence from the diabetes literature indicates it may be premature to assume that controlling glucose to normal or near normal levels completely mitigates the risk of microvascular and macrovascular events. While it is more likely than not that this is true, conclusive proof is lacking, and the point is still debated in the diabetes literature.

Another limitation is the dearth of high quality studies. Randomized controlled trials (RCTs) are considered the highest level of medical evidence. We found three RCTs of surgery versus nonsurgical treatment (one of these also compared two procedures) and another RCT comparing surgical procedures. This was expected given the difficulty in conducting randomized trials of surgery. Still, we identified only two observational studies comparing surgical procedures and two small cohort studies comparing surgery with nonsurgical approaches. The rest of our data come from studies with no comparison group, with data submitted primarily by the practicing surgeons. The sample sizes, regardless of methodological design, are far smaller than those of most trials of diet, exercise, and medications.

Applicability of this research to the larger treatment population of diabetes and IGT patients with BMI between 30.0 kg/m^2 and 34.9 kg/m^2 is important in interpreting the results. The participation rate, population characteristics, representativeness of the setting, and representativeness of the individuals are used to assess applicability. One RCT comparing surgery with non-surgery was performed in the United States and included two of the more commonly performed procedures – Roux-en-Y gastric bypass (RYGB) and sleeve gastrectomy (SG). However, it was of modest size and was conducted in an academic setting in a select group of patients with uncontrolled type II diabetes at baseline. Two RCTs of LAGB versus nonsurgical interventions conducted in Australia were comprised primarily of Caucasian patients. However, the RCT comparing laparoscopic adjustable gastric banding (LAGB) with SG was conducted in Taiwan, where diets and lifestyle may differ considerably from the West. One of the cohort studies comparing procedures was conducted in the U.S, but only three of the remaining observational studies were conducted here. The others were conducted in Western Europe, South America, India, Asia, and Australia. Diet, behavior, and culture in many of these locations may differ dramatically from that in the United States. In addition, there may be biological or genetic differences. Thus, the results seen in non-U.S. studies may not be directly applicable to American patients.

Data reported on adverse events have several limitations. Most studies were not designed to assess these outcomes and reflect surgeon or surgery-team reported events. Additionally, followup times and rates were variable, and many studies did not state exactly when adverse events occurred, other than "within a year post surgery." As such, the rates of adverse events may be biased and lower than actual. Comparisons between procedure types are limited for the same reasons. We found almost no long-term adverse events data for our target population.

Key stakeholders, especially consumers, expressed interest in quality of life (QOL) and psychological outcomes post-surgery. These were rarely reported in the studies we identified.

Finally, although our literature search procedures were extensive and included canvassing experts for studies we may have missed, the possibility of publication bias still exists. For all surgical procedures there is the concern that published studies usually come from academic medical centers with high performing surgical teams and careful patients selection. Outcomes reported for such patients may not be representative of the outcomes achieved in the wider community. The difference between complication rates seen in the major clinical trials of carotid endarterectomy and those observed in the general Medicare population is one well-known example of this phenomenon. In addition, there are media reports (Los Angeles Times) on a number of deaths following LAGB surgery. Whether there is any causal relationship between the surgery and the deaths has not yet been assessed in a peer-reviewed publication, so no conclusions can be drawn. Still, it illustrates the potential for there to exist adverse events and/or beneficial outcomes in as-yet-undescribed populations.

Conclusions

Short-Term Outcomes

Based on glucose control outcomes, there is moderate strength evidence of efficacy of bariatric surgery in treating diabetes in patients with BMI of at least 30 but less than 35 kg/m^2 in the short term. At one year, surgery patients show much greater weight loss than usually seen in studies of diet, exercise, or other behavioral interventions. With the exception of GLP-1T agonists, diabetes medications do not cause significant weight loss. While both behavioral interventions and various medications lower HbA1c levels significantly, the decreases reported in bariatric surgery patients at one year are greater. Improvements in glucose control outcomes have been reported as early as one month post-surgery. Several studies report improvement in hypertension and cholesterol at one year. We rated the overall evidence as moderate due to sparseness of data - three RCTs directly compared surgery with nonsurgical interventions, and two came from the same group of researchers. Observational data, which start as "low" strength evidence, were upgraded due to consistency of results regarding BMI and blood sugar. Thus, the total body of evidence is considered moderate strength, based on moderate strength of evidence for BMI and glucose outcomes. Strength of evidence for cholesterol and blood pressure outcomes is low.

Long-Term Outcomes

There are few long-term data on patients with diabetes or IGT in this weight class who have undergone bariatric surgery. We identified only two studies with followup of more than two years. One, a case series of LAGB patients in Italy, reported followup at five years for 29 of the 210 initial patients, for a followup rate of only 13.8 percent. Another very small Italian study followed seven biliopancreatic diversion with duodenal switch (BPD) patients for at least 5 years Thus, despite promising short term outcomes reported, the evidence that bariatric surgery is an effective way to treat diabetes in patients with BMI of at least 30 kg/m² but less than 35 kg/m² in the long term is insufficient. Strength of evidence is insufficient for all outcomes, including BMI, blood glucose, cholesterol, and hypertension. In contrast, behavior and medication interventions have been studied extensively for decades; several large long-term RCTs have found improved HbA1c continues for 10 years. Several long-term trials and meta-analyses have reported clinically significant improvements in microvascular and macrovascular outcomes as a result of behavioral or medication interventions.

Specific Bariatric Procedures

We found two head to head trials comparing bariatric procedures (one also had a medication only group). An average size trial (N=60) conducted in Taiwan compared RYGB with SG; the RYGB group had better weight and diabetes outcomes at one year post surgery. A recent United States trial comparing these same procedures found similar results.

We also found two observational studies that compared procedures. One conducted in the United States compared RYGB with LAGB. This study was fairly large (N = 235), and had an adequate followup rate (61.9 percent for RYGB, 69.2 percent for LAGB) at 6 to 12 months. Some patients were followed for two years. Weight loss was similar among groups; diabetes outcomes were generally better for RYGB patients. The other study, conducted in Germany, compared results for twelve BPD patients with four RYGB patients. Both groups lost a significant amount of weight. At one year, decrease in HbA1c was significantly greater in the BPD group.

Observational studies of surgical procedures without a comparison arm reported clinically meaningful decreases in BMI with all types of bariatric surgery at less than one year. Clinically meaningful diabetes outcomes were also reported at less than a year for all surgery types. At a year or more, weight loss was maintained or improved in all groups; RYGB patients had the greatest decrease in BMI.

Taking into consideration the entire body of evidence, we rate the strength of evidence of efficacy as moderate for RYGB, LAGB, and SG in treating diabetes and IGT in patients with a BMI of between 30 kg/m² and 35 kg/m², in the short term (up to two years) based primarily on glucose control outcomes. For BPD, both the number of studies and their sample sizes are much lower; thus the strength of evidence of efficacy is rated low. Evidence on comparative effectiveness of surgical procedures is insufficient.

Adverse Events

We rate the strength of evidence for overall short term harms as low for all four procedure types. In the two RCTs comparing SG with RYGB complications were minor and rates were similar between groups. The surgical complications reported for RYGB and LAGB in observational studies were fairly consistent; they differ due to the nature of the procedures. Complications related to LABG include band slippage, tube problems, and band erosion, while those related to RYGB include stricture, ulcer, and on rare occasions, hemorrhage.

The low strength of evidence reflects several limitations in the data. The majority of the adverse events data were submitted by surgeons, and thus subject to possible publication bias. Few studies were clear exactly when adverse events took place, and patients who were lost followup had no adverse events data. In addition, definitions of complications varied from study to study.

We found no data on long term adverse events of bariatric surgery in diabetes or IGT patients in our specific BMI range. Thus, strength of evidence for long term adverse events is rated insufficient.

Future Research

Future research should focus on long-term outcomes of bariatric surgery in U.S. patients with diabetes or impaired glucose tolerance and a body mass index of 30 kg/m^2 to 34.9 kg/m^2. For this population there is no evidence that bariatric surgery is effective in preventing the clinical consequences of diabetes – microvascular and macrovascular endpoints such as diabetic retinopathy, kidney failure, and myocardial infarction. Studies with followup of five to ten years are needed. Studies in other populations have led to concern about potential for long-term nutritional complications in bariatric surgery patients, so nutritional endpoints should also be measured.

We found only one U.S. cohort study comparing procedures; this study used the BOLD (Bariatric Outcomes Longitudinal Database), a resource created by the Surgical Review Corporation to monitor outcomes from the Bariatric Surgery Center of Excellence (BSCOE) program. As of June 2009, there were 235 patients with diabetes within our BMI range in the BOLD database. The study we identified reported outcomes at 6 to 12 months. Outcomes at 12 to 24 months were reported for only a small number of patients (6.8 percent) presumably because that followup time had not expired for most of the patients. Continued followup of these patients and publication of findings is needed to assess the degree to which bariatric surgery mitigates long-term sequelae of diabetes.

In addition, according to the U.S. clinical trials database, there are several bariatric surgery trials currently being conducted in the target population. In addition to monitoring weight loss, these studies will frequently collect important metabolic data including measures of blood sugar, cholesterol, triglycerides, and blood pressure. Long-term followup of the research subjects, if funded, could add to our knowledge base on the effects of bariatric surgery and cardiovascular morbidity and mortality. Collection and reporting of psychological and quality of life outcomes will also help inform prospective patients and providers.

References

1. Nguyen NT, Nguyen XM, Lane J, et al. Relationship between obesity and diabetes in a US adult population: findings from the National Health and Nutrition Examination Survey, 1999-2006. Obes Surg. 2011 Mar;21(3):351-5. PMID: 21128002.

2. Sjostrom CD, Lissner L, Wedel H, et al. Reduction in incidence of diabetes, hypertension and lipid disturbances after intentional weight loss induced by bariatric surgery: the SOS Intervention Study. Obes Res. 1999 Sep;7(5):477-84. PMID: 10509605.

3. Mingrone G, Panunzi S, De Gaetano A, et al. Bariatric surgery versus conventional medical therapy for type 2 diabetes. N Engl J Med. 2012 Mar 26;366(17):1577-85. PMID: 22449317.

4. Okay DM, Jackson PV, Marcinkiewicz M, et al. Exercise and obesity. Prim Care. 2009 Jun;36(2):379-93. PMID: 19501249.

5. James WP, Caterson ID, Coutinho W, et al. Effect of sibutramine on cardiovascular outcomes in overweight and obese subjects. N Engl J Med. 2010 Sep 2;363(10):905-17. PMID: 20818901.

6. Li Z, Maglione M, Tu W, et al. Meta-analysis: pharmacologic treatment of obesity. Ann Intern Med. 2005 Apr 5;142(7):532-46. PMID: 15809465.

7. Gardner CD, Kiazand A, Alhassan S, et al. Comparison of the Atkins, Zone, Ornish, and LEARN diets for change in weight and related risk factors among overweight premenopausal women: the A TO Z Weight Loss Study: a randomized trial. JAMA. 2007 Mar 7;297(9):969-77. PMID: 17341711.

8. Kelley DE, Bray GA, Pi-Sunyer F X, et al. Clinical efficacy of orlistat therapy in overweight and obese patients with insulin-treated type 2 diabetes: a 1-year randomized controlled trial. Diabetes Care. 2002 Jun;25(6):1033-41. PMID: 12032111.

9. Pi-Sunyer FX. The effects of pharmacologic agents for type 2 diabetes mellitus on body weight. Postgrad Med. 2008 Jul;120(2):5-17. PMID: 18654064.

10. Bode B. An overview of the pharmacokinetics, efficacy and safety of liraglutide. Diabetes Res Clin Pract. 2012 Jan 14;97(1):27-42. PMID: 22245694.

11. Vilsboll T, Christensen M, Junker AE, et al. Effects of glucagon-like peptide-1 receptor agonists on weight loss: systematic review and meta-analyses of randomised controlled trials. BMJ. 2012;344:d7771. PMID: 22236411.

12. Executive summary of the clinical guidelines on the identification, evaluation, and treatment of overweight and obesity in adults. Arch Intern Med. 1998 Sep 28;158(17):1855-67. PMID: 9759681.

13. Medicare National Coverage Determinations Manual Chapter 1, Part 2 (Sections 90-160.26). In: Centers for Medicare & Medicaid Services, editor; 2006.

14. Buchwald H, Estok R, Fahrbach K, et al. Weight and type 2 diabetes after bariatric surgery: systematic review and meta-analysis. Am J Med. 2009 Mar;122(3):248-56 e5. PMID: 19272486.

15. Phurrough S, Salive ME, Brechner R, et al. Decision Memo for Surgery for Diabetes (CAG-00397N). The Centers for Medicare & Medicaid Services, DHHS: December 2, 2010.

16. International Diabetes Federation Taskforce on Epidemiology and Prevention. Bariatric surgical and procedural interventions in the treatment of obese patients with type 2 diabetes. March 28, 2011. www.idf.org/webdata/docs/IDF-Position-Statement-Bariatric-Surgery.pdf. Accessed on January 31 2012.

17. FDA expands use of banding system for weight loss. U.S. Food and Drug Administration; 2011. www.fda.gov/NewsEvents/Newsroom/Press Announcements/ucm245617.htm.

18. Shekelle PG, Morton SC, Maglione M, et al. Pharmacological and surgical treatment of obesity. Agency for Healthcare Research and Quality. 1530-440X (Print) 1530-440X (Linking). Rockville, MD: July 2004. www.ncbi.nlm.nih.gov/entrez/query.fcgi?cmd=Retrieve&db=PubMed&dopt=Citation&list_uids=15526396.

19. Jadad AR, Moore RA, Carroll D, et al. Assessing the quality of reports of randomized clinical trials: is blinding necessary? Control Clin Trials. 1996 Feb;17(1):1-12. PMID: 8721797.

20. Moher D, Pham B, Jones A, et al. Does quality of reports of randomised trials affect estimates of intervention efficacy reported in meta-analyses? Lancet. 1998 Aug 22;352(9128):609-13. PMID: 9746022.

21. Shea BJ, Grimshaw JM, Wells GA, et al. Development of AMSTAR: a measurement tool to assess the methodological quality of systematic reviews. BMC Med Res Methodol. 2007;7:10.

22. Shea BJ, Hamel C, Wells GA, et al. AMSTAR is a reliable and valid measurement tool to assess the methodological quality of systematic reviews. J Clin Epidemiol. 2009;62(10):1013-20.

23. Methods Reference Guide for Effectiveness and Comparative Effectiveness Reviews. Rockville, MD: Draft Posted October 2007. www.effectivehealthcare.ahrq.gov/repFiles/2007_10DraftMethodsGuide.pdf.

24. Owens DK, Lohr KN, Atkins D, et al. AHRQ series paper 5: grading the strength of a body of evidence when comparing medical interventions--agency for healthcare research and quality and the effective health-care program. J Clin Epidemiol. 2010 May;63(5):513-23. PMID: 19595577.

25. Atkins D, Best D, Briss PA, et al. Grading quality of evidence and strength of recommendations. BMJ. 2004 Jun 19;328(7454):1490. PMID: 15205295.

26. Cohen R, Pinheiro, JS, Correa J L, et al. Laparoscopic Roux-en-Y gastric bypass for BMI < 35 kg/m(2): a tailored approach. Surg Obes Relat Dis. 2006 May-Jun;2(3):401-4, discussion 4. PMID: 16925363.

27. Lee WJ, Wang W, Lee Y, et al. Effect of laparoscopic mini-gastric bypass for type 2 diabetes mellitus: comparison of BMI>35 and <35 kg/m2. J Gastrointest Surg. 2008 May;12(5):945-52. PMID: 17940829.

28. Demaria EJ, Wineger DA, Pate VW, et al. Early postoperative outcomes of metabolic surgery to treat diabetes from sites participating in the ASMBS bariatric surgery center of excellence program as reported in the Bariatric Outcomes Longitudinal Database. Ann Surg. 2010 Sep;252(3):559-66; discussion 66-7. PMID: 20739857.

29. Shah SS, Todkar JS. Shah PS, et al. Diabetes remission and reduced cardiovascular risk after gastric bypass in Asian Indians with body mass index <35 kg/m(2). Surg Obes Relat Dis. 2010 Jul-Aug;6(4):332-8. PMID: 19846351.

30. Boza C, Gamboa C, Viscido G, et al. Laparoscopic Roux-en-Y gastric bypass for the treatment of type 2 diabetes in patients with BMI below 35. Obesity Surgery. 2010;20(8):1011.

31. de Sa VC, Ferraz AA, Campos JM, et al. Gastric bypass in the treatment of type 2 diabetes in patients with a BMI of 30 to 35 kg/m2. Obes Surg. 2011 Mar;21(3):283-7. PMID: 21153449.

32. Frenken M, Cho EY. Metabolic intestinal bypass surgery for type 2 diabetes in patients with a BMI < 35 kg/m2: comparative analysis of 16 patients undergoing either BPD, BPD-DS, or RYGB. Obesity Facts. 2011;4(SUPPL. 1):13-7.

33. Huang C-K, Shabbir A, Lo C-H, et al. Laparoscopic Roux-en-Y gastric bypass for the treatment of type II diabetes mellitus in Chinese patients with body mass index of 25-35. Obes Surg. 2011 Apr 9;21(9):1344-9. PMID: 21479764.

34. Lee WJ, Chong K, Ser KH, et al. Gastric bypass vs sleeve gastrectomy for type 2 diabetes mellitus: a randomized controlled trial. Arch Surg. 2011 Feb;146(2):143-8. PMID: 21339423.

35. Lee WJ, Chong K, Chen CY, et al. Diabetes remission and insulin secretion after gastric bypass in patients with body mass index <35 kg/m2. Obesity Surgery. 2011;21(7):889-95.

36. Ramos A, Neto MPG, Galvao M, et al. Metabolic bypass. Initial experience with Roux-and-Y gastric bypass on type 2 diabetes treatments for non-morbid obese patients. Obesity Surgery. 2010;20(8):1011-2.

37. Schauer PR, Kashyap SR, Wolski K, et al. Bariatric surgery versus intensive medical therapy in obese patients with diabetes. N Engl J Med. 2012 Mar 26;366(17):1567-76. PMID: 22449319.

38. Serrot FJ, Dorman RB, Miller CJ, et al. Comparative effectiveness of bariatric surgery and nonsurgical therapy in adults with type 2 diabetes mellitus and body mass index <35 kg/m(2). Surgery. 2011 Oct;150(4):684-91. PMID: 22000180.

39. Angrisani LF, Furbetta F, Iuppa F, et al. Italian Group for Lap-Band System®: Results of multicenter study on patients with BMI ≤35 kg/m2. Obes Surg. 2004;14(3):415-8.

40. O'Brien PE, Dixon JB, Laurie C, et al. Treatment of mild to moderate obesity with laparoscopic adjustable gastric banding or an intensive medical program: a randomized trial. Ann Intern Med. 2006 May 2;144(9):625-33. PMID: 16670131.

41. Parikh M, Duncombe J, Fielding GA. Laparoscopic adjustable gastric banding for patients with body mass index of <or=35 kg/m2. Surg Obes Relat Dis. 2006 Sep-Oct;2(5):518-22. PMID: 17015204.

42. Dixon JB, O'Brien PE, Playfair J, et al. Adjustable gastric banding and conventional therapy for type 2 diabetes: a randomized controlled trial. JAMA. 2008 Jan 23;299(3):316-23. PMID: 18212316.

43. Sultan S, Parikh M, Youn H, et al. Early U.S. outcomes after laparoscopic adjustable gastric banding in patients with a body mass index less than 35 kg/m2. Surg Endosc. 2009 Jul;23(7):1569-73. PMID: 19263156.

44. Choi J, Digiorgi M, Milone L, et al. Outcomes of laparoscopic adjustable gastric banding in patients with low body mass index. Surg Obes Relat Dis. 2010 Jul-Aug;6(4):367-71. PMID: 20185374.

45. Lembach H, Lanzarini E, Csendes A, et al. Metabolic outcomes of sleeve gastrectomy in patients with impaired glucose metabolism. Obes Surg. 2010;20(8):988.

46. Noya G, Cossu ML, Coppola M, et al. Biliopancreatic diversion preserving the stomach and pylorus in the treatment of hypercholesterolemia and diabetes type II: results in the first 10 cases. Obes Surg. 1998 Feb;8(1):67-72. PMID: 9562490.

47. Scopinaro N, Papadia F, Marinari G, et al. Long-term control of type 2 diabetes mellitus and the other major components of the metabolic syndrome after biliopancreatic diversion in patients with BMI < 35 kg/m2. Obes Surg. 2007 Feb;17(2):185-92. PMID: 17476869.

48. Chiellini C, Rubino F, Castagneto M, et al. The effect of bilio-pancreatic diversion on type 2 diabetes in patients with BMI <35 kg/m2. Diabetologia. 2009 Jun;52(6):1027-30. PMID: 19308351.

49. Scopinaro N, Adami GF, Papadia FS, et al. The effects of biliopancreatic diversion on type 2 diabetes mellitus in patients with mild obesity (BMI 30-35 kg/m(2)) and simple overweight (BMI 25-30 kg/m (2)): a prospective controlled study. Obes Surg. 2011 Jul;21(7):880-8. PMID: 21541815.

50. Geloneze B, Geloneze SR, Fiori C, et al. Surgery for nonobese type 2 diabetic patients: an interventional study with duodenal-jejunal exclusion. Obes Surg. 2009 Aug;19(8):1077-83. PMID: 19475464.

51. Whitlock EP, Lin JS, Chou R, et al. Using existing systematic reviews in complex systematic reviews. Ann Intern Med. 2008 May 20;148(10):776-82. PMID: 18490690.

52. Norris SL, Zhang X, Avenell A, et al. Long-term effectiveness of lifestyle and behavioral weight loss interventions in adults with type 2 diabetes: a meta-analysis. Am J Med. 2004 Nov 15;117(10):762-74. PMID: 15541326.

53. Kirk JK, Graves DE, Craven TE, et al. Restricted-carbohydrate diets in patients with type 2 diabetes: a meta-analysis. J Am Diet Assoc. 2008 Jan;108(1):91-100. PMID: 18155993.

54.   Dyson PA. A review of low and reduced carbohydrate diets and weight loss in type 2 diabetes. J Hum Nutr Diet. 2008 Dec;21(6):530-8. PMID: 18759958.

55.   Kodama S, Saito K, Tanaka S, et al. Influence of fat and carbohydrate proportions on the metabolic profile in patients with type 2 diabetes: a meta-analysis. Diabetes Care. 2009 May;32(5):959-65. PMID: 19407076.

56.   Norris SL, Zangh X, Avenell A, et al. Long-term effectiveness of weight-loss interventions in adults with pre-diabetes: a review. Am J Prev Med. 2005 Jan;28(1):126-39. PMID: 15626569.

57.   Gillies CL, Abrams KR, Lambert PC, et al. Pharmacological and lifestyle interventions to prevent or delay type 2 diabetes in people with impaired glucose tolerance: systematic review and meta-analysis. BMJ. 2007 February 10, 2007;334(7588):299. PMID: 17237299.

58.   Fakhoury WK, Lereun C, Wright D. A meta-analysis of placebo-controlled clinical trials assessing the efficacy and safety of incretin-based medications in patients with type 2 diabetes. Pharmacology. 2010;86(1):44-57. PMID: 20616619.

59.   Bolen S, Feldman L, Vassy J, et al. Systematic review: comparative effectiveness and safety of oral medications for type 2 diabetes mellitus. Ann Intern Med. 2007 Sep 18;147(6):386-99. PMID: 17638715.

60.   Waugh N, Cummins E, Royle P, et al. Newer agents for blood glucose control in type 2 diabetes: systematic review and economic evaluation. Health Technol Assess. 2010 Jul;14(36):1-248. PMID: 20646668.

61.   Li G, Zhang P, Wang J, et al. The long-term effect of lifestyle interventions to prevent diabetes in the China Da Qing Diabetes Prevention Study: a 20-year follow-up study. The Lancet. 2008;371(9626):1783-9. PMID: 18502303.

62.   Ilanne-Parikka P, Eriksson JG, Lindstrom, J, et al. Effect of lifestyle intervention on the occurrence of metabolic syndrome and its components in the Finnish Diabetes Prevention Study. Diabetes Care. 2008 Apr;31(4):805-7. PMID 18184907.

63.   Knowler WC, Fowler SE, Hamman RF, et al. 10-year follow-up of diabetes incidence and weight loss in the Diabetes Prevention Program Outcomes Study. Lancet. 2009 Nov 14;374(9702):1677-86. PMID: 19878986.

64.   Holman RR, Paul SK, Bethel MA, et al. 10-year follow-up of intensive glucose control in type 2 diabetes. N Engl J Med. 2008 Oct 9;359(15):1577-89. PMID 18784090.

65.   Ramachandran A, Snehalatha C, Mary S, et al. Indian Diabetes Prevention, Programme. The Indian Diabetes Prevention Programme shows that lifestyle modification and metformin prevent type 2 diabetes in Asian Indian subjects with impaired glucose tolerance (IDPP-1). Diabetologia. 2006;49(2):289-97. PMID: 16391903.

66.   Salas-Salvado J, Fernandez-Ballart J, Ros E, et al. Effect of a Mediterranean diet supplemented with nuts on metabolic syndrome status: one-year results of the PREDIMED randomized trial. Arch Intern Med. 2008 Dec 8;168(22):2449-58. PMID: 19064829.

67.   Davies MJ, Heller S, Skinner TC, et al. Effectiveness of the diabetes education and self management for ongoing and newly diagnosed (DESMOND) programme for people with newly diagnosed type 2 diabetes: cluster randomised controlled trial. BMJ. 2008 Mar 1;336(7642):491-5. PMID: 18276664.

68.   DePaula AL, Stival A, Halpern A, et al. Thirty-day morbidity and mortality of the laparoscopic ileal interposition associated with sleeve gastrectomy for the treatment of type 2 diabetic patients with BMI <35: an analysis of 454 consecutive patients. World J Surg. 2011 Jan;35(1):102-8. PMID: 21052999.

69.   Snyder B, Nguyen A, Scarbourough T, et al. Comparison of those who succeed in losing significant excessive weight after bariatric surgery and those who fail. Surg Endosc. 2009 Oct;23(10):2302-6. PMID: 19184204.

70.   Chevallier JM Paita M, Rodde-Dunet MH, et al. Predictive factors of outcome after gastric banding: a nationwide survey on the role of center activity and patients' behavior. Ann Surg. 2007 Dec;246(6):1034-9. PMID: 18043107.

71.   Dixon JB,Dixon ME, O'Brien PE. Pre-operative predictors of weight loss at 1-year after Lap-Band surgery. Obes Surg. 2001 Apr;11(2):200-7. PMID: 11355027.

72.   Livhits M, Mercado C, Yermilov I, et al. Exercise following bariatric surgery: systematic review. Obes Surg. 2010 May;20(5):657-65. PMID: 20180039.

73.   Livhits M, Mercado C, Yermilov I, et al. Is social support associated with greater weight loss after bariatric surgery?: a systematic review. Obes Rev. 2011 Feb;12(2):142-8. PMID 20158617.

74.   Livhits M, Mercado C, Yermilov I, et al. Does weight loss immediately before bariatric surgery improve outcomes: a systematic review. Surg Obes Relat Dis. 2009 Nov-Dec;5(6):713-21. PMID: 19879814.

75.   Hildebrandt SE. Effects of participation in bariatric support group after Roux-en-Y gastric bypass. Obes Surg. 1998 Oct;8(5):535-42. PMID: 9819086.

76.   Elakkary E, Gazayerli MM. Laparoscopic adjustable gastric band: do support groups add to the weight loss? Obes Surg. 2004 Sep;14(8):1139-40. PMID: 15479609.

77.   Elakkary E, Elhorr A, Aziz F, et al. Do support groups play a role in weight loss after laparoscopic adjustable gastric banding? Obes Surg. 2006 Mar;16(3):331-4. PMID: 16545165.

78.   Himpens J, Cadiere GB, Bazi M, et al. Long-term outcomes of laparoscopic adjustable gastric banding. Arch Surg. 2011 July;146(7):802-7. PMID: 21422330.

Abbreviations/Acronyms

AHRQ	Agency for Healthcare Research and Quality
AMSTAR	Measurement tool created to assess the methodological quality of systematic reviews
BL	Baseline
BMI	Body Mass Index
BPD	Biliopancreatic Diversion
cc	Cubic Centimeters
CCTs	Controlled Clinical Trials
CDQDPS	China Da Qing Diabetes Prevention Study
CENTRAL	Cochrane Central Register of Controlled Trials
CER	Comparative Effectiveness Review
CHIP	Children's Health Insurance Program
CINAHL	Cumulative Index to Nursing and Allied Health Literature
CMS	Center for Medicare & Medicaid Services
CPAP	Continuous Positive Airway Pressure
CV	Cardiovascular
CVD	Cardiovascular Disease
DARE	Cochrane Database of Abstracts of Reviews of Effects
DM	Diabetes Mellitus
DPP	Diabetes Prevention Program
EPC	Evidence-based Practice Center
EWL	Excess Weight Loss
FDA	Food and Drug Administration
GERD	Gastroesophageal Reflux Disease
GHb	Glycated Hemoglobin
GI	Gastrointestinal
HbA1c	Glycosylated Hemoglobin
HDL	High-Density Lipoprotein
HFLC	High-Fat Low-Carbohydrate Diet
IDPP	Indian Diabetes Prevention Programme
IGT	Impaired Glucose Tolerance
LAGB	Laparoscopic Adjustable Gastric Banding
LDL	Low-Density Lipoprotein
LFHC	Low-Fat High-Carbohydrate Diet
N	Sample Size

OSA	Obstructive Sleep Apnea
QOL	Quality of Life
RCTs	Randomized Controlled Trials
RYGB	Roux-en-Y Gastric Bypass
SE	Standard Error
SG	Sleeve Gastrectomy
TEP	Technical Expert Panel
UKPDS	United Kingdom Prospective Diabetes Study
VBG	Vertical Banded Gastroplasty
VLCDs	Very-Low-Calorie Diets
WMD	Weighted Mean Difference

Appendix A. Search Methodology

BARIATRIC SURGERY & METABOLIC CONDITIONS – SEARCH METHODOLOGIES

Search performed 3/5/2010:

DATABASE SEARCHED & TIME PERIOD COVERED:
PubMed - All years

SEARCH STRATEGY:
diabetes OR diabetic* OR diabetes mellitus
AND
lifestyle* OR life style* OR life style OR exercis*[tiab] OR exercise therapy OR physical activity OR diet, reducing OR diet OR diets OR dieting OR nutrition
AND
obese OR obesity OR (weight AND reduce) OR (weight AND reducing) OR (weight AND reduction) OR weight-reducing OR (decreas* AND weight) OR "weight loss" OR (weight AND lost) OR overweight
AND
intervention OR patient education as topic OR "look ahead" OR prevent*[tiab] OR prevention[sh] OR psychology[sh]
AND
follow-up studies OR follow-up[tiab] OR followup[tiab] OR longitudinal studies OR longitudinal[tiab] OR outcome assessment (health care) OR treatment outcome OR randomi* OR randomized controlled trial[pt] OR double-blind OR double blind OR prospective studies

NUMBER OF RESULTS: 1413

Search performed 3/10/2010:

DATABASE SEARCHED & TIME PERIOD COVERED:
PubMed - All years

SEARCH STRATEGY:
[diabetes[tiab] OR diabetic* OR diabetes mellitus
AND
patient utilities OR "quality of life" OR "standard gamble" OR "time tradeoff" OR "time trade-off" OR cost-utilit* OR patient utilit* OR utility OR utilities]
AND
bariatric OR obesity/su OR (obesity AND (surgery OR surgical)]

NUMBER OF RESULTS: 161

Search performed 3/11/2010:

DATABASE SEARCHED & TIME PERIOD COVERED:
PubMed - All years

SEARCH STRATEGY:
diabetes[tiab] OR diabetic* OR diabetes mellitus
AND
cost-utilit* OR patient utilit* OR "standard gamble" OR "time tradeoff" OR "time trade-off"
OR bariatric OR obesity/su OR (obesity AND (surgery OR surgical))

NUMBER OF RESULTS: 108

Search performed 3/25/2010:

DATABASE SEARCHED & TIME PERIOD COVERED:
PubMed - All years

SEARCH STRATEGY:
diabetes[tiab] OR diabetic* OR diabetes mellitus
AND
obese OR obesity OR (weight AND reduce) OR (weight AND reducing) OR (weight AND
reduction) OR weight-reducing OR (decreas* AND weight) OR "weight loss" OR (weight
AND lost) OR overweight
AND
lifestyle* OR life style* OR life style OR exercis*[tiab] OR exercise therapy OR physical
activity OR diet, reducing OR diet OR diets OR dieting OR nutrition
AND
systematic[sb] OR systematic review* OR meta-analy* OR meta analy* OR metaanaly*
OR meta-analysis[pt] OR randomized controlled trial* OR rct* OR randomized controlled
trial[pt] OR controlled clinical trial* OR cct* OR controlled clinical trial[pt]

NUMBER OF RESULTS: 1766

Appendix B. Data Collection Forms

Short Form Screener

EPC PROJECT: SCREENER FORM BARIATRIC SURGERY/METABOLIC CONDITIONS   FINAL 05-10-2010

ID: _____

Reviewer: _____

Last name, first author: _____

Year of publication: _____

1. Does article report on cases with BMI between 30 and 35?   (Circle one)

    Yes...1
    Other weight determination.................2
    No/Unclear......................................3 (STOP)

2. Does article include cases with type II diabetes or other metabolic conditions?   (Circle one)

    Yes...1
    No ....2 (STOP)

3. Does article report on any of these treatments?   (Check all that apply)

    Non-surgical treatments of metabolic conditions ....☐

    Surgical treatments:
      Lap adjustable banding (LAGB) ....☐
      Roux-en-y gastric bypass.................☐
      Sleeve gastrectomy ....☐

      Other bariatric surgeries ....☐
      Biliopancreatic diversion (BPD/DS)....☐
      (if only BPD/DS, then STOP)

    None of the above...............................☐ (STOP)
    (To flag an article for background go to Q4; to flag duplicate data go to Q9; to order a reference go to Q10.)

4. Study design: (Circle one)

    Background (historical, editorial etc.) .....1 (STOP)
    Non-systematic review ....2 (STOP)
    Systematic review / Meta-analysis......3 (STOP)
    Case Report....................................4 (STOP)

    Case series.....................................5
    Cohort..6
    Case control....................................7
    Controlled trial.................................8
    Other...9

5. Does the study focus on the following outcomes?   (Check all that apply)

    Blood glucose/diabetes related ....☐
    Blood pressure.................................☐
    Lipids/cholesterol ....☐
    Weight loss outcomes.........................☐

    Quality of life measures ....☐
    Removal rates..................................☐
    Band-to-RYGB conversion rates...........☐
    Mortality ....☐

    Healthcare utilization/economics..........☐
    Adverse events/complications..............☐
    Other relevant outcomes....................☐

6. Total sample size entering study. If entering sample not reported then enter total completing: (Enter # or 999 if no sample reported)

    [_____]

7. Total duration of follow up:

    Duration #   Units Code

    [_____]   [_____]

Unit Codes		
01. Hour	03. Week	05. Year
02. Day	04. Month	99. NR

8. Language of article: (Circle one)

    English..1
    Other..2

    Language (specify): _____

9. Do you think that this article might be a duplicate or include the same data as another study? (Circle one)

    Yes 1
    No...2
    If YES, which one(s) :

    _____
    (Enter study ID #, author or 9999 if don't know.)

10. Is there a reference that needs to be checked?   (Circle one)

    Yes 1
    No...2
    If YES, which one(s) :

    _____
    (Enter reference # and/or author or 9999 if don't know.)

Notes:

Detailed Abstraction Form

Submit Form and go to ☐ or Skip to Next

Participants

Country

☐ US ☐ UK ☐ Japan ☐ Unclear

☐ Canada ☐ Western Europe ☐ Asia (not Japan) ☐ Other _____

☐ South/Central America ☐ Eastern Europe ☐ India

☐ Australia/NZ ☐ Middle East

Race

% Caucasian % Black/African Ancestry % Asian _____ % Hispanic % Middle-eastern % American Indian/Alaskan Native % other race _____ ☐ Race not reported

Instructions: If study has only one arm, please put data into the "Arm 1" box, rather than the "Overall" box.

	Arm 1	Arm 2	Overall
Sample Size			
Intervention			
Sex - % female			

Ages - Min

Max

Mean

Median

Std Dev

Baseline weight

BMI:	Min	Max	Mean	Median	Std Dev

Weight:	Min	Max	Mean	Median	Std Dev

Select an Answer

Diabetes

	Overall	Arm 1	Arm 2

B-2

% with Diabetes

Severity

- Years since dx
- Need for Meds (%)
- hgbA1c
- Pre-diabetes/IGT

Severity of Diabetes-Other   Label   Data

- Years since dx
- Need for Meds (%)
- hgbA1c
- Pre-diabetes/IGT

Label   Data

- Years since dx
- Need for Meds (%)
- hgbA1c
- Pre-diabetes/IGT

Label   Data

Comorbidities

	%		
	0	1	2
Asthma			Hypertension
Osteoarthritis			Depression
Elevated lipids			Metabolic syndrome
Oth			

Comorbidities

	%		
	0	1	2
			Sleep apnea
			GERD

Study Characteristics

Surgery type   □ LAGB   □ RYGB   □ Sleeve   □ BPD   □ Other Surgical   □ Other non-Surgical

If RYGB, characterize the type

- Lap
- Open
- Mixed
- Unknown
- Other

Duration

Study   Select an Answer

Outcomes

Outcomes	Arm	Baseline	1st Follow-up	2nd Follow-up	3rd Follow-up	4th Follow-up	5th Follow-up	6th Follow-up	Units
		t0	t1	t2	t3	t4	t5	t6	Select an Answer
N	Arm 1								
N	Arm 2								
BMI	Arm 1								
BMI	Arm 2								

B-3

Weight	Arm 1	Select an Answer
Weight	Arm 2	Select an Answer
HbA1c	Arm 1	
HbA1c	Arm 2	
Fasting Glucose	Arm 1	Select an Answer
Fasting Glucose	Arm 2	Select an Answer
% on Diabetes meds	Arm 1	
% on Diabetes meds	Arm 2	Select an Answer
Cholesterol	Arm 1	Select an Answer
Cholesterol	Arm 2	Select an Answer
Hypertension	Arm 1	Select an Answer
Hypertension	Arm 2	Select an Answer

Select an Answer
Select an Answer
Select an Answer
Select an Answer
Select an Answer
Select an Answer
Select an Answer
Select an Answer
Select an Answer

Select an Answer

And finally, please do not forget to answer these last questions:

Does this study report adverse events?

☐ Yes
☐ No

Is this article / abstract related to others? If so, please enter ID.

This form was filled out using...

☐ Abstract only
☐ Full text

Comments:

Submit Form and go to or Skip to Next

B-5

Bariatric surgery & metabolic conditions
Author, year _____
ID _____

AMSTAR Quality Assessment ANSWER EACH QUESTION

A/1 Was an 'a priori' design provided?

Yes 1
No 2
Not reported 8
Not applicable 9

A/2 Was there duplicate study selection and data extraction?

Yes 1
No 2
Not reported 8
Not applicable 9

A/3 Was a comprehensive literature search performed?

Yes 1
No 2
Not reported 8
Not applicable 9

A/4 Was the status of publication (i.e. grey literature) used as an inclusion criterion?

Yes 1
No 2
Not reported 8
Not applicable 9

A/5 Was a list of included studies provided?

Yes 1
No 2
Not reported 8
Not applicable 9

A/6 Were the characteristics of the included studies provided?

Yes 1
No 2

Not reported 8
Not applicable 9

A/7 Was the scientific quality of the included studies assessed and documented?

Yes 1
No 2
Not reported 8
Not applicable 9

A/8 Was the scientific quality of the included studies used appropriately in formulating conclusions?

Yes 1
No 2
Not reported 8
Not applicable 9

A/9 Were the methods used to combine the findings of studies appropriate?

Yes 1
No 2
Not reported 8
Not applicable 9

A/10 Was the likelihood of publication bias assessed?

Yes 1
No 2
Not reported 8
Not applicable 9

A/11 Was the conflict of interest stated?

Yes 1
No 2
Not reported 8
Not applicable 9

Appendix C. Evidence Tables

Appendix C Evidence Tables For Surgical Treatment v. Non-Surgical Treatment Trials

Author, Year	Study Design	Patient Population	Procedures	Weight Loss Outcomes	Resolution or improvement in diabetes	Other Outcomes	Adverse Events
Schauer 2012[37] US	RCT	50 T2DM patients with mean age 48.3 (SD=8.4), BMI 37.0 (SD=3.3)	RYGB	**Mean Weight (kg):** 12mths: 77.3 (SD=13.0) **Mean BMI:** 3mth: 31.8 (SD NR) 6mths: 28.2 (SD NR) 9mths: 26.9 (SD NR) 12mths: 26.8 (SD NR)	**Fasting plasma glucose, mg/dl:** 3mths: 109(SD NR) 6mths: 96 (SD NR) 9mths: 96 (SD NR) 12mths: 99 (SD NR) **HbA1c, %:** 3mths: 6.8 (SD NR) 6mths: 6.3 (SD NR) 9mths: 6.4 (SD NR) 12mths: 6.4 (SD=0.9) **HbA1c<6.0%:** 12mths: 42% **HbA1c<6.0%, no meds:** 12mths: 42% **# of DM meds:** Baseline: 2.6 (SD NR) 3mths: 1.1 (SD NR) 6mths: 0.6 (SD NR) 9mths: 0.4 (SD NR) 12mths: 0.3 (SD NR)	Median Percentage Change in: Triglyceride level: -44 (IQR -65- to -16) Mean Percentage Change in: HDL cholesterol level: -28.5 (SD=22.7)	

Appendix C Evidence Tables For Surgical Treatment v. Non-Surgical Treatment Trials

Author, Year	Study Design	Patient Population	Procedures	Weight Loss Outcomes	Resolution or improvement in diabetes	Other Outcomes	Adverse Events
Schauer 2012[37] US	RCT	50 T2DM patients with mean age 47.9 (SD=8.0), BMI 36.2 (SD=3.9)	Sleeve	**Mean Weight (kg):** 12mths: 75.5 (SD=12.9) **Mean BMI:** 3mth: 31.3 (SD NR) 6mths: 28.3 (SD NR) 9mths: 27.3 (SD NR) 12mths: 27.2 (SD NR)	**Fasting plasma glucose, mg/dl:** 3mths: 118(SD NR) 6mths: 104 (SD NR) 9mths: 102 (SD NR) 12mths: 97 (SD NR) **HbA1c, %:** 3mths: 7.1 (SD NR) 6mths: 6.7 (SD NR) 9mths: 6.7 (SD NR) 12mths: 6.6 (SD=1.0) **HbA1c<6.0%:** 12mths: 37% **HbA1c<6.0%, no meds:** 12mths: 27% **# of DM meds:** Baseline: 2.4 (SD NR) 3mths: 1.1 (SD NR) 6mths: 0.9 (SD NR) 9mths: 0.8 (SD NR) 12mths: 0.9 (SD NR)	Median Percentage Change in: Triglyceride level: -42 (IQR -56- to 0) Mean Percentage Change in: HDL cholesterol level: 28.4 (SD=21.9)	

Appendix C Evidence Tables For Surgical Treatment v. Non-Surgical Treatment Trials

Author, Year	Study Design	Patient Population	Procedures	Weight Loss Outcomes	Resolution or improvement in diabetes	Other Outcomes	Adverse Events
Schauer 2012[37] US	RCT	50 T2DM patients with mean age 49.7 (SD=7.4), BMI 36.8 (SD=3.0)	Medical Therapy	**Mean Weight (kg):** 12mths: 99.0 (SD=16.4) **Mean BMI:** 3mth: 35.4 (SD NR) 6mths: 34.8(SD NR) 9mths: 34.5 (SD NR) 12mths: 34.4 (SD NR)	**Fasting plasma glucose, mg/dl:** 3mths: 122(SD NR) 6mths: 113 (SD NR) 9mths: 120 (SD NR) 12mths: 120 (SD NR) **HbA1c, %:** 3mths: 7.7 (SD NR) 6mths: 7.1 (SD NR) 9mths: 7.4 (SD NR) 12mths: 7.5 (SD=1.8) **HbA1c<6.0%:** 12mths: 12% **HbA1c<6.0%, no meds:** 12mths: 0% **# of DM meds:** Baseline: 2.8 (SD NR) 3mths: 3.1 (SD NR) 6mths: 3.1 (SD NR) 9mths: 3.0 (SD NR) 12mths: 3.0 (SD NR)	Median Percentage Change in: Triglyceride level: -14 (IQR -40- to 3) Mean Percentage Change in: HDL cholesterol level: 11.3 (SD=25.7)	
Dixon 2008[42] Australia/ New Zealand	RCT	30 T2DM patients with mean age 46.6 (SD=7.4), BMI 36.9 (SD NR)	LABG	**Mean Weight (kg):** 24mths: 84.6 (SD=15.8) **Mean BMI:** 24mths: 29.4 (SD NR)	**Fasting blood glucose, mg/dL:** 24mths: 105.6 (SD=30.3) **HbA1c, %:** 24mths: 6.0 (SD=0.8) **HbA1c<6.2%:** 24mths: 80% **Taking DM meds, %:** Baseline: 28/30 (93.3%) 24mths: 4/30 (13.3%) **Metabolic Syndrome, %:** Baseline: 29/30 (96.7%) 24mths: 9/30 (30.0%)	Blood pressure, mm Hg: Systolic: 130.4 (SD=19.0) Diastolic: 85.4 (SD=7.0) Total Cholestrol, mg/dL:205.4 (SD=46.6) Triglycerides, mg/dL:118.9 (SD=79.7) HDL-C, mg/dL: 59.7 (SD=13.6)	**GI:** Feeding difficulties, 1/30 (3.3%) Other, 1/30 (3.3%) **Hepatobiliary:** Acute cholecystitis or CBD obstruction, 4/40 (10%) **Metabolic:** Hypoglycemia, 1/30 (3.3%) **Other:** Constitutional, 1/30 (3.3%) **Pouch/anastomosis:** Pouch dilation: 2/30 (6.7%) **Wound:** Infection: 1/30 (3.3%)

Appendix C Evidence Tables For Surgical Treatment v. Non-Surgical Treatment Trials

Author, Year	Study Design	Patient Population	Procedures	Weight Loss Outcomes	Resolution or improvement in diabetes	Other Outcomes	Adverse Events
Dixon 2008[42] Australia/ New Zealand	RCT	30 T2DM patients with mean age 47.1(SD=8.7), BMI 37.1 (SD NR)	Non-surgical treatment- Diet, pharmocothe rapy & lifestyle change	**Mean Weight (kg):** 24mths: 104.8 (SD=15.3) **Mean BMI:** 24mths: 36. (SD NR)	**Fasting blood glucose, mg/dL:** 24mths: 139.6 (SD=38.1) **HbA1c, %:** 24mths: 7.2 (SD=1.4) **HbA1c<6.2%:** 24mths: 20% **Taking DM meds, %:** Baseline: 26/30 (86.7%) 24mths: 22/30 (73.3%) **Metabolic Syndrome, %:** Baseline: 29/30 (96.7%) 24mths: 26/30 (86.7%)	Blood pressure, mm Hg: Systolic: 132.6 (SD=17.7) Diastolic: 83.1 (SD=8.5) Total Cholestrol, mg/dL:197.8 (SD=59.3) Triglycerides, mg/dL:186.7 (SD=127.2) HDL-C, mg/dL: 50.7 (SD=12.1)	**GI:** Diarrhea, 1/30 (3.3%) Feeding difficulties, 2/30 (6.7%) Other, 2/30 (6.7%) **Hepatobiliary:** Acute cholecystitis or CBD obstruction, 4/40 (10%) **Metabolic:** Hypoglycemia, 1/30 (3.3%) **Other:** Constitutional, 1/30 (3.3%) TIA, 1/30 (3.3%)
O'Brien 2006[40] Australia/ New Zealand	RCT	40 patients with mean age 41.8 (SD=6.4), BMI 33.7 (32.9-34.4) kg/m2	LABG	**Mean Weight (kg):** 6mth: 81.6 (79.4-83.7) 12mths: 76.3 (74.1-78.5) 18mths: 75.2 (73.1-77.4) 24mths: 74.5 (72.4-76.7) **Mean BMI:** 1mth: 28.9 (28.1-29.7) 12mths: 27.0 (26.2-27.8) 18mths: 26.7 (25.9-27.5) 24mths: 26.4 (25.6-27.2) **Mean EWL, %:** 1mth: 57.2 (47.8-66.6) 12mths: 78.6 (69.2-88.1) 18mths: 83.6 (74.2-93.1) 24mths: 87.2 (77.7-96.6)	**Metabolic Syndrome, %:** Baseline: 15/40 (37.5%) 24mths: 1/39 (2.7%)	Percentage Change in: Systolic BP: -10.8 (SD=10.8) Diastolic BP: -10.9 (SD=12.5) Total cholesterol level: -0.4 (SD=18.1) Triglyceride level: -19.1 (SD=35.7) HDL cholesterol level: 30.0 (SD=28.9) LDL cholesterol level: -6.5 (19.0)	**Band related:** Band slippage, 4/40 (10%) Port infection, 1/40 (2.5%) **Hepatobiliary:** Acute cholecystitis or CBD obstruction, 1/40 (2.5%) **Major surgical complications:** NOS, 5/40 (12.5%)

Appendix C Evidence Tables For Surgical Treatment v. Non-Surgical Treatment Trials

Author, Year	Study Design	Patient Population	Procedures	Weight Loss Outcomes	Resolution or improvement in diabetes	Other Outcomes	Adverse Events
O'Brien 2006[40] Australia/ New Zealand	RCT	40 patients with mean age 40.7 (SD=7.0), BMI 33.5(32.7-34.3) kg/m2	Non-surgical treatment- Diet, pharmacotherapy & lifestyle change	**Mean Weight (kg):** 6mth: 81.6 (79.4-83.7) 12mths: 85.3 (83.0-87.5) 18mths: 87.7 (79.9-83.0) 24mths: 89.5 (80.5-83.6) **Mean BMI:** 1mth: 28.7 (27.9-29.6) 12mths: 29.9 (29.1-30.8) 18mths: 30.9 (30.0-31.8) 24mths: 31.5 (30.6-32.4) **Mean EWL, %:** 1mth: 57.4 (47.6-66.4) 12mths: 41.1 (31.1-50.9) 18mths: 29.0 (19.0-38.9) 24mths: 21.8 (11.9-31.6)	**Metabolic Syndrome, %:** Baseline: 15/40 (37.5%) 24mths: 8/33 (24.0%)	Percentage Change in: Systolic BP: -7.2 (SD=9.7) Diastolic BP: -1.6 (SD=11.2) Total cholesterol level: -3.0 (SD=17.0) Triglyceride level: -3.7 (SD=39.4) HDL cholesterol level: 6.9 (SD=18.9) LDL cholesterol level: -5.2 (21.6)	**GI:** Feeding difficulties, 1/40 (2.5%) Other, 8/40 (20.0%) **Hepatobiliary:** Acute cholecystitis or CBD obstruction, 4/40 (10%) **Major surgical complications:** NOS, 4/40 (10%)
Chiellini, 2009[48] Western Europe	Matched Cohort	5 T2DM patients with mean age 48 years (SE=3), BMI 30.9 (SE=1.1) kg/m2	Non-surgical treatment- Diet, pharmacotherapy & lifestyle change	**Mean Weight (kg):** 1mth: 92.6 (SE=6.4) 12mths: 77.8 (SE=3.5) 18mths: 76.8 (SE=3.0) **Mean BMI:** 1mth: 30.0(SE=0.8) 12mths: 25.4 (SE=0.01) 18mths: 25.1 (SE=0.01)	**2 hr Fasting Blood Glucose,mmol/L:** 1mth: 6.2 (SE=0.5) **HbA1c, %:** 1mth: 7.2 (SE=0.3) 12mths: 5.6 (SE=0.2) 18mth: 5.7 (SE=0.2)		No Mention of Adverse Events
Chiellini, 2009[48] Western Europe	Matched Cohort	7 T2DM patients with mean age 51 years (SE=3), BMI 30.0 (SE=1.7) kg/m2	Non-surgical treatment- Diet	**Mean Weight (kg):** 1mth: 83.7 (SE=5.5) **Mean BMI:** 1mth: 29.2 (SE=1.8)	**2 hr Fasting Blood Glucose, mmol/L:** 1mth: 15.2 TO 6.2 **HbA1c, %:** 1mth: 8.6 (SE=0.3)		No Mention of Adverse Events

Appendix C Evidence Tables For Surgical Treatment v. Non-Surgical Treatment Trials

Author, Year	Study Design	Patient Population	Procedures	Weight Loss Outcomes	Resolution or improvement in diabetes	Other Outcomes	Adverse Events
Serrot, 2011[38] US	Cohort	17 T2DM patients with median age 56.0 years (IQR=7.0), median BMI 34.6 (IQR=0.8) kg/m²	RYGB	**Median BMI:** 12mths: 25.8 (IQR=2.5) **%EWL:** 12mths: 70 (IQR=21) **%WL:** 12mths: 25 (IQR=6)	**Median HbA1c,%:** 12mths: 6.1 (IRQ=2.7) **Off anti-diabetic meds:** 12mths: 9/17 (52.9%) **Resolution of DM:** 12mths: 11/17 (64.7%)	Systolic blood pressure,mm Hg: 12mths: 132 (IQR=27)) LDL,mg/dL: 12mths: 92 (IQR=62))	**Other major surgical complications** Incisional hernia 2/17 (11.8%) **Metabolic:** Hypoglycemia, 0/17 (0%) **GI:** Ulcers, 2/17 (11.8%) **Death:** NOS, 0/17 (0%)
Serrot, 2011[38] US	Cohort	17 T2DM patients with median age 62.0 years (IQR=12.0), median BMI 34.0 (IQR=1.0) kg/m²	Non-surgical treatment - routine medical management	**Median BMI:** 12mths: 34.2 (IQR=2.1) **%EWL:** 12mths: -4 (IQR=10) **%WL:** 12mths: -1 (IQR=4)	**Median HbA1c,%:** 12mths: 7.1 (IRQ=1.8) **Off anti-diabetic meds:** 12mths: 0/17 (0%)	Systolic blood pressure,mm Hg: 12mths: 124 (IQR=26)) LDL,mg/dL: 12mths: 100 (IQR=66))	**Death:** NOS, 0/17 (0%)

Appendix C Evidence Tables For Surgical Treatment v. Surgical Treatment Trials

Author, Year	Study Design	Patient Population	Procedures	Weight Loss Outcomes	Resolution or improvement in diabetes	Other Outcomes	Adverse Events
DeMaria, 2010[28] US	Cohort	109 T2DM patients with mean age 52.8 years (SD=9.5), BMI 33.7 (SE=1.1) kg/m²	RYGB	**Mean BMI:** 0-3mths: 30.6(SD=3.0) 3-6mths: 27.2(SD=3.8) 6-12mths: 27.1(SD=4.5) 12-24mths: 23.0(SD=2.0) **% EBW:** 0-3mths: 41.7(SD=15.0) 3-6mths: 26.8(SD=17.4) 6-12mths: 26.9(SD=19.7) 12-24mths: 7.6(SD=7.6)	**Number of T2DM meds:** 0-3mths: 0.8(SD=1.0) 3-6mths: 0.4(SD=0.7) 6-12mths: 0.5(SD=0.7) 12-24mths: 0(SD=0) **% off T2DM meds:** 0-3mths: 37.5 3-6mths: 50.0 6-12mths: 55.2 12-24mths: 75.0	**Number of meds:** 0-3mths: 3.9(SD=3.2) 3-6mths: 3.5(SD=3.2) 6-12mths: 3.0(SD=2.5) 12-24mths: 1.5(SD=1.9)	**Bleeding/hematoma:** Band slippage, 1/109 (0.9%) **Cardiovascular/Respiratory:** Arrhythmia, 1/109 (0.9%) Atelectasis, 1/109 (0.9%) Pneumonia, 2/109 (1.8%) **Death:** NOS, 0/40 (0%) **GI:** Feeding difficulties, 1/109 (0.9%) Vomiting and/or nausea, 4/109 (3.7%) **Hepatobiliary:** Acute cholecystitis or CBD obstruction, 1/109 (0.9%) **Major Surgical Complications:** Internal hernia, 1/109 (0.9%) **Metabolic:** Vitamin def, 1/109 (0.9%) **Other:** NOS, 1/109 (0.9%) **Pouch/anastomosis:** Anastomotic leak, 1/109 (0.9%) Stricture, 4/109 (3.7%) **Wound:** Infection, 1/109 (0.9%)
DeMaria, 2010[28] US	Cohort	109 T2DM patients with mean age 52.0 years (SD=11.2), BMI 33.9 (SE=1.1) kg/m²	LABG	**Mean BMI:** 0-3mths: 31.6(SD=2.5) 3-6mths: 31.0(SD=2.7) 6-12mths: 30.9(SD=2.9) 12-24mths: 29.9(SD=2.2) **% EBW:** 0-3mths: 40.6(SD=46.8) 3-6mths: 45.5(SD=12.9) 6-12mths: 45.4(SD=13.6) 12-24mths: 41.8(SD=10.2)	**Number of T2DM meds:** 0-3mths: 1.0(SD=1.1) 3-6mths: 0.8(SD=1.0) 6-12mths: 0.6(SD=0.8) 12-24mths: 0.8 (SD=1.1) **% off T2DM meds:** 0-3mths: 21.1 3-6mths: 31.8 6-12mths: 27.5 12-24mths: 36.4	**Number of meds:** 0-3mths: 4.2(SD=3.8) 3-6mths: 3.5(SD=3.7) 6-12mths: 3.1(SD=3.7) 12-24mths: 3.0(SD=3.3)	**Band related:** Band slippage, 1/109 (0.9%) **Death:** NOS, 0/40 (0%) **GI:** Ileus, 1/109 (0.9%) Vomiting and/or nausea, 1/109 (0.9%)

Appendix C Evidence Tables For Surgical Treatment v. Surgical Treatment Trials

Author, Year	Study Design	Patient Population	Procedures	Weight Loss Outcomes	Resolution or improvement in diabetes	Other Outcomes	Adverse Events
Frenken, 2011[32] Western Europe	Case Series	4 T2DM patients with mean age 50 years (range 37-63), BMI 32 (range 31-34) kg/m²	RYGB	Mean BMI: 12mths: 27 (range 26-28)	HbA1c, %: 12mth: 6.7 (range 5.8-7.8)		GI: Anorexia/excessive weight loss, 0/4 (0%)
Frenken, 2011[32] Western Europe	Case Series	12 T2DM patients with mean age 57.3 years (range 36-68), BMI 32 (range 26-34.5) kg/m²	BPD	Mean BMI: 12mths: 24.6(range 19-30)	HbA1c, %: 12mth: 5.2 (range 4.1-6.4)		GI: Anorexia/excessive weight loss, 0/12 (0%)
Lee, 2011[34] Taiwan	RCT	30 T2DM patients with mean age 45 years (range 34-58), BMI 30.3 (range 25.0-34.0) kg/m²*	RYGB	Mean BMI: 12mths: 22.8(SD=2.2) Weight, kg: 12mths: 60.7(SD=10.1) % EWL: 12mths: 94.4(SD=33.1)	Remission of DM: 12mths: 28/30 (93%) Sucessful treatment of DM: 12mths: 17/30 (57%) Metabolic syndrome: 12mths: 2/30 (7%)	C-peptides: 12 mths: 1.6(SD=1.1) Systolic BP: 12 mths: 119.6 (SD=17.3) Diastolic BP: 12 mths: 74.2(SD=12.3) Total cholesterol: 12 mths: 162.2(SD=26.6) Triglycerides: 12 mths: 104.9(SD=62.0) HDL-C: 12 mths: 49.3(SD=7.7) LDL-C: 12 mths: 96.9(SD=21.5)	Death: NOS, 0/30 (0%) Major surgical complications: NOS, 0/30 (0%) Other: Minor surgical complications 3/30 (10%) Readmission: Conservative treatment, 1/30 (3.3%)

Appendix C Evidence Tables For Surgical Treatment v. Surgical Treatment Trials

Author, Year	Study Design	Patient Population	Procedures	Weight Loss Outcomes	Resolution or improvement in diabetes	Other Outcomes	Adverse Events
Lee, 2011[34] Taiwan	RCT	30 T2DM patients with mean age 45 years (range 34-58), BMI 30.3 (range 25.0-34.0) kg/m[2]*	Sleeve	**Mean BMI:** 12mths: 24.4(SD=2.4) **Weight, kg:** 12mths: 65.7(SD=7.9) **% EWL:** 12mths: 76.3(SD=38.9)	**Remission of DM:** 12mths: 14/30 (47%) **Sucessful treatment of DM:** 12mths: 0 (0%) **Metabolic syndrome:** 12mths: 18 (60%)	C-peptides: 12 mths: 1.6(SD=0.5) Systolic BP: 12 mths: 123.5(SD=9.8) Diastolic BP: 12 mths: 75.4(SD=8.5) Total cholesterol: 12 mths: 207.8(SD=67.0) Triglycerides: 12 mths: 144.2(SD=58.9) HDL-C: 12 mths: 45.4(SD=7.9) LDL-C: 12 mths: 136.6(SD=40.8)	**Death:** NOS, 0/30 (0%) **Major surgical complications:** NOS, 0/30 (0%) **Other:** Minor surgical complications 3/30 (10%) **Readmission:** Conservative treatment, 1/30 (3.3%)

Appendix C Evidence Tables For Observational Studies and Controlled Trials with 1 surgical arm**

Author, Year	Study Design	Patient Population	Procedures	Weight Loss Outcomes	Resolution or improvement in diabetes	Other Outcomes	Adverse Events
Boza, 2011[30] South America	Cohort	80 T2DM patients with mean age 47.7 years (SD=8.9), BMI 33 (SD=1.4) kg/m2*	RYGB	**% EWL:** 6mths: 93.8(SD=25.4) 12mths: 103.2(SD=29.4) 24mths: 112.3(SD=30.5)	**% Resolution of DM:** 12mths: 61/80 (76%)	Resolution of Hypertension: 12mths: 46.7% Resolution of Dyslipidemia: 12mths: 80.1%	**Other major surgical complication:** Reoperation,0/80 (0%) **Pouch/anastomosis:** Stricture, 9/80 (12.3%) Leak, 0/80 (0%) **Death:** NOS,0/80 (0%)
Cohen, 2006[26] South America	Case Series	37 T2DM patients with mean age 34 years (range 28-45), BMI 32.5 (range 23.4-34.9) kg/m2*	RYGB	**%EWL:** 6mths: 44 (SD NR) 12mths: 71.6 (SD NR) 18mths: 78.4 (SD NR) 36mths: 77 (SD NR) 48mths: 81 (SD NR)	**% off DM meds:** 20mths: 37/37 (100%) **% DM Remission:** 6mths: 36/37 (97.29%) **Mean Fasting Glucose, mg/dL:** 20mths: 88 (range 60-94)	Cholesterol,mg/dL: 20mths: 172 (range 161-190) Triglycerides,mg/dL: 20mths: 156 (range 172-163) LDL,mg/dL: 20mths: 115 (range 101-127) HDL men,mg/dL: 20mths: 41 (range 40-51) HDL women,mg/dL: 20mths: 50 (range 49-58)	**Death:** NOS,0/37 (0%) **GI:** GERD, 0/37 (0%)
de Sa, 2011[31] South America	Cohort	27 T2DM patients with mean age 50.3 years (SD=8.3), BMI 33.6 (SD=1.5) kg/m2*	RYGB	**Mean BMI:** 20mths: 25.7(SD=2.9) **Weight, kg:** 20mths: 68.5(SD=12.4)	**Mean Fasting Glucose, mg/dL:** 20mths: 93.9 (SD=17.0) **Mean HbA1c:** 20mths: 6.0 (SD=0.7) **% Resolution of DM:** 20mths: 13/27 (48.1%) **% Glycemic Control without Medication:** 20mths: 20/47 (74.1%)		**Major surgical complication:** NOS,0/27 (0%) **Pouch/anastomosis:** Stricture, 1/27 (3.7%) **Death:** NOS,0/27 (0%) **Metabolic:** Malnutrition,0/27 (0%) **Wound:** Seroma,4/27 (14.8%) Infection/abscess, 2/27 (7.4%)
Huang, 2011[33] Asia	Case Series	22 T2DM patients with mean age 47 years (range 28-63), BMI 30.8 (SD=2.9) kg/m²	RYGB	**Mean BMI:** 6mths: 24.4 (SD=2.6) 12mths: 23.7 (SD=1.6)	**% off DM meds:** 12mths: 20/22 (90.3%) **% Remission of DM:** 12mths: 14/22 (63.6%) **Fasting plasma glucose,mg/dL** 6mths: 113.5 (SD=42.5) 12mths: 103.5 (SD=27.6) **HbA1c,%:** 6mths: 6.3 (SD NR) 12mths: 5.9 (SD NR)	**Fasting C-peptide, ng/ml (for 10 patients with mean BMI 29.4):** 1mth: 1.94 (SD=1.29) 3mths: 1.90 (SD=0.92) 6mths: 1.88 (SD=0.82) 12mths: 1.88 (SD=1.07)	**Death:** NOS,0/22 (0%) **GI:** Diarrhea, 1/22 (4.6%) **Bleeding/hematoma:** Anastomotic hemorrage: 1/22 (4.6%)

C-11

Appendix C Evidence Tables For Observational Studies and Controlled Trials with 1 surgical arm**

Author, Year	Study Design	Patient Population	Procedures	Weight Loss Outcomes	Resolution or improvement in diabetes	Other Outcomes	Adverse Events
Lee, 2008[27] Asia	Cohort	44 T2DM patients with mean age 39.0 years (SD=8.9), BMI 31.7 (SD=2.7) kg/m2*	RYGB	**Change in BMI:** 12mths: 8.5 (SD=2.2) **Change in Body Weight,kg:** 12mths: 23.1 (SD=6.7)	**% Metabolic Syndrome:** 12mths: 42.7% **Change in Glucose,mg/dl:** 12mths: 80.1 (SD=56.2) **Change in Insulin,pmol/l:** 20.6 (SD=27.1) **Change in HbA1c:** 1.7 (SD=2.3)	Change in HDL-C, mg/dl: 8.3 (SD=11.2) Change in LDL,mg/dl: 53.8 (SD=29) Triglyceride,mg/dl: 147.4 (SD=150.4) C-peptide,mmol/l: 2.6 (SD=2.3)	**Death:** NOS, 0/44, (0%) **Other:** Morbidity major, 2/44, (4.6%)
Lee, 2011[35] Asia	Case Series	62 T2DM patients with mean age 43.1 years (SD=10.8), BMI 30.1 (SD=3.3) kg/m2*	RYGB	**Mean BMI:** .25mths: 28.9 (SD=3.1) 1mths: 26.7 (SD=2.9) 3mths: 23.4 (SD=2.6) 6mths: 23.8 (SD=2.4) 12mths: 22.6 (SD=2.3) 24mths: 23.0 (SD=2.7) **%EWL:** .25mths: 22.9(SD=30.2) 1mths: 47.9 (SD=36.1) 3mths: 78.2 (SD=41.2) 6mths: 102.5 (SD=71.3) 12mths: 113 (SD=37.3) 24mths: 82.8 (SD=28.8)	**Blood glucose level,mg/dL:** .25mths: 168.9 (SD=52.0) 1mths: 140.2 (SD=41.6) 3mths: 116.6 (SD=25.9) 6mths: 103.2 (SD=19.2) 12mths: 100.2 (SD=19.4) 24mths: 106.3 (SD=18.8) **Insulin, uIU/mL:** .25mths: 4.6(SD=3.2) 1mths: 4.5(SD=2.6) 3mths: 5.0 (SD=3.1) 6mths: 5.2 (SD=4.7) 12mths: 4.6 (SD=3.8) 24mths: 2.8 (SD=1.6) **Mean HbA1c:** .25mths: 9.1 (SD=1.1) 1mths: 7.2 (SD=1.2) 3mths: 6.0 (SD=0.8) 6mths: 5.7 (SD=0.6) 12mths: 5.8 (SD=0.5) 24mths: 5.9 (SD=0.5) **% DM Remission:** .25mths: 0/62 (0%) 1mths: 7/62 (11%) 3mths: 17/45 (37%) 6mths: 21/40 (53%) 12mths: 17/30(57%) 24mths: 11/20 (55%)		**Other major surgical:** NOS, 0/62, (0%) **Minor surgical:** NOS, 7/62, (11.3%)
Ramos, 2011[36] South America	Cohort	147 T2DM patients with mean age 46.9 years (range 34-60), BMI 29.1 (range	RYGB	**Not Reported**	**HbA1c,%:** 18mths: 6.4 (SD=range 5.4-7.2), 31 patients **% T2DM Control (no med + glucose control):** 18mths: 124/147 (84.3%) **% on oral diabeties meds ONLY:** 18mths: 23/147 (15.6%)		**Pouch/anastomosis:** Stricture, 3/147 (2.0%) Fistula, 1/147 (0.7%) **Death:** NOS,0/147 (0%)

Appendix C Evidence Tables For Observational Studies and Controlled Trials with 1 surgical arm**

Author, Year	Study Design	Patient Population	Procedures	Weight Loss Outcomes	Resolution or improvement in diabetes	Other Outcomes	Adverse Events
		26-33) kg/m²					
Shah, 2010[29] India	Case Series	15 T2DM patients with mean age 45.6 years (SD=12), BMI 28.9 (SD=4.0) kg/m²*	RYGB	**Mean BMI:** 9mths: 23.0 (SD=3.6) **Mean Body Weight,kg:** 62.7 (SD NR)	**% off DM meds:** 1mths: 12/15 (80%) 3mths: 15/15 (100%) 6mths: 15/15 (100%) 9mths: 15/15 (100%) **Fasting blood glucose,mg/dL:** 1mths: 106.7 (SD NR) 3mths: 112.3 (SD NR) 6mths: 100.2 (SD NR) 9mths: 89.2 (SD=12) **Mean HbA1c,%:** 1mths: 8.3 (SD NR) 3mths: 7.4 (SD NR) 6mths: 6.6 (SD NR) 9mths: 6.1 (SD=0.6)	Systolic blood pressure,mm Hg: 9mths: 116 (SD NR) Total cholesterol,mg/dL: 9mths: 135 (SD NR) High-density lipoprotein,mg/dL.: 9mths: 50 (SD NR)	**Death:** NOS, 0/15 (0%) **Major surgical complications:** NOS, 0/15 (0%) **GI:** Anorexia/excessive weight loss, 0/15 (0%)
Angrisani, 2004[39] Western Europe	Cohort	210 patients (1.9% with DM) with mean age 38.2 years (range 17-66), BMI 33.9 (range 25.1-35.0) kg/m²*	LABG	**Mean BMI:** 6mths: 31.1(SD=2.2) 12mths: 29.7(SD=2.2) 24mths: 28.7(SD=3.8) 36mths: 26.7(SD=4.3) 48mths: 27.9(SD=3.2) 60mths: 28.2(SD=0.9) **% EWL:** 6mths: 28.1(SD=20.7) 12mths: 52.5(SD=13.2) 24mths: 61.3(SD=14.7) 36mths: 64.7(SD=12.2) 48mths: 68.8(SD=15.3) 60mths: 71.9(SD=10.7)	**Resolution of DM:** 12mths: 210/210 (100%)	Hypertension: Baseline: 9/210 (4.3%) 12mth: 1/210 (0.5%) GERD: Baseline: 5/210 (2.4%) 12mth: 0/210 (0%)	**Band related:** Band slippage, 2/210 (1.0%) Port tube leak, 4/210 (1.9%) Removal, 7/210 (3.3%) **Death:** Band related - gastric perforation, 1/210 (0.5%) **Pouch/anastomosis:** Pouch dilation, 11/210 (5.2%)

Appendix C Evidence Tables For Observational Studies and Controlled Trials with 1 surgical arm**

Author, Year	Study Design	Patient Population	Procedures	Weight Loss Outcomes	Resolution or improvement in diabetes	Other Outcomes	Adverse Events
Choi, 2010[44] US	Cohort	66 patients (6.5% with T2DM) with mean age 40.7 years (SD=11.0), BMI 36.1 (SD=2.6) kg/m[2]*	LABG	**% EWL:** 3mths: 20.3 (SD=9.0) 6mths: 28.5 (SD=14.0) 12mths: 44.7 (SD=19.3) 18mths: 42.2 (33.7)	**DM improved/resolved:** 12mths: 22/66 (33.3%)	Hypertension Improved/resolved: 28.6% Hyperlipidemia inproved/resolved: 15.4% Apnea improved/resolved: 33.3% Arthritis improved/resolved: 36.7% GERD improved/resolved: 31.3% Stress incontinence improved/resolved: 46.6%	**Band related:** Band slippage, 2/66 (3.0%) Erosion, 1/66 (1.5%) Port site seroma, 1/66 (1.5%) **Death:** NOS, 0/66 (0%)
Parikh 2006[41] Australia/ New Zealand	Case Series	93 patients (8.6% with T2DM) with mean age 44.6 years (range 16-76), BMI 32.7 (range 30-34) kg/m[2]*	LABG	**Mean BMI:** 12mths: 27 (SD=2) 24mths: 27 (SD=3) 36mths: 27 (SD=3) **%EWL:** 12mths: 58 (SD=24) 24mths: 57 (SD=29) 36mths: 54 (SD=32)	**% off DM meds:** Pre-op 8/93 took DM meds, Post-op 0/93 needed meds (100%)	Asthma Meds: Pre-op 5/93, Post-op 1/93 Depression Meds: Pre-op 11/93, Post-op 7/93 no meds, 4/93 improved Hypertension Meds: Pre-op 8/93, Post-op 2/93 Sleep apnea Meds: Pre-op 7/93, Post-op 1/93 Arthritis Meds: Pre-op 9/93, Post-op 8/93 improved	**Band Related:** Band slippage, 3/93 (3.2%) Port leak, 1/93 (1.1%) **Death:** NOS, 0/93, (0%) **GI:** Hiatal hernia, 2/93, (2.2%)
Sultan, 2009[43] US	Case Series	53 patients (28.3% with T2DM) with mean age 46.9 years (range 16-68), BMI 33.1 (range 28.2-35) kg/m[2]*	LABG	**Mean BMI:** 6mths: 28.1 (SD=2.4) 12mths: 25.8 (SD=2.9) 24mths: 25.8 (SD=3.1) **%EWL:** 6mths: 48.3 (SD=17.6) 12mths: 69.9 (SD=28.0) 24mths: 69.7 (SD=31.7)	**% off & improved DM meds:** Pre-op 15/53 took DM meds, Post-op 50% meds resolved & improved	Asthma Meds: Pre-op 8/53, Post-op 66.7% resolved, 0% improved Depression Meds: Pre-op 15/53, Post-op 25% resolved, 37.5% improved Hypercholesteremia Meds: Pre-op 25/53, Post-op 33.3% resolved, 0% improved Hypertension Meds: Pre-op 21/53, Post-op 45.5% resolved, 27.3% improved Hypertriglyceridemia Meds: Pre-op 11/53, Post-op 40% resolved, 20% improved Obstructive sleep apnea Meds: Pre-op 19/53, Post-op 50% resolved, 30% improved Osteoarthritis Meds: Pre-op 11/53, Post-op 100% resolved, 0% improved	**Band Related:** Band slippage, 1/53 (1.9%) Port leak, 2/53 (3.8%) **Death:** NOS, 0/53, (0%) **GI:** Esophagitis 2/53 (3.8%) Feeding difficulties 2/53 (3.8%)

Appendix C Evidence Tables For Observational Studies and Controlled Trials with 1 surgical arm**

Author, Year	Study Design	Patient Population	Procedures	Weight Loss Outcomes	Resolution or improvement in diabetes	Other Outcomes	Adverse Events
Lembach, 2011[45] South America	Cohort	12 patients with T2DM with mean age NR, BMI 35.8 kg/m2 (SD NR); And 9 Insulin Resistant patients with mean age NR, BMI 33.6 kg/m2 (SD NR)	Sleeve	**Mean BMI:** 12mths,T2DM: 28.2 (SD NR) 12mths,IR: 23.4 (SD NR)	**Blood glucose level,mg/dL:** 12mths,T2DM: 88(SD NR) 12mths,IR: 76 (SD NR) **Mean HbA1c:** 12mths,T2DM: 4.1 (SD NR)	Triglyceride,mg/dl: 12mths,T2DM: 150 (SD NR) 12mths,IR: 88 (SD NR)	No Mention of Adverse Events
Noya, 1998[46] Western Europe	Case Series	10 T2DM patients with mean age 52.1 years (range 40-62), BMI 33.2 (range 24-39) kg/m2*	BPD	**Mean BMI:** 7mths: 27.2 (SD=3.6) **Mean Excess Weight,kg:** 7mths: 11.9 (SD=7.9)	**% off DM meds:** 8mths: 9/10 (90%)	Cholesterol: 7mths: 165.1 (sd=8.7)	**Cardiovascular:** PE,1/10 (10%0 **Major surgical complications** Reoperation NOS 1/10 (10%)
Scopinaro, 2007[47] Western Europe	Case Series	7 T2DM patients with mean age 49 years (range 39-60), BMI 33.4 (range 32.0-34.6) kg/m2*	BPD	**Mean Weight, kg:** 12mths: 71.2 (SD=9.5) 24mths: 74.7 (SD=9.8) **Mean BMI:** 12mths: 26.2 (SD=2.1) 24mths: 26.9 (SD=2.1)	**Mean serum glucose:** 12mths: 87.0 (SD=8.1) 24mths: 90.4 (SD=7.4) **% off DM meds:** 24mths: 7/7 (100%)	Triglycerides: 12mths: 156.5 (SD=67.5) 24mths: 144.1 (SD=62.2) Cholesterol: 12mths: 140.5 (SD=38.3) 24mths: 138.3 (SD=18.0)	No Mention of Adverse Events

Appendix C Evidence Tables For Observational Studies and Controlled Trials with 1 surgical arm**

Author, Year	Study Design	Patient Population	Procedures	Weight Loss Outcomes	Resolution or improvement in diabetes	Other Outcomes	Adverse Events
Scopinaro, 2011[49] Western Europe	Case Control	15 T2DM obese (OB) patients with mean age 55.1 years (SD=8.0), BMI 33.1 (SD=1.5) kg/m2; And 15 T2DM overweight (OW) patients with mean age 57.8 years (SD=6.7), BMI 28.0 (SD=1.3) kg/m2	BPD	**Mean BMI, OB:** 1mth: 29.1(SD=2.4) 4mths: 27.2(SD=1.6) 8mths: 26.9(SD=2.3) 12mths: 26.4(SD=2.4) 24mths: 27.4(SD=2.3) **Mean BMI, OW:** 1mth: 24.3(SD=0.9) 4mths: 24.2(SD=1.0) 8mths: 24.3(SD=1.3) 12mths: 24.2(SD=1.6) 24mths: 24.6(SD=1.8) **Weight, kg, OB:** 1mth: 78.2(SD=9.9) 4mths: 73.2(SD=9.1) 8mths: 72.4(SD=10.4) 12mths: 71.1(SD=10.4) 24mths: 73.7(SD=10.5) **Weight, kg, OB:** 1mth: 70.4(SD=8.7) 4mths: 70.0(SD=9.5) 8mths: 70.0(SD=8.2) 12mths: 70.3(SD=9.2) 24mths: 70.9(SD=9.6)	**Mean fasting serum glucose, mg/dl,OB:** 1mth: 154(SD=49) 4mths: 129(SD=32) 8mths: 133(SD=39) 12mths: 131(SD=32) 24mths: 134(SD=41) **Mean fasting serum glucose, mg/dl,OW:** 1mth: 176(SD=75) 4mths: 165(SD=58) 8mths: 171(SD=42) 12mths: 167(SD=48) 24mths: 154(SD=41) **HbA1c,%, OB:** 1mth: 7.3(SD=1.1) 4mths: 6.3(SD=0.8) 8mths: 5.9(SD=1.1) 12mths: 5.9(SD=0.6) 24mths: 5.9(SD=0.9) **HbA1c,%, OW:** 1mth: 7.3(SD=1.2) 4mths: 7.3(SD=1.3) 8mths: 6.9(SD=1.1) 12mths: 7.1(SD=1.1) 24mths: 6.9(SD=1.1) **% Patients HbA1c<=7%, OB:** 1mth: 8/15 (53%) 4mths: 13/15 (87%) 8mths: 13/15 (87%) 12mths: 15/15 (100%) 24mths: 12/15 (80%) **% Patients HbA1c<=7%,OW:** 1mth: 4/15 (27%) 4mths: 9/15 (60%) 8mths: 11/15 (73%) 12mths: 10/15 (67%) 24mths: 9/15 (60%)	**Serum Triglyceride,mg/dL, OB:** 1mth: 223(SD=258) 4mths: 174(SD=85) 8mths: 208(SD=123) 12mths: 181(SD=123) 24mths: 177(SD=82) **Serum Triglyceride,mg/dL, OW:** 1mth: 137(SD=52) 4mths: 240(SD=170) 8mths: 222(SD=85) 12mths: 227(SD=104) 24mths: 225(SD=116) **Serum Total Cholesterol,OB:** 1mth: 134(SD=35.4) 4mths: 138(SD=33.8) 8mths: 146(SD=35.5) 12mths: 153(SD=35) 24mths: 156(SD=28) **Serum Total Cholesterol, OW:** 1mth: 116(SD=31) 4mths: 158(SD=40) 8mths: 150(SD=29) 12mths: 141(SD=36) 24mths: 146(SD=29) **Serum HDL Cholesterol,OB:** 1mth: 37(SD=8.8) 4mths: 36(SD=6.6) 8mths: 39(SD=6.9) 12mths: 47(SD=10.4) 24mths: 47(SD=10.1) **Serum HDL Cholesterol, OW:** 1mth: 29(SD=8.1) 4mths: 38(SD=7.2) 8mths: 41(SD=6) 12mths: 41(SD=16) 24mths: 38(SD=7.3)	**Bleeding/hematoma:** Intraperitoneal bleeding, 1/30 (3.3%) **Other major surgical complications** NOS 0/30 (0%) **GI:** Gastroplegia, 4/30 (13.3%) Revision secondary to diarrhea, 1/30 (3.3%) **Death:** Sudden cardiac, 0/30 (0%)

* Demographic characteristics only reported overall, not for each group. No statistically significant differences found between demographic characteristics.
** Comparison arm did not receive non-surgical treatment

Appendix D. Excluded Studies

Reject Background:

1. Blackburn GL, Wollner SB, Jones DB. Bariatric surgery as treatment for type 2 diabetes. Curr Diab Rep. 2010 Aug;10(4):261-3. PMID 20440583.

2. Caballero MG. [Surgery of type 2 diabetes mellitus: the great discovery of bariatric surgery]. Nutr Hosp. 2010 Sep-Oct;25(5):693-4. PMID 21336421.

3. Campos GM, Rabl C, Roll GR, et al. Better Weight Loss, Resolution of Diabetes, and Quality of Life for Laparoscopic Gastric Bypass vs Banding: Results of a 2-Cohort Pair-Matched Study. Arch Surg. 2011 Feb;146(2):149-55. PMID 21339424.

4. Clifton P. Diabetes: treatment of type 2 diabetes mellitus with bariatric surgery. Nat Rev Endocrinol. 2010 Apr;6(4):191-3. PMID 20336164.

5. Cummings DEF, D. R. Gastrointestinal surgery as a treatment for diabetes. JAMA. 2008 Jan 23;299(3):341-3. PMID 18212321.

6. Deitel M. Surgery for diabetes at lower BMI: some caution. Obes Surg. 2008 Oct;18(10):1211-4. PMID 18758867.

7. Ferrannini EM, G. Impact of different bariatric surgical procedures on insulin action and beta-cell function in type 2 diabetes. Diabetes Care. 2009 Mar;32(3):514-20. PMID 19246589.

8. Gagner M. Laparoscopic sleeve gastrectomy with ileal interposition (SGIT): a modified duodenal switch for resolution of type 2 diabetes mellitus in lesser obese patients (BMI < 35). World J Surg. 2011 Jan;35(1):109-10. PMID 21052995.

9. Gagner M. Surgical treatment of nonseverely obese patients with type 2 diabetes mellitus: sleeve gastrectomy with ileal transposition (SGIT) is the same as the neuroendocrine brake (NEB) procedure or ileal interposition associated with sleeve gastrectomy (II-SG), but ileal interposition with diverted sleeve gastrectomy (II-DSG) is the same as duodenal switch. Surg Endosc. 2011 Feb;25(2):655-6. PMID 20614137.

10. Gary TLB-T, M. Bone, L. R. Yeh, H. C. Wang, N. Y. Hill-Briggs, F. Levine, D. M. Powe, N. R. Hill, M. N. Saudek, C. McGuire, M. Brancati, F. L. A randomized controlled trial of the effects of nurse case manager and community health worker team interventions in urban African-Americans with type 2 diabetes. Control Clin Trials. 2004 Feb;25(1):53-66. PMID 14980748.

11. Gill RS, Sharma AM, Al-Adra DP, et al. The impact of bariatric surgery in patients with type-2 diabetes mellitus. Curr Diabetes Rev. 2011 May;7(3):185-9. PMID 21488837.

12. Inabnet WB. Comment on: Prospective randomized controlled trial comparing 2 versions of laparoscopic ileal interposition associated with sleeve gastrectomy for patients with type 2 diabetes with BMI 2134 kg/m2. Surgery for Obesity and Related Diseases. 2010;6(3):304-5.

13. Keating CLD, J. B. Moodie, M. L. Peeters, A. Playfair, J. O'Brien, P. E. Cost-efficacy of surgically induced weight loss for the management of type 2 diabetes: a randomized controlled trial. Diabetes Care. 2009 Apr;32(4):580-4. PMID 19171726.

14. Lautz D, Halperin F, Goebel-Fabbri A, et al. The great debate: Medicine or surgery: What is best for the patient with type 2 diabetes? Diabetes Care. 2011;34(3):763-70.

15. Lynis Dohm G, Pories WJ. Bypass of metabolic diseases with surgery. Obesity. 2011;19(7):1323-4.

16. Nathan DMB, M. Trials that matter: rosiglitazone, ramipril, and the prevention of type 2 diabetes. Ann Intern Med. 2007 Mar 20;146(6):461-3. PMID 17371892.

17. Pories WJ, Mehaffey JH, Staton KM. The surgical treatment of type two diabetes mellitus. Surg Clin North Am. 2011 Aug;91(4):821-36. PMID 21787970.

18. Shikora SA. Comment on: diabetes remission and reduced cardiovascular risk after gastric bypass in Asian Indians with body mass index <35 kg/m(2). Surg Obes Relat Dis. 2010 Jul-Aug;6(4):338-9. PMID 19914146.

19. Spector D, Shikora S. Neuro-modulation and bariatric surgery for type 2 diabetes mellitus. Int J Clin Pract Suppl. 2010 Feb(166):53-8. PMID 20377665.

Reject Case Report:

1. Friedman MNS, A. J. Magovern, G. J. The amelioration of diabetes mellitus following subtotal gastrectomy. Surg Gynecol Obstet. 1955 Feb;100(2):201-4. PMID 13238177.

2. Palanivelu C, Praveen Raj P, Senthilnathan P, et al. Surgery for type II diabetes mellitus: Laparoscopic ileal interposition (TYPEI). Surgical Endoscopy and Other Interventional Techniques. 2011;25:S224.

3. Velez JP, Arias RH, Olaya P. Laparoscopic sleeve gastrectomy on heart transplant recipient with body mass index of 34 kg/m(2) and metabolic syndrome. Surg Obes Relat Dis. 2010 Dec 4PMID 21212027.

Reject No Diabetes or Impaired Glucose Tolerance:

1. Al-Sarraj TS, H. Calle, M. C. Volek, J. S. Fernandez, M. L. Carbohydrate restriction, as a first-line dietary intervention, effectively reduces biomarkers of metabolic syndrome in Emirati adults. J Nutr. 2009 Sep;139(9):1667-76. PMID 19587123.

2. Andersen TB, O. G. Stokholm, K. H. Quaade, F. Randomized trial of diet and gastroplasty compared with diet alone in morbid obesity. N Engl J Med. 1984 Feb 9;310(6):352-6. PMID 6690963.

3. Andersen TS, K. H. Backer, O. G. Quaade, F. Long-term (5-year) results after either horizontal gastroplasty or very-low-calorie diet for morbid obesity. Int J Obes. 1988;12(4):277-84. PMID 3058614.

4. Anderson AES, R. T. Scott, D. H. Gastric bypass for morbid obesity in children and adolescents. J Pediatr Surg. 1980 Dec;15(6):876-81. PMID 7463289.

5. Ashley SB, D. L. Sugden, G. Royston, C. M. Vertical banded gastroplasty for the treatment of morbid obesity. Br J Surg. 1993 Nov;80(11):1421-3. PMID 8252354.

6. Aude YWA, A. S. Lopez-Jimenez, F. Lieberman, E. H. Marie, Almon Hansen, M. Rojas, G. Lamas, G. A. Hennekens, C. H. The national cholesterol education program diet vs a diet lower in carbohydrates and higher in protein and monounsaturated fat: a randomized trial. Arch Intern Med. 2004 Oct 25;164(19):2141-6. PMID 15505128.

7. Bacci VB, M. S. Greco, F. Lamberti, R. Elmore, U. Restuccia, A. Perrotta, N. Silecchia, G. Bucci, A. Modifications of metabolic and cardiovascular risk factors after weight loss induced by laparoscopic gastric banding. Obes Surg. 2002 Feb;12(1):77-82. PMID 11868304.

8. Benfield JRG, F. L. Bray, G. A. Barry, R. E. Lechago, J. Mena, I. Schedewie, H. Experience with jejunoileal bypass for obesity. Surg Gynecol Obstet. 1976 Sep;143(3):401-10. PMID 1085495.

9. Berrevoet FP, P. Cardon, A. de Ryck, F. Hesse, U. J. de Hemptinne, B. Retrospective analysis of laparoscopic gastric banding technique: short-term and mid-term follow-up. Obes Surg. 1999 Jun;9(3):272-5. PMID 10484315.

10. Bradley US, Michelle Courtney, C. Hamish McKinley, Michelle C. Ennis, Cieran N. McCance, David R. McEneny, Jane Bell, Patrick M. Young, Ian S. Hunter, Steven J. Low-Fat Versus Low-Carbohydrate Weight Reduction Diets. Diabetes. 2009 December 2009;58(12):2741-8.

11. Bravata DMS-S, C. Sundaram, V. Gienger, A. L. Lin, N. Lewis, R. Stave, C. D. Olkin, I. Sirard, J. R. Using pedometers to increase physical activity and improve health: a systematic review. JAMA. 2007 Nov 21;298(19):2296-304. PMID 18029834.

12. Brekke HKJ, P. A. Lenner, R. A. Long-term (1- and 2-year) effects of lifestyle intervention in type 2 diabetes relatives. Diabetes Res Clin Pract. 2005 Dec;70(3):225-34. PMID 15885845.

13. Brown TA, A. Edmunds, L. D. Moore, H. Whittaker, V. Avery, L. Summerbell, C. Systematic review of long-term lifestyle interventions to prevent weight gain and morbidity in adults. Obesity Reviews. 2009;10(6):627-38.

14. Buckwalter JA. A prospective comparison of the jejunoileal and gastric bypass operations for morbid obesity. World J Surg. 1977 Nov;1(6):757-68. PMID 607594.

15. Charles MAE, E. Grandmottet, P. Isnard, F. Cohen, J. M. Bensoussan, J. L. Berche, H. Chapiro, O. Andre, P. Vague, P. Juhan-Vague, I. Bard, J. M. Safar, M. Treatment with metformin of non-diabetic men with hypertension, hypertriglyceridaemia and central fat distribution: the BIGPRO 1.2 trial. Diabetes Metab Res Rev. 2000 Jan-Feb;16(1):2-7. PMID 10707032.

16. Charuzi IL, P. Peiser, J. Peled, R. Bariatric surgery in morbidly obese sleep-apnea patients: short- and long-term follow-up. Am J Clin Nutr. 1992 Feb;55(2 Suppl):594S-6S. PMID 1733135.

17. Chua TYM, R. M. Laparoscopic Vertical Banded Gastroplasty: The Milwaukee Experience. Obes Surg. 1995 Feb;5(1):77-80. PMID 10733799.

18. Claessens MvB, M. A. Monsheimer, S. Saris, W. H. M. The effect of a low-fat, high-protein or high-carbohydrate ad libitum diet on weight loss maintenance and metabolic risk factors. Int J Obes. 2009;33(3):296-304.

19. Colles SLD, J. B. O'Brien, P. E. Hunger control and regular physical activity facilitate weight loss after laparoscopic adjustable gastric banding. Obes Surg. 2008 Jul;18(7):833-40. PMID 18408982.

20. Contreras J, Villao D, Bravo J, et al. Medium term results of laparoscopic vertical sleeve gastrectomy in 300 obese patients. Obesity Surgery. 2010;20(8):1063.

21. Dansinger MLT, A. Wong, J. B. Chung, M. Balk, E. M. Meta-analysis: the effect of dietary counseling for weight loss. Ann Intern Med. 2007 Jul 3;147(1):41-50. PMID 17606960.

22. Dastjerdi MSK, F. Najafian, A. Mohammady, M. Aminorroaya, A. Amini, M. An open-label pilot study of the combination therapy of metformin and fluoxetine for weight reduction. Int J Obes (Lond). 2007 Apr;31(4):713-7. PMID 16969361.

23. Davis JNV, E. E. Alexander, K. E. Salguero, L. E. Weigensberg, M. J. Crespo, N. C. Spruijt-Metz, D. Goran, M. I. Feasibility of a home-based versus classroom-based nutrition intervention to reduce obesity and type 2 diabetes in Latino youth. Int J Pediatr Obes. 2007;2(1):22-30. PMID 17763007.

24. de Rougemont AN, S. Nazare, J. A. Skilton, M. R. Sothier, M. Vinoy, S. Laville, M. Beneficial effects of a 5-week low-glycaemic index regimen on weight control and cardiovascular risk factors in overweight non-diabetic subjects. Br J Nutr. 2007 Dec;98(6):1288-98. PMID 17617942.

25. de Zwaan ML, K. L. Mitchell, J. E. Howell, L. M. Monson, N. Roerig, J. L. Crosby, R. D. Health-related quality of life in morbidly obese patients: effect of gastric bypass surgery. Obes Surg. 2002 Dec;12(6):773-80. PMID 12568181.

26. Derosa GC, A. F. Murdolo, G. Piccinni, M. N. Fogari, E. Bertone, G. Ciccarelli, L. Fogari, R. Efficacy and safety comparative evaluation of orlistat and sibutramine treatment in hypertensive obese patients. Diabetes Obes Metab. 2005 Jan;7(1):47-55. PMID 15642075.

27. DeWind LTP, J. H. Intestinal bypass surgery for morbid obesity. Long-term results. JAMA. 1976 Nov 15;236(20):2298-301. PMID 989831.

28. Dhabuwala AC, R. J. Stubbs, R. S. Improvement in co-morbidities following weight loss from gastric bypass surgery. Obes Surg. 2000 Oct;10(5):428-35. PMID 11054247.

29. Ditschuneit HHF-M, Marion Johnson, Timothy D Adler, Guido. Metabolic and weight-loss effects of a long-term dietary intervention in obese patients. Am J Clin Nutr. 1999 February 1, 1999;69(2):198-204.

30. Dolan KF, G. A comparison of laparoscopic adjustable gastric banding in adolescents and adults. Surg Endosc. 2004 Jan;18(1):45-7. PMID 14625730.

31. Due AL, T. M. Mu, H. Hermansen, K. Stender, S. Astrup, A. Comparison of 3 ad libitum diets for weight-loss maintenance, risk of cardiovascular disease, and diabetes: a 6-mo randomized, controlled trial. Am J Clin Nutr. 2008 Nov;88(5):1232-41. PMID 18996857.

32. Eckhout GVW, O. L. Moore, J. T. Vertical ring gastroplasty for morbid obesity. Five year experience with 1,463 patients. Am J Surg. 1986 Dec;152(6):713-6. PMID 3789301.

33. Farnsworth EL, N. D. Noakes, M. Wittert, G. Argyiou, E. Clifton, P. M. Effect of a high-protein, energy-restricted diet on body composition, glycemic control, and lipid concentrations in overweight and obese hyperinsulinemic men and women. Am J Clin Nutr. 2003 Jul;78(1):31-9. PMID 12816768.

34. Flechtner-Mors MD, Herwig H. Johnson, Timothy D. Suchard, Mark A. Adler, Guido. Metabolic and Weight Loss Effects of Long-Term Dietary Intervention in Obese Patients: Four-Year Results. Obesity. 2000;8(5):399-402.

35. Fobi ML, H. Igwe, D. Felahy, B. James, E. Stanczyk, M. Fobi, N. Gastric bypass in patients with BMI < 40 but > 32 without life-threatening co-morbidities: preliminary report. Obes Surg. 2002 Feb;12(1):52-6. PMID 11868299.

36. Foley EFB, P. N. Borlase, B. C. Hollingshead, J. Blackburn, G. L. Impact of gastric restrictive surgery on hypertension in the morbidly obese. Am J Surg. 1992 Mar;163(3):294-7. PMID 1539761.

37. Forsell PH, G. The Swedish Adjustable Gastric Banding (SAGB) for morbid obesity: 9 year experience and a 4-year follow-up of patients operated with a new adjustable band. Obes Surg. 1997 Aug;7(4):345-51. PMID 9730522.

38. Frank LLS, B. E. Yasui, Y. Tworoger, S. S. Schwartz, R. S. Ulrich, C. M. Irwin, M. L. Rudolph, R. E. Rajan, K. B. Stanczyk, F. Bowen, D. Weigle, D. S. Potter, J. D. McTiernan, A. Effects of exercise on metabolic risk variables in overweight postmenopausal women: a randomized clinical trial. Obes Res. 2005 Mar;13(3):615-25. PMID 15833948.

39. Fransis KD, F. Vanrykel, J. P. Aelvoet, C. Experience with laparoscopic adjustable gastric banding (la-band system) up to 8 years. Acta Chir Belg. 2005 Feb;105(1):69-73. PMID 15790206.

40. Freeman JBB, H. J. A comparison of gastric bypass and gastroplasty for morbid obesity. Surgery. 1980 Sep;88(3):433-44. PMID 7414518.

41. Frey H. [An investigation of the effect of biguanides on glucose tolerance and body weight in overweight individuals without diabetes mellitus]. Tidsskr Nor Laegeforen. 1972 May 30;92(15):1036-8. PMID 4555163.

42. Galani CS, H. Prevention and treatment of obesity with lifestyle interventions: review and meta-analysis. Int J Public Health. 2007;52(6):348-59. PMID 18368998.

43. Gleysteen JJ. Four-year weight loss Roux-Y gastric bypass: anastomotic reinforcement not additive. Gastroenterol Clin North Am. 1987 Sep;16(3):525-7. PMID 3325428.

44. Gomez CA. Gastroplasty in morbid obesity. Surg Clin North Am. 1979 Dec;59(6):1113-20. PMID 531744.

45. Grey NK, D. M. Effect of diet composition on the hyperinsulinemia of obesity. N Engl J Med. 1971 Oct 7;285(15):827-31. PMID 5570845.

46. Hafner RJW, J. M. Rogers, J. Quality of life after gastric bypass for morbid obesity. Int J Obes. 1991 Aug;15(8):555-60. PMID 1938099.

47. Hajdukovic ZJ, A. Zivotic-Vanovic, M. Raden, S. [Influence of orlistat therapy on serum insulin level and morphological and functional parameters of peripheral arterial circulation in obese patients]. Vojnosanit Pregl. 2005 Nov;62(11):803-10. PMID 16375203.

48. Hall WDF, Z. George, V. A. Lewis, C. E. Oberman, A. Huber, M. Fouad, M. Cutler, J. A. Low-fat diet: effect on anthropometrics, blood pressure, glucose, and insulin in older women. Ethn Dis. 2003 Summer;13(3):337-43. PMID 12894958.

49. Harrison RAR, C. Elton, P. J. Does primary care referral to an exercise programme increase physical activity one year later? A randomized controlled trial. J Public Health (Oxf). 2005 Mar;27(1):25-32. PMID 15564275.

50. Herbst CA, Jr. Buckwalter, J. A. Weight loss and complications after four gastric operations for morbid obesity. South Med J. 1982 Nov;75(11):1324-8. PMID 7146960.

51. Kakoulidis TP, Karringer A, Gloaguen T, et al. Initial results with sleeve gastrectomy for patients with class I obesity (BMI 30-35 kg/m2). Surg Obes Relat Dis. 2009 Jul-Aug;5(4):425-8. PMID 18996758.

52. Kasama K, Seki Y, Shimizu H, et al. Anti diabetic effect of laparoscopic sleeve gastrectomy with duodenal jejunal bypass. Obesity Surgery. 2010;20(8):990.

53. Kellum JMK, J. F. O'Dorisio, T. M. Rayford, P. Martin, D. Engle, K. Wolf, L. Sugerman, H. J. Gastrointestinal hormone responses to meals before and after gastric bypass and vertical banded gastroplasty. Ann Surg. 1990 Jun;211(6):763-70; discussion 70-1. PMID 2192696.

54. Kukkonen-Harjula KTB, P. T. Nenonen, A. M. Fogelholm, M. G. Effects of a weight maintenance program with or without exercise on the metabolic syndrome: a randomized trial in obese men. Prev Med. 2005 Sep-Oct;41(3-4):784-90. PMID 16125218.

55. Larsen JFK, J. P. [Laparoscopic adjustable gastric banding for the treatment of morbid obesity. Six years' experiences]. Ugeskr Laeger. 2005 May 2;167(18):1946-9. PMID 15929267.

56. Lee WJL, Y. C. Ser, K. H. Chen, J. C. Chen, S. C. Improvement of insulin resistance after obesity surgery: a comparison of gastric banding and bypass procedures. Obes Surg. 2008 Sep;18(9):1119-25. PMID 18317853.

57. Lee WJW, W. Yu, P. J. Wei, P. L. Huang, M. T. Gastrointestinal quality of life following laparoscopic adjustable gastric banding in Asia. Obes Surg. 2006 May;16(5):586-91. PMID 16687026.

58. Lucas CPB, M. N. Reaven, G. M. Effect of orlistat added to diet (30% of calories from fat) on plasma lipids, glucose, and insulin in obese patients with hypercholesterolemia. Am J Cardiol. 2003 Apr 15;91(8):961-4. PMID 12686336.

59. Martinez-Gonzalez MAdlF-A, C. Nunez-Cordoba, J. M. Basterra-Gortari, F. J. Beunza, J. J. Vazquez, Z. Benito, S. Tortosa, A. Bes-Rastrollo, M. Adherence to Mediterranean diet and risk of developing diabetes: prospective cohort study. BMJ. 2008 Jun 14;336(7657):1348-51. PMID 18511765.

60. McMahon FGF, K. Singh, B. N. Mendel, C. M. Rowe, E. Rolston, K. Johnson, F. Mooradian, A. D. Efficacy and safety of sibutramine in obese white and African American patients with hypertension: a 1-year, double-blind, placebo-controlled, multicenter trial. Arch Intern Med. 2000 Jul 24;160(14):2185-91. PMID 10904462.

61. Melchionda NB, L. Di Domizio, S. Pasqui, F. Nuccitelli, C. Migliorini, S. Baraldi, L. Natale, S. Manini, R. Bellini, M. Belsito, C. Forlani, G. Marchesini, G. Cognitive behavioural therapy for obesity: one-year follow-up in a clinical setting. Eat Weight Disord. 2003 Sep;8(3):188-93. PMID 14649781.

62. Moon Han SK, W. W. Oh, J. H. Results of laparoscopic sleeve gastrectomy (LSG) at 1 year in morbidly obese Korean patients. Obes Surg. 2005 Nov-Dec;15(10):1469-75. PMID 16354529.

63. Morino MT, M. Garrone, C. Disappointing long-term results of laparoscopic adjustable silicone gastric banding. Br J Surg. 1997 Jun;84(6):868-9. PMID 9189114.

64. Morino MT, M. Garrone, C. Morino, F. Laparoscopic adjustable silicone gastric banding for the treatment of morbid obesity. Br J Surg. 1994 Aug;81(8):1169-70. PMID 7953351.

65. Narayan KMH, M. Kozak, D. Kriska, A. M. Hanson, R. L. Pettitt, D. J. Nagi, D. K. Bennett, P. H. Knowler, W. C. Randomized clinical trial of lifestyle interventions in Pima Indians: a pilot study. Diabet Med. 1998 Jan;15(1):66-72. PMID 9472866.

66. Nedelnikova KS, S. Haas, T. Matoulek, M. Fried, M. Influence of metabolic state and diabetes on the outcome at the end of first year after gastric banding. Obes Surg. 2000 Aug;10(4):372-5. PMID 11007633.

67. Nicklas BJD, K. E. Berman, D. M. Sorkin, J. Ryan, A. S. Goldberg, A. P. Lifestyle intervention of hypocaloric dieting and walking reduces abdominal obesity and improves coronary heart disease risk factors in obese, postmenopausal, African-American and Caucasian women. J Gerontol A Biol Sci Med Sci. 2003 Feb;58(2):181-9. PMID 12586858.

68. Nilsson PML, L. H. Schersten, B. F. Life style changes improve insulin resistance in hyperinsulinaemic subjects: a one-year intervention study of hypertensives and normotensives in Dalby. J Hypertens. 1992 Sep;10(9):1071-8. PMID 1328367.

69. Olsson SAN-E, P. Pettersson, B. G. Sorbris, R. Gastroplasty as a treatment for massive obesity. A clinical and biochemical evaluation. Scand J Gastroenterol. 1985 Mar;20(2):215-21. PMID 3992180.

70. Olsson SAR, O. Danielsson, A. Nilsson-Ehle, P. Weight reduction after gastroplasty: the predictive value of surgical, metabolic, and psychological variables. Int J Obes. 1984;8(3):245-58. PMID 6746192.

71. Owen ERA, R. Kark, A. E. Gastroplasty for morbid obesity: technique, complications and results in 60 cases. Br J Surg. 1989 Feb;76(2):131-5. PMID 2702443.

72. Payne JHD, L. Schwab, C. E. Kern, W. H. Surgical treatment of morbid obesity. Sixteen years of experience. Arch Surg. 1973 Apr;106(4):432-7. PMID 4696715.

73. Peiser JL, P. Ovnat, A. Charuzi, I. Sleep apnea syndrome in the morbidly obese as an indication for weight reduction surgery. Ann Surg. 1984 Jan;199(1):112-5. PMID 6691724.

74. Pereira MAS, J. Goldfine, A. B. Rifai, N. Ludwig, D. S. Effects of a low-glycemic load diet on resting energy expenditure and heart disease risk factors during weight loss. JAMA. 2004 Nov 24;292(20):2482-90. PMID 15562127.

75. Peterson CMJ-P, L. Randomized crossover study of 40% vs. 55% carbohydrate weight loss strategies in women with previous gestational diabetes mellitus and non-diabetic women of 130-200% ideal body weight. J Am Coll Nutr. 1995 Aug;14(4):369-75. PMID 8568114.

76. Pittas AGR, S. B. Das, S. K. Gilhooly, C. H. Saltzman, E. Golden, J. Stark, P. C. Greenberg, A. S. The effects of the dietary glycemic load on type 2 diabetes risk factors during weight loss. Obesity (Silver Spring). 2006 Dec;14(12):2200-9. PMID 17189547.

77. Rabast US, J. Kasper, H. Dietetic treatment of obesity with low and high-carbohydrate diets: comparative studies and clinical results. Int J Obes. 1979;3(3):201-11. PMID 395115.

78. Ramsey-Stewart G. Vertical banded gastroplasty for morbid obesity: weight loss at short and long-term follow up. Aust N Z J Surg. 1995 Jan;65(1):4-7. PMID 7818421.

79. Reinhold RB. Critical analysis of long term weight loss following gastric bypass. Surg Gynecol Obstet. 1982 Sep;155(3):385-94. PMID 7051382.

80. Rokling-Andersen MHR, J. E. Veierod, M. B. Anderssen, S. A. Jacobs, D. R., Jr. Urdal, P. Jansson, J. O. Drevon, C. A. Effects of long-term exercise and diet intervention on plasma adipokine concentrations. Am J Clin Nutr. 2007 Nov;86(5):1293-301. PMID 17991638.

81. Ross RD, D. Jones, P. J. Smith, H. Paddags, A. Hudson, R. Janssen, I. Reduction in obesity and related comorbid conditions after diet-induced weight loss or exercise-induced weight loss in men. A randomized, controlled trial. Ann Intern Med. 2000 Jul 18;133(2):92-103. PMID 10896648.

82. Ross RJ, I. Physical activity, total and regional obesity: dose-response considerations. Med Sci Sports Exerc. 2001 Jun;33(6 Suppl):S521-7; discussion S8-9. PMID 11427779.

83. Rucker RD, Jr. Horstmann, J. Schneider, P. D. Varco, R. L. Buchwald, H. Comparisons between jejunoileal and gastric bypass operations for morbid obesity. Surgery. 1982 Aug;92(2):241-9. PMID 7101125.

84. Ryden OO, S. A. Danielsson, A. Nilsson-Ehle, P. Weight loss after gastroplasty: psychological sequelae in relation to clinical and metabolic observations. J Am Coll Nutr. 1989 Feb;8(1):15-23. PMID 2538497.

85. Schwarz AB, M. Usinger, K. Rieger, H. Glasbrenner, B. Friess, H. Kunz, R. Beger, H. G. Importance of the duodenal passage and pouch volume after total gastrectomy and reconstruction with the Ulm pouch: prospective randomized clinical study. World J Surg. 1996 Jan;20(1):60-6; discussion 6-7. PMID 8588415.

86. Shah MS, V. Garg, A. Review: long-term impact of bariatric surgery on body weight, comorbidities, and nutritional status. J Clin Endocrinol Metab. 2006 Nov;91(11):4223-31. PMID 16954156.

87. Toft UNK, L. H. Aadahl, M. von Huth Smith, L. Pisinger, C. Jorgensen, T. Diet and exercise intervention in a general population--mediators of participation and adherence: the Inter99 study. Eur J Public Health. 2007 Oct;17(5):455-63. PMID 17170019.

88. Tweddle EAW, S. Blamey, S. Laparoscopic gastric banding: safe and modestly successful. ANZ J Surg. 2004 Apr;74(4):191-4. PMID 15043723.

89. Vishne THR, E. Alper, D. Avraham, Z. Seror, D. Dreznik, Z. Long-term follow-up and factors influencing success of silastic ring vertical gastroplasty. Dig Surg. 2004;21(2):134-40; discussion 40-1. PMID 15044814.

90. Weiner RA. Surgical treatment of the metabolic syndrome. Viszeralmedizin: Gastrointestinal Medicine and Surgery. 2010;26(1):8-12.

91. Weissgerber TLW, L. A. Davies, G. A. Mottola, M. F. Exercise in the prevention and treatment of maternal-fetal disease: a review of the literature. Appl Physiol Nutr Metab. 2006 Dec;31(6):661-74. PMID 17213880.

92. Wickremesekera KM, G. Naotunne, T. D. Knowles, G. Stubbs, R. S. Loss of insulin resistance after Roux-en-Y gastric bypass surgery: a time course study. Obes Surg. 2005 Apr;15(4):474-81. PMID 15946424.

93. Wing RRJ, R. W. Effect of modest weight loss on changes in cardiovascular risk factors: are there differences between men and women or between weight loss and maintenance? Int J Obes Relat Metab Disord. 1995 Jan;19(1):67-73. PMID 7719395.

94. Yates BT. Survey comparison of success, morbidity, mortality, fees and psychological benefits and costs of 3,146 patients receiving jejunoileal or gastric bypass. Am J Clin Nutr. 1980 Feb;33(2 Suppl):518-22. PMID 7355832.

Reject BMI > 35:

1. Abbatini F, Rizzello M, Casella G, et al. Long-term effects of laparoscopic sleeve gastrectomy, gastric bypass, and adjustable gastric banding on type 2 diabetes. Surg Endosc. 2010 May;24(5):1005-10. PMID 19866235.

2. Adami GFC, R. Camerini, G. Marinari, G. M. Scopinaro, N. Long-term normalization of insulin sensitivity following biliopancreatic diversion for obesity. Int J Obes Relat Metab Disord. 2004 May;28(5):671-3. PMID 15024397.

3. Adams TDG, R. E. Smith, S. C. Halverson, R. C. Simper, S. C. Rosamond, W. D. Lamonte, M. J. Stroup, A. M. Hunt, S. C. Long-term mortality after gastric bypass surgery. N Engl J Med. 2007 Aug 23;357(8):753-61. PMID 17715409.

4. Agren GN, K. Naslund, I. Sjostrom, L. Peltonen, M. Long-term effects of weight loss on pharmaceutical costs in obese subjects. A report from the SOS intervention study. Int J Obes Relat Metab Disord. 2002 Feb;26(2):184-92. PMID 11850749.

5. Agren GN, I. A prospective randomized comparison of vertical banded gastroplasty (VBG), loop gastric bypass (GBY) and gastric banding (GB). Int J Obes 1989;13:595.

6. Alekseeva RIS, KhKh Plotnikova, O. A. Meshcheriakova, V. A. Mal'tsev, GIu Kulakova, S. N. [Effects of diet therapy including eiconol on clinical and metabolic parameters in patients with type 2 diabetes mellitus]. Vopr Pitan. 2000;69(5):36-9. PMID 11247166.

7. Almbrand BJ, M. Sjostrand, B. Malmberg, K. Ryden, L. Cost-effectiveness of intense insulin treatment after acute myocardial infarction in patients with diabetes mellitus; results from the DIGAMI study. Eur Heart J. 2000 May;21(9):733-9. PMID 10739728.

8. Anderson JWC, S. B. Nicholas, A. S. One hundred pound weight losses with an intensive behavioral program: changes in risk factors in 118 patients with long-term follow-up. Am J Clin Nutr. 2007 Aug;86(2):301-7. PMID 17684198.

9. Angrisani LA, M. Basso, N. Belvederesi, N. Campanile, F. Capizzi, F. D. D'Atri, C. Di Cosmo, L. Doldi, S. B. Favretti, F. Forestieri, P. Furbetta, F. Giacomelli, F. Giardiello, C. Iuppa, A. Lesti, G. Lucchese, M. Puglisi, F. Scipioni, L. Toppino, M. Turicchia, G. U. Veneziani, A. Docimo, C. Borrelli, V. Lorenzo, M. Laparoscopic Italian experience with the Lap-Band. Obes Surg. 2001 Jun;11(3):307-10. PMID 11433906.

10. Angrisani LDL, N. Favretti, F. Furbetta, F. Iuppa, A. Doldi, S. B. Paganelli, M. Basso, N. Lucchese, M. Zappa, M. Lesti, G. Capizzi, F. D. Giardiello, C. Paganini, A. Di Cosmo, L. Veneziani, A. Lacitignola, S. Silecchia, G. Alkilani, M. Forestieri, P. Puglisi, F. Gardinazzi, A. Toppino, M. Campanile, F. Marzano, B. Bernante, P. Perrotta, G. Borrelli, V. Lorenzo, M. The Italian Group for LAP-BAND: predictive value of initial body mass index for weight loss after 5 years of follow-up. Surg Endosc. 2004 Oct;18(10):1524-7. PMID 15791382.

11. Angrisani LF, F. Doldi, S. B. Basso, N. Lucchese, M. Giacomelli, F. Zappa, M. Di Cosmo, L. Veneziani, A. Turicchia, G. U. Alkilani, M. Forestieri, P. Lesti, G. Puglisi, F. Toppino, M. Campanile, F. Capizzi, F. D. D'Atri, C. Sciptoni, L. Giardiello, C. Di Lorenzo, N. Lacitignola, S. Belvederesi, N. Marzano, B. Bernate, P. Iuppa, A. Borrelli, V. Lorenzo, M. Lap Band adjustable gastric banding system: the Italian experience with 1863 patients operated on 6 years. Surg Endosc. 2003 Mar;17(3):409-12. PMID 12457216.

12. Angrisani LL, M. Borrelli, V. Laparoscopic adjustable gastric banding versus Roux-en-Y gastric bypass: 5-year results of a prospective randomized trial. Surg Obes Relat Dis. 2007 Mar-Apr;3(2):127-32; discussion 32-3. PMID 17331805.

13. Aronne LF, K. Aroda, V. Chen, K. Halseth, A. Kesty, N. C. Burns, C. Lush, C. W. Weyer, C. Progressive reduction in body weight after treatment with the amylin analog pramlintide in obese subjects: a phase 2, randomized, placebo-controlled, dose-escalation study. J Clin Endocrinol Metab. 2007 Aug;92(8):2977-83. PMID 17504894.

14. Ashrafian H, Athanasiou T, Li JV, et al. Diabetes resolution and hyperinsulinaemia after metabolic Roux-en-Y gastric bypass. Obes Rev. 2011 May;12(5):e257-72. PMID 20880129.

15. Ashy ARM, A. A. A prospective study comparing vertical banded gastroplasty versus laparoscopic adjustable gastric banding in the treatment of morbid and super-obesity. Int Surg. 1998 Apr-Jun;83(2):108-10. PMID 9851324.

16. Avenell AB, J. Brown, T. J. Poobalan, A. Aucott, L. Stearns, S. C. Smith, W. C. Jung, R. T. Campbell, M. K. Grant, A. M. Systematic review of the long-term effects and economic consequences of treatments for obesity and implications for health improvement. Health Technol Assess. 2004 May;8(21):iii-iv, 1-182. PMID 15147610.

17. Babio NB, M. Salas-Salvado, J. Mediterranean diet and metabolic syndrome: the evidence. Public Health Nutr. 2009 Sep;12(9A):1607-17. PMID 19689829.

18. Balducci SZ, S. Fernando, F. Fallucca, S. Fallucca, F. Pugliese, G. Physical activity/exercise training in type 2 diabetes. The role of the Italian Diabetes and Exercise Study. Diabetes Metab Res Rev. 2009 Sep;25 Suppl 1:S29-33. PMID 19662617.

19. Baltasar AB, R. Miro, J. Et al. Roux-en-Y laparoscopic gastric bypass in patients with morbid obesity. Revista Espanola de Enfermedades Digestivas. 2000;92:661-8.

20. Barnard RJM, M. R. Cherny, S. O'Brien, L. T. Pritikin, N. Long-term use of a high-complex-carbohydrate, high-fiber, low-fat diet and exercise in the treatment of NIDDM patients. Diabetes Care. 1983 May-Jun;6(3):268-73. PMID 6307614.

21. Basdevant AP, M. Rodde-Dunet, M. H. Marty, M. Nogues, F. Slim, K. Chevallier, J. M. A nationwide survey on bariatric surgery in France: two years prospective follow-up. Obes Surg. 2007 Jan;17(1):39-44. PMID 17355767.

22. Basso N, Casella G, Rizzello M, et al. T2DM and sleeve gastrectomy: Diabetes duration as prognostic factor of cure. Obesity Surgery. 2010;20(8):980.

23. Batsis JAR-C, A. Collazo-Clavell, M. L. Sarr, M. G. Somers, V. K. Lopez-Jimenez, F. Effect of bariatric surgery on the metabolic syndrome: a population-based, long-term controlled study. Mayo Clin Proc. 2008 Aug;83(8):897-907. PMID 18674474.

24. Beaser SBH, F. M. Partial remission of diabetes mellitus after oral antidiabetic therapy. Postgrad Med. 1971 Mar;49(3):101-5. PMID 5547891.

25. Belachew MJ, P. Lardinois, F. Karler, C. Vertical Banded Gastroplasty vs Adjustable Silicone Gastric Banding in the Treatment of Morbid Obesity: a Preliminary Report. Obes Surg. 1993 Aug;3(3):275-8. PMID 10757933.

26. Belachew ML, M. J. Vincent, V. Defechereux, T. H. Jourdan, J.L. Monami, B. Jacquet, N. Laparoscopic placement of adjustable silicone gastric banding in the treatment of morbid obesity. Obes Surg. 1992;5:66-9.

27. Belalcazar LMR, David M. Haffner, Steven M. Reeves, Rebecca S. Schwenke, Dawn C. Hoogeveen, Ron C. Pi-Sunyer, F. Xavier Ballantyne, Christie M. Marine ω-3 Fatty Acid Intake. Diabetes Care. 2010 January 2010;33(1):197-9.

28. Benaiges Boix D, Goday Arno A, Pedro-Botet J. [Bariatric surgery for the treatment of type 2 diabetes mellitus.]. Med Clin (Barc). 2011 Jun 20PMID 21696780.

29. Berry M, Lionel U, Guixe C, et al. Sleeve gastrectomy in type 2 diabetic obese patients. Surgical Endoscopy and Other Interventional Techniques. 2011;25:S254.

30. Best JHB, K. S. Rubin, R. R. Cao, D. Kim, T. H. Peyrot, M. Improved treatment satisfaction and weight-related quality of life with exenatide once weekly or twice daily. Diabet Med. 2009 Jul;26(7):722-8. PMID 19573122.

31. Bischoff SC, Damms-Machado A, Betz C, et al. Multicenter evaluation of an interdisciplinary 52-week weight loss program for obesity with regard to body weight, comorbidities and quality of life-a prospective study. Int J Obes (Lond). 2011 Jun 14PMID 21673653.

32. Bjorntorp PK, M. Exercise treatment in diabetes mellitus. Acta Med Scand. 1985;217(1):3-7. PMID 3883702.

33. Boule NGH, E. Kenny, G. P. Wells, G. A. Sigal, R. J. Effects of exercise on glycemic control and body mass in type 2 diabetes mellitus: a meta-analysis of controlled clinical trials. JAMA. 2001 Sep 12;286(10):1218-27. PMID 11559268.

34. Boza C, Gamboa C, Awruch D, et al. Laparoscopic Roux-en-Y gastric bypass versus laparoscopic adjustable gastric banding: Five years of follow-up. Surgery for Obesity and Related Diseases. 2010;6(5):470-5.

35. Boza C, Gamboa C, Viscido G, et al. Laparoscopic sleeve gastrectomy as a primary bariatric procedure. Results in 1000 consecutive patients. Obesity Surgery. 2010;20(8):989.

36. Bradshaw C, Collins W, Hakky S, et al. Surgical morbidity associated with laparoscopic bariatric surgery in type 1 and type 2 diabetics. Obesity Surgery. 2010;20(8):1010.

37. Bray GA. Baseline characteristics of the randomised cohort from the Look AHEAD (Action for Health in Diabetes) study. Diabetes and Vascular Disease Research. 2006 December 1, 2006;3(3):202-15.

38. Bray GA. Lifestyle and pharmacological approaches to weight loss: efficacy and safety. J Clin Endocrinol Metab. 2008 Nov;93(11 Suppl 1):S81-8. PMID 18987274.

39. Brehm BJL, B. L. Summer, S. S. Boback, J. A. Gilchrist, G. M. Jandacek, R. J. D'Alessio, D. A. One-year comparison of a high-monounsaturated fat diet with a high-carbohydrate diet in type 2 diabetes. Diabetes Care. 2009 Feb;32(2):215-20. PMID 18957534.

40. Breum LB, U. Bak, J. F. Jacobsen, S. Astrup, A. Long-term effects of fluoxetine on glycemic control in obese patients with non-insulin-dependent diabetes mellitus or glucose intolerance: influence on muscle glycogen synthase and insulin receptor kinase activity. Metabolism. 1995 Dec;44(12):1570-6. PMID 8786726.

41. Briatore LS, B. Andraghetti, G. Danovaro, C. Sferrazzo, E. Scopinaro, N. Adami, G. F. Maggi, D. Cordera, R. Restoration of acute insulin response in T2DM subjects 1 month after biliopancreatic diversion. Obesity (Silver Spring). 2008 Jan;16(1):77-81. PMID 18223616.

42. Brolin RE. Bariatric surgery and long-term control of morbid obesity. JAMA. 2002 Dec 11;288(22):2793-6. PMID 12472304.

43. Brolin REK, H. A. Wilson, A. C. Kuo, P. T. Cody, R. P. Serum lipids after gastric bypass surgery for morbid obesity. Int J Obes. 1990 Nov;14(11):939-50. PMID 2276855.

44. Buchwald HE, R. Fahrbach, K. Banel, D. Jensen, M. D. Pories, W. J. Bantle, J. P. Sledge, I. Weight and type 2 diabetes after bariatric surgery: systematic review and meta-analysis. Am J Med. 2009 Mar;122(3):248-56 e5. PMID 19272486.

45. Buchwald HV, R. L. A bypass operation for obese hyperlipidemic patients. Surgery. 1971 Jul;70(1):62-70. PMID 5092117.

46. Buchwald HV, R. L. Matts, J. P. Long, J. M. Fitch, L. L. Campbell, G. S. Pearce, M. B. Yellin, A. E. Edmiston, W. A. Smink, R. D., Jr. et al.,. Effect of partial ileal bypass surgery on mortality and morbidity from coronary heart disease in patients with hypercholesterolemia. Report of the Program on the Surgical Control of the Hyperlipidemias (POSCH). N Engl J Med. 1990 Oct 4;323(14):946-55. PMID 2205799.

47. Buffington CKC, G. S., Jr. Smith, H. Significant Changes in the Lipid-Lipoprotein Status of Premenopausal Morbidly Obese Females following Gastric Bypass Surgery. Obes Surg. 1994 Nov;4(4):328-35. PMID 10742796.

48. Buffington CKM, R. T. Ethnic differences in obesity and surgical weight loss between African-American and Caucasian females. Obes Surg. 2006 Feb;16(2):159-65. PMID 16469217.

49. Busetto LP, C. Rinaldi, D. Longhin, P. L. Segato, G. De Marchi, F. Foletto, M. Favretti, F. Lise, M. Enzi, G. Variation in lipid levels in morbidly obese patients operated with the LAP-BAND adjustable

gastric banding system: effects of different levels of weight loss. Obes Surg. 2000 Dec;10(6):569-77. PMID 11175968.

50. Butner KN-R, Sharon Clark, Susan Ramp, Warren Herbert, William. A Review of Weight Loss Following Roux-en-Y Gastric Bypass vs Restrictive Bariatric Surgery: Impact on Adiponectin and Insulin. Obesity Surgery. 2010;20(5):559-68.

51. Cabrera A, Sabench F, Hernandez M, et al. Analysis of the weight-reducing and metabolic efficacy of laparascopic sleeve gastrectomy. Surgical Endoscopy and Other Interventional Techniques. 2011;25:S124.

52. Caiazzo R, Arnalsteen L, Pigeyre M, et al. Long-term metabolic outcome and quality of life after laparoscopic adjustable gastric banding in obese patients with type 2 diabetes mellitus or impaired fasting glucose. Br J Surg. 2010 Jun;97(6):884-91. PMID 20473998.

53. Carey DGP, G. J. Raymond, R. L. Body composition and metabolic changes following bariatric surgery: effects on fat mass, lean mass and basal metabolic rate: six months to one-year follow-up. Obes Surg. 2006 Dec;16(12):1602-8. PMID 17217636.

54. Cariani SN, D. Grani, S. Vittimberga, G. Lucchi, A. Amenta, E. Complications after gastroplasty and gastric bypass as a primary operation and as a reoperation. Obes Surg. 2001 Aug;11(4):487-90. PMID 11501361.

55. Carlson LAO, J. Effect of chlorpropamide treatment on serum lipid levels in diabetes mellitus. Acta Med Scand. 1961 Nov;170:561-4. PMID 13876642.

56. Caro JJK, W. S. Raggio, G. Kavanagh, P. L. O'Brien, J. A. Shomphe, L. A. Flegel, K. M. Copley-Merriman, C. Sigler, C. Economic assessment of troglitazone as an adjunct to sulfonylurea therapy in the treatment of type 2 diabetes. Clin Ther. 2000 Jan;22(1):116-27. PMID 10688395.

57. Carson JLR, M. E. Duff, A. E. Holmes, N. J. Cody, R. P. Brolin, R. E. The effect of gastric bypass surgery on hypertension in morbidly obese patients. Arch Intern Med. 1994 Jan 24;154(2):193-200. PMID 8285814.

58. Case CCJ, P. H. Nelson, K. O'Brian Smith, E. Ballantyne, C. M. Impact of weight loss on the metabolic syndrome. Diabetes Obes Metab. 2002 Nov;4(6):407-14. PMID 12406040.

59. Catona AG, M. Mussini, G. La Manna, L. De Bastiani, T. Armeni, E. Videolaparoscopic Vertical Banded Gastroplasty. Obes Surg. 1995 Aug;5(3):323-6. PMID 10733820.

60. CDC Diabetes Cost-effectiveness Group Research Support. Cost-effectiveness of intensive glycemic control, intensified hypertension control, and serum cholesterol level reduction for type 2 diabetes. JAMA. 2002 May 15;287(19):2542-51. PMID 12020335.

61. Ceelen WW, J. Cardon, A. Van Renterghem, K. Hesse, U. El Malt, M. Pattyn, P. Surgical treatment of severe obesity with a low-pressure adjustable gastric band: experimental data and clinical results in 625 patients. Ann Surg. 2003 Jan;237(1):10-6. PMID 12496524.

62. Champagne CM. Magnesium in hypertension, cardiovascular disease, metabolic syndrome, and other conditions: a review. Nutr Clin Pract. 2008 Apr-May;23(2):142-51. PMID 18390781.

63. Champagne CM. The usefulness of a Mediterranean-based diet in individuals with type 2 diabetes. Curr Diab Rep. 2009 Oct;9(5):389-95. PMID 19793509.

64. Chapman AEK, G. Game, P. Foster, B. O'Brien, P. Ham, J. Maddern, G. J. Laparoscopic adjustable gastric banding in the treatment of obesity: a systematic literature review. Surgery. 2004 Mar;135(3):326-51. PMID 14976485.

65. Charbonnel BK, A. Liu, J. Wu, M. Meininger, G. Efficacy and safety of the dipeptidyl peptidase-4 inhibitor sitagliptin added to ongoing metformin therapy in patients with type 2 diabetes inadequately controlled with metformin alone. Diabetes Care. 2006 Dec;29(12):2638-43. PMID 17130197.

66. Chau WYS, H. J. Kouli, W. Davis, D. Wasielewski, A. Ballantyne, G. H. Patient characteristics impacting excess weight loss following laparoscopic adjustable gastric banding. Obes Surg. 2005 Mar;15(3):346-50. PMID 15826467.

67. Chen JF. A hemorrheological study on the effect of acupuncture in treating diabetes mellitus. J Tradit Chin Med. 1987 Jun;7(2):95-100. PMID 3448402.

68. Chen KML, W. J. Lai, H. S. Chen, W. J. Fifteen years' experience with gastric partitioning for obesity treatment. J Formos Med Assoc. 1998 Jun;97(6):381-6. PMID 9650465.

69. Cheskin LJM, A. M. Jhaveri, A. D. Mitola, A. H. Davis, L. M. Lewis, R. A. Yep, M. A. Lycan, T. W. Efficacy of meal replacements versus a standard food-based diet for weight loss in type 2 diabetes: a controlled clinical trial. Diabetes Educ. 2008 Jan-Feb;34(1):118-27. PMID 18267998.

70. Chevallier JMP, M. Rodde-Dunet, M. H. Marty, M. Nogues, F. Slim, K. Basdevant, A. Predictive factors of outcome after gastric banding: a nationwide survey on the role of center activity and patients' behavior. Ann Surg. 2007 Dec;246(6):1034-9. PMID 18043107.

71. Chiasson JL. Acarbose for the prevention of diabetes, hypertension, and cardiovascular disease in subjects with impaired glucose tolerance: the Study to Prevent Non-Insulin-Dependent Diabetes Mellitus (STOP-NIDDM) Trial. Endocr Pract. 2006 Jan-Feb;12 Suppl 1:25-30. PMID 16627376.

72. Chiasson JLG, R. Hanefeld, M. Josse, R. G. Karasik, A. Laakso, M. The STOP-NIDDM Trial: an international study on the efficacy of an alpha-glucosidase inhibitor to prevent type 2 diabetes in a population with impaired glucose tolerance: rationale, design, and preliminary screening data. Study to Prevent Non-Insulin-Dependent Diabetes Mellitus. Diabetes Care. 1998 Oct;21(10):1720-5. PMID 9773737.

73. Chikunguwo SD, Patricia W. Meador, Jill G. Wolfe, Luke G. Baugh, Nancy Kellum, John M. Maher, James W. PL-101: Durable resolution of diabetes after Roux-en-Y gastric bypass is associated with maintenance of weight loss. Surgery for Obesity and Related Diseases. 2009;5(3, Supplement 1):S1-S.

74. Christou NVS, J. S. Liberman, M. Look, D. Auger, S. McLean, A. P. MacLean, L. D. Surgery decreases long-term mortality, morbidity, and health care use in morbidly obese patients. Ann Surg. 2004 Sep;240(3):416-23; discussion 23-4. PMID 15319713.

75. Clegg AS, M. Colquitt, J. Et al. Clinical and cost effectiveness of surgery for people with morbid obesity Wessex Institute for Health and Research and Development. Southhampton: 2001.

76. Closset JM, A. Barea, M. Buedts, K. Gelin, M. Houben, J. J. Results of silastic ring vertical gastroplasty more than 6 years after surgery: analysis of a cohort of 214 patients. Obes Surg. 2004 Oct;14(9):1233-6. PMID 15527640.

77. Cohen BEC, A. A. Grady, D. Kanaya, A. M. Restorative yoga in adults with metabolic syndrome: a randomized, controlled pilot trial. Metab Syndr Relat Disord. 2008 Fall;6(3):223-9. PMID 18710330.

78. Coleman J, Phillips S. Bariatric surgery: a cutting-edge cure for Type 2 diabetes? N Z Med J. 2010 Mar 19;123(1311):65-8. PMID 20360798.

79. Colle BB, S. [Cardiovascular risk reduction: impact of an international project]. Ann Ig. 2008 May-Jun;20(3 Suppl 1):43-8. PMID 18773604.

80. Collet DR, A. Sa Cunha, A. Larroude, D. Masson, B. Laparoscopic adjustable gastric banding results after 2 years with two different band types. Obes Surg. 2005 Jun-Jul;15(6):853-7. PMID 15978158.

81. Contreras J, Villao D, Bravo J, et al. Improvement and remission in type 2 diabetes mellitus after laparoscopic vertical sleeve gastrectomy in obese patients. Obesity Surgery. 2010;20(8):981-2.

82. Cottam DRA, J. Anderson, A. Grace, B. Fisher, B. A case-controlled matched-pair cohort study of laparoscopic Roux-en-Y gastric bypass and Lap-Band patients in a single US center with three-year follow-up. Obes Surg. 2006 May;16(5):534-40. PMID 16687018.

83. Cowan GS, Jr. Buffington, C. K. Significant changes in blood pressure, glucose, and lipids with gastric bypass surgery. World J Surg. 1998 Sep;22(9):987-92. PMID 9717426.

84. Cramer JSS, R. F. Bartlett, D. P. Kahn, L. S. Loffredo, L. An adaptation of the diabetes prevention program for use with high-risk, minority patients with type 2 diabetes. Diabetes Educ. 2007 May-Jun;33(3):503-8. PMID 17570881.

85. Crampton NAI, V. Stubbs, R. S. Silastic ring gastric bypass: a comparison of two ring sizes: a preliminary report. Obes Surg. 1997 Dec;7(6):495-9. PMID 9730507.

86. Cranor CWB, B. A. Christensen, D. B. The Asheville Project: long-term clinical and economic outcomes of a community pharmacy diabetes care program. J Am Pharm Assoc (Wash). 2003 Mar-Apr;43(2):173-84. PMID 12688435.

87. Cremieux PY, Ledoux S, Clerici C, et al. The impact of bariatric surgery on comorbidities and medication use among obese patients. Obes Surg. 2010 Jul;20(7):861-70. PMID 20440579.

88. Cummings DEW, D. S. Frayo, R. S. Breen, P. A. Ma, M. K. Dellinger, E. P. Purnell, J. Q. Plasma ghrelin levels after diet-induced weight loss or gastric bypass surgery. N Engl J Med. 2002 May 23;346(21):1623-30. PMID 12023994.

89. Cunneen SA. Review of meta-analytic comparisons of bariatric surgery with a focus on laparoscopic adjustable gastric banding. Surg Obes Relat Dis. 2008 May-Jun;4(3 Suppl):S47-55. PMID 18501315.

90. Cunneen SAP, E. Fielding, G. Banel, D. Estok, R. Fahrbach, K. Sledge, I. Studies of Swedish adjustable gastric band and Lap-Band: systematic review and meta-analysis. Surg Obes Relat Dis. 2008 Mar-Apr;4(2):174-85. PMID 18243061.

91. Dan D, Harnanan D, Singh Y, et al. Effects of bariatric surgery on Type-2 Diabetes Mellitus in a Caribbean setting. Int J Surg. 2011;9(5):386-91. PMID 21420513.

92. Dapri GC, G. B. Himpens, J. Reinforcing the staple line during laparoscopic sleeve gastrectomy: prospective randomized clinical study comparing three different techniques. Obes Surg. 2010 Apr;20(4):462-7. PMID 20012507.

93. Dasgupta KG, S. A. Da Costa, D. Lowensteyn, I. Yale, J. F. Rahme, E. Impact of modified glucose target and exercise interventions on vascular risk factors. Diabetes Res Clin Pract. 2006 Apr;72(1):53-60. PMID 16256242.

94. Davidson JAS, A. J. Howlett, H. C. Tolerability profile of metformin/glibenclamide combination tablets (Glucovance): a new treatment for the management of type 2 diabetes mellitus. Drug Saf. 2004;27(15):1205-16. PMID 15588116.

95. Davila-Cervantes AB, D. Dominguez-Cherit, G. Gamino, R. Vargas-Vorackova, F. Gonzalez-Barranco, J. Herrera, M. F. Open versus laparoscopic vertical banded gastroplasty: a randomized controlled double blind trial. Obes Surg. 2002 Dec;12(6):812-8. PMID 12568187.

96. Davis-Smith YMB, J. M. Seale, J. P. Shellenberger, S. Blalock, T. Tobin, B. Implementing a diabetes prevention program in a rural African-American church. J Natl Med Assoc. 2007 Apr;99(4):440-6. PMID 17444435.

97. Davis NJT, N. Schechter, C. Isasi, C. R. Segal-Isaacson, C. J. Stein, D. Zonszein, J. Wylie-Rosett, J. Comparative study of the effects of a 1-year dietary intervention of a low-carbohydrate diet versus a low-fat diet on weight and glycemic control in type 2 diabetes. Diabetes Care. 2009 Jul;32(7):1147-52. PMID 19366978.

98. Davis TM, Coleman C. Laparoscopic adjustable gastric banding in patients with insulin-treated type 2 diabetes. Med J Aust. 2011 Apr 18;194(8):427-8. PMID 21495950.

99. de Gordejuela AG, Pujol Gebelli J, Garcia NV, et al. Is sleeve gastrectomy as effective as gastric bypass for remission of type 2 diabetes in morbidly obese patients? Surg Obes Relat Dis. 2011 Jul-Aug;7(4):506-9. PMID 21411376.

100. de la Cruz-Munoz N, Messiah SE, Arheart KL, et al. Bariatric surgery significantly decreases the prevalence of type 2 diabetes mellitus and pre-diabetes among morbidly obese multiethnic adults: long-term results. J Am Coll Surg. 2011 Apr;212(4):505-11; discussion 12-3. PMID 21463779.

101. de Paula ALM, A. L. Prudente, A. S. Queiroz, L. Schraibman, V. Pinus, J. Laparoscopic sleeve gastrectomy with ileal interposition ("neuroendocrine brake")--pilot study of a new operation. Surg Obes Relat Dis. 2006 Jul-Aug;2(4):464-7. PMID 16925382.

102. Deakin TM, C. E. Cade, J. E. Williams, R. D. Group based training for self-management strategies in people with type 2 diabetes mellitus. Cochrane Database Syst Rev. 2005(2):CD003417. PMID 15846663.

103. Del Castillo D. Analysis of the weight-reducing and metabolic efficacy of laparascopic sleeve gastrectomy. Obesity Surgery. 2010;20(8):1047-8.

104. Delea TEE, J. S. Hagiwara, M. Oster, G. Phillips, L. S. Use of thiazolidinediones and risk of heart failure in people with type 2 diabetes: a retrospective cohort study. Diabetes Care. 2003 Nov;26(11):2983-9. PMID 14578227.

105. Delgado HL, T. Bobbioni-Harsch, E. Ybarra, J. Golay, A. Acarbose improves indirectly both insulin resistance and secretion in obese type 2 diabetic patients. Diabetes Metab. 2002 Jun;28(3):195-200. PMID 12149599.

106. DeMaria EJS, H. J. A critical look at laparoscopic adjustable silicone gastric banding for surgical treatment of morbid obesity: does it measure up? Surg Endosc. 2000 Aug;14(8):697-9. PMID 10954811.

107. Demssie YN, Jawaheer J, Farook S, et al. Weight and glycaemic outcomes following bariatric surgery in people with type 2 diabetes. Endocrine Abstracts. 2010;21:P161.

108. DePaula AL, Stival AR, Halpern A, et al. Surgical treatment of morbid obesity: mid-term outcomes of the laparoscopic ileal interposition associated to a sleeve gastrectomy in 120 patients. Obes Surg. 2011 May;21(5):668-75. PMID 20652440.

109. Desaive C. A critical review of a personal series of 1000 gastroplasties. Int J Obes Relat Metab Disord. 1995 Sep;19 Suppl 3:S56-60. PMID 8581079.

110. Dibble CTG, E. V. Cannon, C. P. Rimonabant: the role of endocannabinoid type 1 receptor antagonism in modulating the weight and lipid profile of obese patients. Curr Atheroscler Rep. 2007 Nov;9(5):359-66. PMID 18001618.

111. Dietary measures for type 2 diabetes. Weight loss and a Mediterranean-type diet, with no foods off-limits. Prescrire Int. 2009 Oct;18(103):224. PMID 19882798.

112. DiGiorgi M, Rosen DJ, Choi JJ, et al. Re-emergence of diabetes after gastric bypass in patients with mid- to long-term follow-up. Surg Obes Relat Dis. 2010 May-Jun;6(3):249-53. PMID 20510288.

113. DiGiorgi MC, Jenny Jee-Eun Milone, Luca Schrope, Beth Olivero-Rivera, Lorraine Restuccia, Nancy Urban-Skuro, Meredith C. Inabnet, William B. Bessler, Marc. PL-213: Recurrence of diabetes after gastric bypass in patients with mid to long-term follow up. Surgery for Obesity and Related Diseases. 2009;5(3, Supplement 1):S13-S.

114. Dixon J, Oefelein M, Okersonf T. Resolution of hypertension after adjustable gastric banding - 1 year interim results of the lap-band AP(registered trademark) experience (APEX) study. Journal of Clinical Hypertension. 2011;13(4):A150-A1.

115. Dixon JBD, M. E. O'Brien, P. E. Quality of life after lap-band placement: influence of time, weight loss, and comorbidities. Obes Res. 2001 Nov;9(11):713-21. PMID 11707538.

116. Dixon JBOB, P. E. Changes in comorbidities and improvements in quality of life after LAP-BAND placement. Am J Surg. 2002 Dec;184(6B):51S-4S. PMID 12527352.

117. Dixon JBOB, P. E. Health outcomes of severely obese type 2 diabetic subjects 1 year after laparoscopic adjustable gastric banding. Diabetes Care. 2002 Feb;25(2):358-63. PMID 11815510.

118. Dixon JBOB, P. E. Lipid profile in the severely obese: changes with weight loss after lap-band surgery. Obes Res. 2002 Sep;10(9):903-10. PMID 12226139.

119. Dixon JBP, W. J. O'Brien, P. E. Schauer, P. R. Zimmet, P. Surgery as an effective early intervention for diabesity: why the reluctance? Diabetes Care. 2005 Feb;28(2):472-4. PMID 15677819.

120. Doar JWW, C. E. Thompson, M. E. Sewell, P. F. Influence of treatment with diet alone on oral glucose-tolerance test and plasma sugar and insulin levels in patients with maturity-onset diabetes mellitus. Lancet. 1975 Jun 7;1(7919):1263-6. PMID 48896.

121. Dolan KB, R. Fielding, G. Treating diabetes in the morbidly obese by laparoscopic gastric banding. Obes Surg. 2003 Jun;13(3):439-43. PMID 12841908.

122. Dowse GKG, H. Alberti, K. G. Zimmet, P. Tuomilehto, J. Purran, A. Fareed, D. Chitson, P. Collins, V. R. Changes in population cholesterol concentrations and other cardiovascular risk factor levels after five years of the non-communicable disease intervention programme in Mauritius. Mauritius Non-communicable Disease Study Group. BMJ. 1995 Nov 11;311(7015):1255-9. PMID 7496233.

123. Durbin RJ. Thiazolidinedione therapy in the prevention/delay of type 2 diabetes in patients with impaired glucose tolerance and insulin resistance. Diabetes Obes Metab. 2004 Jul;6(4):280-5. PMID 15171752.

124. Dyson PAB, S. Matthews, D. R. A low-carbohydrate diet is more effective in reducing body weight than healthy eating in both diabetic and non-diabetic subjects. Diabet Med. 2007 Dec;24(12):1430-5. PMID 17971178.

125. Eastman RCJ, J. C. Herman, W. H. Dasbach, E. J. Copley-Merriman, C. Maier, W. Dong, F. Manninen, D. Zbrozek, A. S. Kotsanos, J. Garfield, S. A. Harris, M. Model of complications of NIDDM. II.

Analysis of the health benefits and cost-effectiveness of treating NIDDM with the goal of normoglycemia. Diabetes Care. 1997 May;20(5):735-44. PMID 9135935.

126. Edelson PK, Dumon KR, Sonnad SS, et al. Robotic vs. conventional laparoscopic gastric banding: A comparison of 407 cases. Surgical Endoscopy and Other Interventional Techniques. 2011;25(5):1402-8.

127. Egan R, Higgs SM, Mason K, et al. Mmotility and weight loss after gastric banding is comparible between diabetics and thier non-diabetic counterparts at one year. Obesity Surgery. 2010;20(8):1045.

128. Elmore UR, A. Perrotta, N. Et al. Laparoscopic adjustable silicone gastric banding (LASGB) - analysis of 64 consecutive patients. Obes Surg. 1998;8:399 (abstract).

129. Encinosa WEB, D. M. Chen, C. C. Steiner, C. A. Healthcare utilization and outcomes after bariatric surgery. Med Care. 2006 Aug;44(8):706-12. PMID 16862031.

130. Encinosa WEB, D. M. Du, D. Steiner, C. A. Recent improvements in bariatric surgery outcomes. Med Care. 2009 May;47(5):531-5. PMID 19318997.

131. Favretti FS, G. Ashton, D. Busetto, L. De Luca, M. Mazza, M. Ceoloni, A. Banzato, O. Calo, E. Enzi, G. Laparoscopic adjustable gastric banding in 1,791 consecutive obese patients: 12-year results. Obes Surg. 2007 Feb;17(2):168-75. PMID 17476867.

132. Fayez R, Court O, Christou N. Laparscopic adjustable gastric banding: Long term results and complications, a single center experiance. Surgical Endoscopy and Other Interventional Techniques. 2011;25:S257.

133. Fera TB, B. M. Ellis, W. M. Schaller, C. W. Garrett, D. G. The Diabetes Ten City Challenge: interim clinical and humanistic outcomes of a multisite community pharmacy diabetes care program. J Am Pharm Assoc (2003). 2008 Mar-Apr;48(2):181-90. PMID 18359731.

134. Ferchak CVM, L. F. Obesity, bariatric surgery and type 2 diabetes--a systematic review. Diabetes Metab Res Rev. 2004 Nov-Dec;20(6):438-45. PMID 15386803.

135. Fernandez AZ, Jr. DeMaria, E. J. Tichansky, D. S. Kellum, J. M. Wolfe, L. G. Meador, J. Sugerman, H. J. Experience with over 3,000 open and laparoscopic bariatric procedures: multivariate analysis of factors related to leak and resultant mortality. Surg Endosc. 2004 Feb;18(2):193-7. PMID 14691697.

136. Fica S, Sirbu A, Copaescu C, et al. Significant improvement in metabolic status 6 months after bariatric surgery. Diabetes Technology and Therapeutics. 2011;13(2):223-4.

137. Fielding GAD, Jennifer E. Laparoscopic adjustable gastric banding in severely obese adolescents. Surgery for Obesity and Related Diseases.1(4):399-405.

138. Finer NR, D. H. Renz, C. L. Hewkin, A. C. Prediction of response to sibutramine therapy in obese non-diabetic and diabetic patients. Diabetes Obes Metab. 2006 Mar;8(2):206-13. PMID 16448525.

139. Fleischman AS, S. E. Bernier, R. Goldfine, A. B. Salsalate improves glycemia and inflammatory parameters in obese young adults. Diabetes Care. 2008 Feb;31(2):289-94. PMID 17959861.

140. Flum DRD, E. P. Impact of gastric bypass operation on survival: a population-based analysis. J Am Coll Surg. 2004 Oct;199(4):543-51. PMID 15454136.

141. Flum DRS, L. Elrod, J. A. Dellinger, E. P. Cheadle, A. Chan, L. Early mortality among Medicare beneficiaries undergoing bariatric surgical procedures. JAMA. 2005 Oct 19;294(15):1903-8. PMID 16234496.

142. Fobi MAL, H. Igwe, D., Jr. Stanczyk, M. Tambi, J. N. Prospective comparative evaluation of stapled versus transected silastic ring gastric bypass: 6-year follow-up. Obes Surg. 2001 Feb;11(1):18-24. PMID 11361162.

143. Fobi MAL, H. SILASTIC ring vertical banded gastric bypass for the treatment of obesity: two years of follow-up in 84 patients [corrected]. J Natl Med Assoc. 1994 Feb;86(2):125-8. PMID 8169987.

144. Fontbonne AA, P. Eschwege, E. BIGPRO (biguanides and the prevention of the risk of obesity): study design. A randomized trial of metformin versus placebo in the correction of the metabolic abnormalities associated with insulin resistance. Diabete Metab. 1991 May;17(1 Pt 2):249-54. PMID 1936485.

145. Foster GDB, K. E. Vander Veur, S. S. Leh Shantz, K. Dilks, R. J. Goldbacher, E. M. Oliver, T. L. Lagrotte, C. A. Homko, C. Satz, W. The effects of a commercially available weight loss program among obese patients with type 2 diabetes: a randomized study. Postgrad Med. 2009 Sep;121(5):113-8. PMID 19820280.

146. Foster GDB, Kelley E. Sanders, Mark H. Millman, Richard Zammit, Gary Newman, Anne B. Wadden, Thomas A. Kelley, David Wing, Rena R. Pi-Sunyer, F. Xavier Reboussin, David Kuna, Samuel T. for the Sleep AHEAD Research Group of the Look AHEAD Research Group,. A Randomized Study on the Effect of Weight Loss on Obstructive Sleep Apnea Among Obese Patients With Type 2 Diabetes: The Sleep AHEAD Study. Arch Intern Med. 2009 September 28, 2009;169(17):1619-26.

147. Foster GDW, H. R. Hill, J. O. McGuckin, B. G. Brill, C. Mohammed, B. S. Szapary, P. O. Rader, D. J. Edman, J. S. Klein, S. A randomized trial of a low-carbohydrate diet for obesity. N Engl J Med. 2003 May 22;348(21):2082-90. PMID 12761365.

148. Fox SRO, K. H. Fox, K. Vertical Banded Gastroplasty and Distal Gastric Bypass as Primary Procedures: A Comparison. Obes Surg. 1996 Oct;6(5):421-5. PMID 10729888.

149. Fragasso GPM, P. M. Monti, L. Palloshi, A. Setola, E. Puccetti, P. Calori, G. Lopaschuk, G. D. Margonato, A. Short- and long-term beneficial effects of trimetazidine in patients with diabetes and ischemic cardiomyopathy. Am Heart J. 2003 Nov;146(5):E18. PMID 14597947.

150. Frenken M, Cho EY. Four-year results after BPD-DS in patients with insulin-dependent type 2 diabetes mellitus. Obesity Surgery. 2010;20(8):980-1.

151. Freys SMT, H. Heimbucher, J. Fuchs, K. H. Fein, M. Thiede, A. Quality of life following laparoscopic gastric banding in patients with morbid obesity. J Gastrointest Surg. 2001 Jul-Aug;5(4):401-7. PMID 11985982.

152. Frost GD, A. The relevance of the glycaemic index to our understanding of dietary carbohydrates. Diabet Med. 2000 May;17(5):336-45. PMID 10872531.

153. Frutos MDL, J. Hernandez, Q. Valero, G. Parrilla, P. Results of laparoscopic gastric bypass in patients > or =55 years old. Obes Surg. 2006 Apr;16(4):461-4. PMID 16608611.

154. Furbetta FG, G. Robortella, E. M. 28-month experience with the lap-band technique: results and critical points of the method. Obes Surg. 1999 Feb;9(1):56-8. PMID 10065585.

155. Gaede PHJ, P. V. Larsen, J. N. Jensen, G. V. Parving, H. H. Pedersen, O. B. [The Steno-2 study. Intensive multifactorial intervention reduces the occurrence of cardiovascular disease in patients with type 2 diabetes]. Ugeskr Laeger. 2003 Jun 23;165(26):2658-61. PMID 12886549.

156. Gaede PV, P. Larsen, N. Jensen, G. V. Parving, H. H. Pedersen, O. Multifactorial intervention and cardiovascular disease in patients with type 2 diabetes. N Engl J Med. 2003 Jan 30;348(5):383-93. PMID 12556541.

157. Gan SSHT, Michael L. Jorgensen, John O. EFFICACY OF SURGERY IN THE MANAGEMENT OF OBESITY-RELATED TYPE 2 DIABETES MELLITUS. ANZ Journal of Surgery. 2007;77(11):958-62.

158. Ganesh RL, T. Rao, A. D. Baladas, H. G. Laparoscopic adjustable gastric banding for severe obesity. Singapore Med J. 2006 Aug;47(8):661-9. PMID 16865204.

159. Gannon MCN, F. Q. Saeed, A. Jordan, K. Hoover, H. An increase in dietary protein improves the blood glucose response in persons with type 2 diabetes. Am J Clin Nutr. 2003 Oct;78(4):734-41. PMID 14522731.

160. Garcia-Fuentes EG-A, J. M. Garcia-Arnes, J. Rivas-Marin, J. Gallego-Perales, J. L. Gonzalez-Jimenez, B. Cardona, I. Garcia-Serrano, S. Garriga, M. J. Gonzalo, M. de Adana, M. S. Soriguer, F. Morbidly obese individuals with impaired fasting glucose have a specific pattern of insulin secretion and sensitivity: effect of weight loss after bariatric surgery. Obes Surg. 2006 Sep;16(9):1179-88. PMID 16989702.

161. Garcia RS, R. Diabetes education in the elderly: a 5-year follow-up of an interactive approach. Patient Educ Couns. 1996 Oct;29(1):87-97. PMID 9006225.

162. Garciacaballero M, Martinez-Moreno JM, Mata JM, et al. Diabetes resolution in morbid and non morbid obese after one anastomosis gastric bypass. Obesity Surgery. 2010;20(8):1034.

163. Garg AB, J. P. Henry, R. R. Coulston, A. M. Griver, K. A. Raatz, S. K. Brinkley, L. Chen, Y. D. Grundy, S. M. Huet, B. A. et al.,. Effects of varying carbohydrate content of diet in patients with non-insulin-dependent diabetes mellitus. JAMA. 1994 May 11;271(18):1421-8. PMID 7848401.

164. Garrett DGB, B. M. Patient self-management program for diabetes: first-year clinical, humanistic, and economic outcomes. J Am Pharm Assoc (2003). 2005 Mar-Apr;45(2):130-7. PMID 15868754.

165. Gautier JFS, A. Lefebvre, P. J. Exercise in the management of non-insulin-dependent (type 2) diabetes mellitus. Int J Obes Relat Metab Disord. 1995 Oct;19 Suppl 4:S58-61. PMID 8581097.

166. Geloneze BG, S. R. Fiori, C. Stabe, C. Tambascia, M. A. Chaim, E. A. Astiarraga, B. D. Pareja, J. C. Surgery for nonobese type 2 diabetic patients: an interventional study with duodenal-jejunal exclusion. Obes Surg. 2009 Aug;19(8):1077-83. PMID 19475464

167. Genuth S. Supplemented fasting in the treatment of obesity and diabetes. Am J Clin Nutr. 1979 Dec;32(12):2579-86. PMID 506979.

168. Gerhard GTA, A. Meeuws, K. McMurry, M. P. Duell, P. B. Connor, W. E. Effects of a low-fat diet compared with those of a high-monounsaturated fat diet on body weight, plasma lipids and lipoproteins, and glycemic control in type 2 diabetes. Am J Clin Nutr. 2004 Sep;80(3):668-73. PMID 15321807.

169. Ghiassi S, Morton J, Bellatorre N, et al. Short-term medication cost savings for treating hypertension and diabetes after gastric bypass. Surg Obes Relat Dis. 2011 May 27PMID 21723203.

170. Gill RS, Birch DW, Shi X, et al. Sleeve gastrectomy and type 2 diabetes mellitus: A systematic review. Canadian Journal of Diabetes. 2011;35(2):150.

171. Glasgow REN, C. C. Kearney, K. A. Reid, R. Ritzwoller, D. P. Strecher, V. J. Couper, M. P. Green, B. Wildenhaus, K. Reach, engagement, and retention in an Internet-based weight loss program in a multi-site randomized controlled trial. J Med Internet Res. 2007;9(2):e11. PMID 17513282.

172. Gleysteen JJ. Results of surgery: long-term effects on hyperlipidemia. Am J Clin Nutr. 1992 Feb;55(2 Suppl):591S-3S. PMID 1733134.

173. Gleysteen JJB, J. J. Sasse, E. A. Sustained coronary-risk-factor reduction after gastric bypass for morbid obesity. Am J Clin Nutr. 1990 May;51(5):774-8. PMID 2333834.

174. Gokcel AK, H. Ertorer, E. M. Tanaci, N. Tutuncu, N. B. Guvener, N. Effects of sibutramine in obese female subjects with type 2 diabetes and poor blood glucose control. Diabetes Care. 2001 Nov;24(11):1957-60. PMID 11679464.

175. Gonzalez RL, E. Mattar, S. G. Venkatesh, K. R. Smith, C. D. Gastric bypass for morbid obesity in patients 50 years or older: is laparoscopic technique safer? Am Surg. 2003 Jul;69(7):547-53; discussion 53-4. PMID 12889614.

176. Gorin AAN, H. M. Hogan, P. Coday, M. Davis, C. DiLillo, V. G. Gluck, M. E. Wadden, T. A. West, D. S. Williamson, D. Yanovski, S. Z. Binge eating and weight loss outcomes in overweight and obese individuals with type 2 diabetes: results from the Look AHEAD trial. Arch Gen Psychiatry. 2008 Dec;65(12):1447-55. PMID 19047532.

177. Gray AR, M. McGuire, A. Fenn, P. Stevens, R. Cull, C. Stratton, I. Adler, A. Holman, R. Turner, R. Cost effectiveness of an intensive blood glucose control policy in patients with type 2 diabetes: economic analysis alongside randomised controlled trial (UKPDS 41). United Kingdom Prospective Diabetes Study Group. BMJ. 2000 May 20;320(7246):1373-8. PMID 10818026.

178. Gray DSF, K. Devine, W. Bray, G. A. A randomized double-blind clinical trial of fluoxetine in obese diabetics. Int J Obes Relat Metab Disord. 1992 Dec;16 Suppl 4:S67-72. PMID 1338389.

179. Grey MB, D. Davidson, M. Galasso, P. Gustafson, E. Melkus, G. Preliminary testing of a program to prevent type 2 diabetes among high-risk youth. J Sch Health. 2004 Jan;74(1):10-5. PMID 15022370.

180. Grunberger GJ, K. L. Artiss, J. D. The benefits of early intervention in obese diabetic patients with FBCx: a new dietary fibre. Diabetes Metab Res Rev. 2007 Jan;23(1):56-62. PMID 17013969.

181. Guidone CM, M. Valera-Mora, E. Iaconelli, A. Gniuli, D. Mari, A. Nanni, G. Castagneto, M. Calvani, M. Mingrone, G. Mechanisms of recovery from type 2 diabetes after malabsorptive bariatric surgery. Diabetes. 2006 Jul;55(7):2025-31. PMID 16804072.

182. Gumbiner BL, C. C. Reaven, P. D. Effects of a monounsaturated fatty acid-enriched hypocaloric diet on cardiovascular risk factors in obese patients with type 2 diabetes. Diabetes Care. 1998 Jan;21(1):9-15. PMID 9538963.

183. Gumbiner BW, J. A. McDermott, M. P. Effects of diet composition and ketosis on glycemia during very-low-energy-diet therapy in obese patients with non-insulin-dependent diabetes mellitus. Am J Clin Nutr. 1996 Jan;63(1):110-5. PMID 8604657.

184. Gupta AKB, George A. Greenway, Frank L. Martin, Corby K. Johnson, William D. Smith, Steven R. Pioglitazone, but not metformin, reduces liver fat in Type-2 diabetes mellitus independent of weight changes. Journal of Diabetes and its Complications.In Press, Corrected Proof.

185. Hamilton ECS, T. L. Hamilton, T. T. Mullican, M. A. Jones, D. B. Provost, D. A. Clinical predictors of leak after laparoscopic Roux-en-Y gastric bypass for morbid obesity. Surg Endosc. 2003 May;17(5):679-84. PMID 12618940.

186. Han SHG, C. Mehran, A. Basa, N. Hines, J. Suleman, L. Vira, D. Dutson, E. Improved outcomes using a systematic and evidence-based approach to the laparoscopic Roux-en-Y gastric bypass in a single academic institution. Am Surg. 2007 Oct;73(10):955-8. PMID 17983055.

187. Harland JW, M. Drinkwater, C. Chinn, D. Farr, L. Howel, D. The Newcastle exercise project: a randomised controlled trial of methods to promote physical activity in primary care. BMJ. 1999 Sep 25;319(7213):828-32. PMID 10496829.

187. Hartweg JP, R. Montori, V. Dinneen, S. Neil, H. A. Farmer, A. Omega-3 polyunsaturated fatty acids (PUFA) for type 2 diabetes mellitus. Cochrane Database Syst Rev. 2008(1):CD003205. PMID 18254017.

189. Havas S. The ACCORD Trial and control of blood glucose level in type 2 diabetes mellitus: time to challenge conventional wisdom. Arch Intern Med. 2009 Jan 26;169(2):150-4. PMID 19171811.

190. Hayes CK, A. Role of physical activity in diabetes management and prevention. J Am Diet Assoc. 2008 Apr;108(4 Suppl 1):S19-23. PMID 18358249.

191. Hell EM, K. A. Moorehead, M. K. Norman, S. Evaluation of health status and quality of life after bariatric surgery: comparison of standard Roux-en-Y gastric bypass, vertical banded gastroplasty and laparoscopic adjustable silicone gastric banding. Obes Surg. 2000 Jun;10(3):214-9. PMID 10929151.

192. Henness S. Pharmacological interventions in the prevention of type 2 diabetes. Curr Opin Endocrinol Diabetes Obes. 2007 Apr;14(2):166-9. PMID 17940436.

193. Henry RRS, L. Olefsky, J. M. Glycemic effects of intensive caloric restriction and isocaloric refeeding in noninsulin-dependent diabetes mellitus. J Clin Endocrinol Metab. 1985 Nov;61(5):917-25. PMID 4044780.

194. Herman WHH, T. J. Brandle, M. Hicks, K. Sorensen, S. Zhang, P. Hamman, R. F. Ackermann, R. T. Engelgau, M. M. Ratner, R. E. The cost-effectiveness of lifestyle modification or metformin in preventing type 2 diabetes in adults with impaired glucose tolerance. Ann Intern Med. 2005 Mar 1;142(5):323-32. PMID 15738451.

195. Hermann LSS, B. Melander, A. Antihyperglycaemic efficacy, response prediction and dose-response relations of treatment with metformin and sulphonylurea, alone and in primary combination. Diabet Med. 1994 Dec;11(10):953-60. PMID 7895460.

196. Hertzman P. The cost effectiveness of orlistat in a 1-year weight-management programme for treating overweight and obese patients in Sweden : a treatment responder approach. Pharmacoeconomics. 2005;23(10):1007-20. PMID 16235974.

197. Heymsfield SBS, K. R. Hauptman, J. Lucas, C. P. Boldrin, M. N. Rissanen, A. Wilding, J. P. Sjostrom, L. Effects of weight loss with orlistat on glucose tolerance and progression to type 2 diabetes in obese adults. Arch Intern Med. 2000 May 8;160(9):1321-6. PMID 10809036.

198. Higa KDB, K. B. Ho, T. Complications of the laparoscopic Roux-en-Y gastric bypass: 1,040 patients--what have we learned? Obes Surg. 2000 Dec;10(6):509-13. PMID 11175957.

199. Himpens J, Dobbeleir J, Peeters G. Long-term results of laparoscopic sleeve gastrectomy for obesity. Ann Surg. 2010 Aug;252(2):319-24. PMID 20622654.

200. Himpens JD, G. Cadiere, G. B. A prospective randomized study between laparoscopic gastric banding and laparoscopic isolated sleeve gastrectomy: results after 1 and 3 years. Obes Surg. 2006 Nov;16(11):1450-6. PMID 17132410.

201. Hofstetter AM, Kerr JL. Bariatric surgery for the treatment of type 2 diabetes mellitus: What are the Options?
. U.S. Pharmacist. 2011;36(5).

202. Huisman SdG, V. Maes, S. Schroevers, M. Chatrou, M. Haak, H. Self-regulation and weight reduction in patients with type 2 diabetes: a pilot intervention study. Patient Educ Couns. 2009 Apr;75(1):84-90. PMID 19097740.

203. Hutter MMR, S. Khuri, S. F. Henderson, W. G. Abbott, W. M. Warshaw, A. L. Laparoscopic versus open gastric bypass for morbid obesity: a multicenter, prospective, risk-adjusted analysis from the National Surgical Quality Improvement Program. Ann Surg. 2006 May;243(5):657-62; discussion 62-6. PMID 16633001.

204. Iannelli A, Anty R, Schneck AS, et al. Inflammation, insulin resistance, lipid disturbances, anthropometrics, and metabolic syndrome in morbidly obese patients: a case control study comparing laparoscopic Roux-en-Y gastric bypass and laparoscopic sleeve gastrectomy. Surgery. 2011 Mar;149(3):364-70. PMID 20932542.

205. Inge T, Jenkins T, Dolan L, et al. Improved insulin sensitivity and decreased insulin secretion in adolescents undergoing gastric bypass. Journal of Laparoendoscopic and Advanced Surgical Techniques. 2011;21(4):A14-A5.

206. Iordache NV, R. Iorgulescu, A. Zmeu, B. Iordache, M. [Laparoscopic adjustable gastric-banding treatment for morbid obesity our first year experience]. Chirurgia (Bucur). 2003 Mar-Apr;98(2):135-42. PMID 14992134.

207. James Hanowell E, Pallati PK, Srinivasan A, et al. Laparoscopic versus open bilio-pancreatic diversion with duodenal switch: Comparable weight loss with decreased long term morbidity. Surgical Endoscopy and Other Interventional Techniques. 2011;25:S250.

208. Jones KB, Jr. Afram, J. D. Benotti, P. N. Capella, R. F. Cooper, C. G. Flanagan, L. Hendrick, S. Howell, L. M. Jaroch, M. T. Kole, K. Lirio, O. C. Sapala, J. A. Schuhknecht, M. P. Shapiro, R. P. Sweet, W. A. Wood, M. H. Open versus laparoscopic Roux-en-Y gastric bypass: a comparative study of over 25,000 open cases and the major laparoscopic bariatric reported series. Obes Surg. 2006 Jun;16(6):721-7. PMID 16756731.

209. Jootun N, Filgate R, Munro W, et al. Reversal of metabolic syndrome by laparoscopic gastric banding in patients with type 2 diabetes. Internal Medicine Journal. 2010;40:178.

210. Kalfarentzos FD, A. Kehagias, I. Loukidi, A. Mead, N. Vertical banded gastroplasty versus standard or distal Roux-en-Y gastric bypass based on specific selection criteria in the morbidly obese: preliminary results. Obes Surg. 1999 Oct;9(5):433-42. PMID 10605899.

211. Kalinowski P, Paluszkiewicz R, Remiszewski P, et al. Effect of Roux-en-Y gastric bypass on metabolic syndrome. Obesity Surgery. 2010;20(8):1010-1.

212. Karastergiou KK, J. C. Medical management of the diabetic patient with coronary artery disease. Curr Pharm Des. 2008;14(25):2527-36. PMID 18991670.

213. Karlsson JS, L. Sullivan, M. Swedish obese subjects (SOS)--an intervention study of obesity. Two-year follow-up of health-related quality of life (HRQL) and eating behavior after gastric surgery for severe obesity. Int J Obes Relat Metab Disord. 1998 Feb;22(2):113-26. PMID 9504319.

214. Karter AJM, H. H. Liu, J. Parker, M. M. Ahmed, A. T. Go, A. S. Selby, J. V. Glycemic response to newly initiated diabetes therapies. Am J Manag Care. 2007 Nov;13(11):598-606. PMID 17988185.

215. Kasalicky M, Pohnan R, Haluzikova D, et al. Influence of the laparoscopic sleeve gastrectomy on the metabolic syndrome. Obesity Surgery. 2010;20(6):815-6.

216. Kasalicky M, Pohnan R, Housova J, et al. Effect of the laparoscopic sleeve gastrectomy - 4 years experience. Surgical Endoscopy and Other Interventional Techniques. 2011;25:S123.

217. Kaukua JKP, T. A. Rissanen, A. M. Health-related quality of life in a randomised placebo-controlled trial of sibutramine in obese patients with type II diabetes. Int J Obes Relat Metab Disord. 2004 Apr;28(4):600-5. PMID 14770192.

218. Keating C, Dixon J, Moodie M, et al. Cost-effectiveness of surgically induced weight loss for the management of type 2 diabetes: Modelled lifetime analysis. Obesity Reviews. 2010;11:45.

219. Keech AC, D. Best, J. Kirby, A. Simes, R. J. Hunt, D. Hague, W. Beller, E. Arulchelvam, M. Baker, J. Tonkin, A. Secondary prevention of cardiovascular events with long-term pravastatin in patients with diabetes or impaired fasting glucose: results from the LIPID trial. Diabetes Care. 2003 Oct;26(10):2713-21. PMID 14514569.

220. Keidar A, Hershkop K, Schweiger C, et al. Preliminary results of prospective randomized controlled study of the effect of laparoscopic sleeve gastrectomy versus laparoscopic Roux-en-Y gastric bypass on resolution of type 2 diabetes mellitus. Obesity Surgery. 2010;20(6):810.

221. Kelley DE. Action for health in diabetes: the look AHEAD clinical trial. Curr Diab Rep. 2002 Jun;2(3):207-9. PMID 12643174.

222. Kelley DEB, G. A. Pi-Sunyer, F. X. Klein, S. Hill, J. Miles, J. Hollander, P. Clinical efficacy of orlistat therapy in overweight and obese patients with insulin-treated type 2 diabetes: A 1-year randomized controlled trial. Diabetes Care. 2002 Jun;25(6):1033-41. PMID 12032111.

223. Kelly TMJ, S. B. Changes in serum lipids after gastric bypass surgery. Lack of a relationship to weight loss. Int J Obes. 1986;10(6):443-52. PMID 3804561.

224. Keyserling TCA, A. S. Samuel-Hodge, C. D. Ingram, A. F. Skelly, A. H. Elasy, T. A. Johnston, L. F. Cole, A. S. Henriquez-Roldan, C. F. A diabetes management program for African American women with type 2 diabetes. Diabetes Educ. 2000 Sep-Oct;26(5):796-805. PMID 11140007.

225. Khan MASP, J. V. Breen, G. A. Hartley, G. G. Vessey, J. T. Diabetes disease stage predicts weight loss outcomes with long-term appetite suppressants. Obes Res. 2000 Jan;8(1):43-8. PMID 10678258.

226. Kim DM, L. Zhuang, D. Kothare, P. A. Trautmann, M. Fineman, M. Taylor, K. Effects of once-weekly dosing of a long-acting release formulation of exenatide on glucose control and body weight in subjects with type 2 diabetes. Diabetes Care. 2007 Jun;30(6):1487-93. PMID 17353504.

227. Kim S, Richards WO. Long-term follow-up of the metabolic profiles in obese patients with type 2 diabetes mellitus after Roux-en-Y gastric bypass. Ann Surg. 2010 Jun;251(6):1049-55. PMID 20485144.

228. Kim Z, Hur KY. Laparoscopic mini-gastric bypass for type 2 diabetes: the preliminary report. World J Surg. 2011 Mar;35(3):631-6. PMID 21165621.

229. Kiong KL, Ganesh R, Cheng AK, et al. Early improvement in type 2 diabetes mellitus post Roux-en-Y gastric bypass in Asian patients. Singapore Med J. 2010 Dec;51(12):937-43. PMID 21221498.

230. Klein SS, N. F. Pi-Sunyer, X. Daly, A. Wylie-Rosett, J. Kulkarni, K. Clark, N. G. Weight management through lifestyle modification for the prevention and management of type 2 diabetes: rationale and strategies: a statement of the American Diabetes Association, the North American Association for the

Study of Obesity, and the American Society for Clinical Nutrition. Diabetes Care. 2004 Aug;27(8):2067-73. PMID 15277443.

231. Knowler WCN, K. M. Hanson, R. L. Nelson, R. G. Bennett, P. H. Tuomilehto, J. Schersten, B. Pettitt, D. J. Preventing non-insulin-dependent diabetes. Diabetes. 1995 May;44(5):483-8. PMID 7729603.

232. Knowler WCS, G. Melander, A. Schersten, B. Glucose tolerance and mortality, including a substudy of tolbutamide treatment. Diabetologia. 1997 Jun;40(6):680-6. PMID 9222648.

233. Korenkov MS, S. Sauerland, S. Duenschede, F. Junginger, Th. Impact of Laparoscopic Adjustable Gastric Banding on Obesity Co-morbidities in the Medium- and Long-Term. Obesity Surgery. 2007;17(5):679-83.

234. Korner JI, W. Conwell, I. M. Taveras, C. Daud, A. Olivero-Rivera, L. Restuccia, N. L. Bessler, M. Differential effects of gastric bypass and banding on circulating gut hormone and leptin levels. Obesity (Silver Spring). 2006 Sep;14(9):1553-61. PMID 17030966.

235. Kothari SND, E. J. Sugerman, H. J. Kellum, J. M. Meador, J. Wolfe, L. Lap-band failures: conversion to gastric bypass and their preliminary outcomes. Surgery. 2002 Jun;131(6):625-9. PMID 12075174.

236. Kramer MKM, R. Venditti, E. Orchard, T. Group Lifestyle Intervention for Diabetes Prevention in those with Metabolic Syndrome in Primary Care Practice. Diabetes Care. 2006;55((suppl.)):A517.

237. Kriska AMB, S. N. Pereira, M. A. The potential role of physical activity in the prevention of non-insulin-dependent diabetes mellitus: the epidemiological evidence. Exerc Sport Sci Rev. 1994;22:121-43. PMID 7925541.

238. Kushner RFS, Melissa. Prevention of Weight Gain in Adult Patients With Type 2 Diabetes Treated With Pioglitazone. Obesity. 2009;17(5):1017-22.

239. Kuzmak LIY, I. S. McGuire, L. Dixon, J. S. Young, M. P. Surgery for morbid obesity. Using an inflatable gastric band. AORN J. 1990 May;51(5):1307-24. PMID 2344182.

240. La Londe MAG, C. L. Falko, J. M. Snow, R. J. Spencer, K. Caulin-Glaser, T. Effect of a weight management program on the determinants and prevalence of metabolic syndrome. Obesity (Silver Spring). 2008 Mar;16(3):637-42. PMID 18239562.

241. Lacey LAW, A. O'Shea, D. Erny, S. Ruof, J. Cost-effectiveness of orlistat for the treatment of overweight and obese patients in Ireland. Int J Obes (Lond). 2005 Aug;29(8):975-82. PMID 15852050.

242. Laferrere B, Reilly D, Arias S, et al. Differential metabolic impact of gastric bypass surgery versus dietary intervention in obese diabetic subjects despite identical weight loss. Sci Transl Med. 2011 Apr 27;3(80):80re2. PMID 21525399.

243. Laferrere BT, J. McGinty, J. Tran, H. Egger, J. R. Colarusso, A. Kovack, B. Bawa, B. Koshy, N. Lee, H. Yapp, K. Olivan, B. Effect of weight loss by gastric bypass surgery versus hypocaloric diet on glucose and incretin levels in patients with type 2 diabetes. J Clin Endocrinol Metab. 2008 Jul;93(7):2479-85. PMID 18430778.

244. Lakka TAL, D. E. Physical activity in prevention and treatment of the metabolic syndrome. Appl Physiol Nutr Metab. 2007 Feb;32(1):76-88. PMID 17332786.

245. Lancaster RTH, M. M. Bands and bypasses: 30-day morbidity and mortality of bariatric surgical procedures as assessed by prospective, multi-center, risk-adjusted ACS-NSQIP data. Surg Endosc. 2008 Dec;22(12):2554-63. PMID 18806945.

246. Lankisch ML, P. Rizza, R. A. DiMagno, E. P. Acute postprandial gastrointestinal and metabolic effects of wheat amylase inhibitor (WAI) in normal, obese, and diabetic humans. Pancreas. 1998 Aug;17(2):176-81. PMID 9700950.

247. Lau DCW. Is surgery an option in the treatment of type 2 diabetes? Canadian Journal of Diabetes. 2011;35(2):85-6.

248. Lee AM, J. E. Metformin decreases food consumption and induces weight loss in subjects with obesity with type II non-insulin-dependent diabetes. Obes Res. 1998 Jan;6(1):47-53. PMID 9526970.

249. Lee HJP, K. Y. [Body weight, cardiovascular risk factors, and self-efficacy of diabetic control among obese type II diabetic patients]. Taehan Kanho Hakhoe Chi. 2005 Aug;35(5):787-97. PMID 16208074.

250. Lee WJH, M. T. Wang, W. Lin, C. M. Chen, T. C. Lai, I. R. Effects of obesity surgery on the metabolic syndrome. Arch Surg. 2004 Oct;139(10):1088-92. PMID 15492149.

251. Lee WJL, I. R. Huang, M.T. Et al. Laparoscopic versus open vertical banded gastroplasty for the treatment of morbid obesity. Surg Laparosc Endosc Percut Techn. 2001;11:9-13.

252. Lee WJW, W. Bariatric surgery: Asia-Pacific perspective. Obes Surg. 2005 Jun-Jul;15(6):751-7. PMID 15978141.

253. Lee WJW, W. Wei, P. L. Huang, M. T. Weight loss and improvement of obesity-related illness following laparoscopic adjustable gastric banding procedure for morbidly obese patients in Taiwan. J Formos Med Assoc. 2006 Nov;105(11):887-94. PMID 17098690.

254. Leichman JGA, D. King, T. M. Mehta, S. Majka, C. Scarborough, T. Wilson, E. B. Taegtmeyer, H. Improvements in systemic metabolism, anthropometrics, and left ventricular geometry 3 months after bariatric surgery. Surg Obes Relat Dis. 2006 Nov-Dec;2(6):592-9. PMID 17138229.

255. Levy PF, M. Santini, F. Finer, N. The comparative effects of bariatric surgery on weight and type 2 diabetes. Obes Surg. 2007 Sep;17(9):1248-56. PMID 18074502.

256. Li YX. [Role of gastric surgery in treating obese patients with type 2 diabetes]. Zhongguo Yi Xue Ke Xue Yuan Xue Bao. 2010 Feb;32(1):13-5. PMID 20236580.

257. Lim PK, O. T. Metformin compared with tolbutamide in the treatment of maturity-onset diabetes mellitus. Med J Aust. 1970 Feb 7;1(6):271-3. PMID 5440868.

258. Livingston EHH, S. Arthur, D. Lee, S. De Shields, S. Heber, D. Male gender is a predictor of morbidity and age a predictor of mortality for patients undergoing gastric bypass surgery. Ann Surg. 2002 Nov;236(5):576-82. PMID 12409663.

259. Lonroth HD, J. Haglind, E. Josefsson, K. Olbe, L. Fagevik Olsen, M. Lundell, L. Vertical banded gastroplasty by laparoscopic technique in the treatment of morbid obesity. Surg Laparosc Endosc. 1996 Apr;6(2):102-7. PMID 8680631.

260. Look AHEAD Research Group Reduction in Weight and Cardiovascular Disease Risk Factors in Individuals With Type 2 Diabetes. Diabetes Care. 2007 June 2007;30(6):1374-83.

261. Low CCG, E. B. Gumbiner, B. Potentiation of effects of weight loss by monounsaturated fatty acids in obese NIDDM patients. Diabetes. 1996 May;45(5):569-75. PMID 8621005.

262. Lujan JAF, M. D. Hernandez, Q. Liron, R. Cuenca, J. R. Valero, G. Parrilla, P. Laparoscopic versus open gastric bypass in the treatment of morbid obesity: a randomized prospective study. Ann Surg. 2004 Apr;239(4):433-7. PMID 15024302.

263. Ma JK, Abby Wilson, Sandra Xiao, Lan Stafford, Randall. Evaluation of lifestyle interventions to treat elevated cardiometabolic risk in primary care (E-LITE): a randomized controlled trial. BMC Family Practice. 2009;10(1):71. PMID doi:10.1186/1471-2296-10-71.

264. Ma YO, B. C. Merriam, P. A. Chiriboga, D. E. Culver, A. L. Li, W. Hebert, J. R. Ockene, I. S. Griffith, J. A. Pagoto, S. L. A randomized clinical trial comparing low-glycemic index versus ADA dietary education among individuals with type 2 diabetes. Nutrition. 2008 Jan;24(1):45-56. PMID 18070658.

265. MacDonald KG, Jr. Long, S. D. Swanson, M. S. Brown, B. M. Morris, P. Dohm, G. L. Pories, W. J. The gastric bypass operation reduces the progression and mortality of non-insulin-dependent diabetes mellitus. J Gastrointest Surg. 1997 May-Jun;1(3):213-20; discussion 20. PMID 9834350.

266. Macgregor AMR, C. S. Gastric surgery in morbid obesity. Outcome in patients aged 55 years and older. Arch Surg. 1993 Oct;128(10):1153-7. PMID 8215875.

267. Maciejewski ML, Livingston EH, Kahwati LC, et al. Discontinuation of diabetes and lipid-lowering medications after bariatric surgery at Veterans Affairs medical centers. Surg Obes Relat Dis. 2010 Nov-Dec;6(6):601-7. PMID 20965791.

268. MacLean LDR, B. M. Nohr, C. W. Late outcome of isolated gastric bypass. Ann Surg. 2000 Apr;231(4):524-8. PMID 10749613.

269. Madan AKO, W. Ternovits, C. A. Tichansky, D. S. Metabolic syndrome: yet another co-morbidity gastric bypass helps cure. Surg Obes Relat Dis. 2006 Jan-Feb;2(1):48-51; discussion PMID 16925317.

270. Madan AKW, J. D. Fain, J. N. Beech, B. M. Ternovits, C. A. Menachery, S. Tichansky, D. S. Are African-Americans as successful as Caucasians after laparoscopic gastric bypass? Obes Surg. 2007 Apr;17(4):460-4. PMID 17608257.

271. Maetzel AR, J. Covington, M. Wolf, A. Economic evaluation of orlistat in overweight and obese patients with type 2 diabetes mellitus. Pharmacoeconomics. 2003;21(7):501-12. PMID 12696990.

272. Maggio CAP-S, F. X. The prevention and treatment of obesity. Application to type 2 diabetes. Diabetes Care. 1997 Nov;20(11):1744-66. PMID 9353619.

273. Makary MA, Clarke JM, Shore AD, et al. Medication utilization and annual health care costs in patients with type 2 diabetes mellitus before and after bariatric surgery. Arch Surg. 2010 Aug;145(8):726-31. PMID 20713923.

274. Marceau PH, F. S. Simard, S. Lebel, S. Bourque, R. A. Potvin, M. Biron, S. Biliopancreatic diversion with duodenal switch. World J Surg. 1998 Sep;22(9):947-54. PMID 9717420.

275. Marinari GMP, F. S. Briatore, L. Adami, G. Scopinaro, N. Type 2 diabetes and weight loss following biliopancreatic diversion for obesity. Obes Surg. 2006 Nov;16(11):1440-4. PMID 17132408.

276. Marjanovic G, Winkler K, Schewe T, et al. [Metabolic surgery and remission of type 2 diabetes]. Dtsch Med Wochenschr. 2010 May;135(20):1020-4. PMID 20461659.

277. Mason EEP, K. J. Blommers, T. J. Scott, D. H. Gastric bypass for obesity after ten years experience. Int J Obes. 1978;2(2):197-206. PMID 711364.

278. Masoudi FAI, S. E. Wang, Y. Havranek, E. P. Foody, J. M. Krumholz, H. M. Thiazolidinediones, metformin, and outcomes in older patients with diabetes and heart failure: an observational study. Circulation. 2005 Feb 8;111(5):583-90. PMID 15699279.

279. Mathus-Vliegen EM. Long-term health and psychosocial outcomes from surgically induced weight loss: results obtained in patients not attending protocolled follow-up visits. Int J Obes (Lond). 2007 Feb;31(2):299-307. PMID 16755282.

280. Mattar SGV, L. M. Rabinovitz, M. Demetris, A. J. Krasinskas, A. M. Barinas-Mitchell, E. Eid, G. M. Ramanathan, R. Taylor, D. S. Schauer, P. R. Surgically-induced weight loss significantly improves nonalcoholic fatty liver disease and the metabolic syndrome. Ann Surg. 2005 Oct;242(4):610-7; discussion 8-20. PMID 16192822.

281. Matvienko OAH, James D. A Lifestyle Intervention Study in Patients with Diabetes or Impaired Glucose Tolerance: Translation of a Research Intervention into Practice. J Am Board Fam Med. 2009 September 1, 2009;22(5):535-43.

282. Mayer-Davis EJDA, A. Martin, M. Wandersman, A. Parra-Medina, D. Schulz, R. Pilot study of strategies for effective weight management in type 2 diabetes: Pounds Off with Empowerment (POWER). Fam Community Health. 2001 Jul;24(2):27-35. PMID 11373164.

283. Mayer-Davis EJDA, A. M. Smith, S. M. Kirkner, G. Levin Martin, S. Parra-Medina, D. Schultz, R. Pounds off with empowerment (POWER): a clinical trial of weight management strategies for black and white adults with diabetes who live in medically underserved rural communities. Am J Public Health. 2004 Oct;94(10):1736-42. PMID 15451743.

284. McAuley KAH, C. M. Smith, K. J. McLay, R. T. Williams, S. M. Taylor, R. W. Mann, J. I. Comparison of high-fat and high-protein diets with a high-carbohydrate diet in insulin-resistant obese women. Diabetologia. 2005 Jan;48(1):8-16. PMID 15616799.

285. McNabb WLQ, M. T. Rosing, L. Weight loss program for inner-city black women with non-insulin-dependent diabetes mellitus: PATHWAYS. J Am Diet Assoc. 1993 Jan;93(1):75-7. PMID 8417099.

286. McNeely WG, K. L. Sibutramine. A review of its contribution to the management of obesity. Drugs. 1998 Dec;56(6):1093-124. PMID 9878996.

287. McNulty SJU, E. Williams, G. A randomized trial of sibutramine in the management of obese type 2 diabetic patients treated with metformin. Diabetes Care. 2003 Jan;26(1):125-31. PMID 12502668.

288. McTigue KMC, Molly B. Bigi, Lori Murphy, Cynthia McNeil, Melissa. Weight Loss Through Living Well: Translating an Effective Lifestyle Intervention Into Clinical Practice. The Diabetes Educator. 2009 March 1, 2009;35(2):199-208.

289. McTigue KMH, R. Ziouras, J. Obesity in older adults: a systematic review of the evidence for diagnosis and treatment. Obesity (Silver Spring). 2006 Sep;14(9):1485-97. PMID 17030958.

290. Meece J. Pancreatic islet dysfunction in type 2 diabetes: a rational target for incretin-based therapies. Curr Med Res Opin. 2007 Apr;23(4):933-44. PMID 17407650.

291. Meijer RI, van Wagensveld BA, Siegert CE, et al. Bariatric surgery as a novel treatment for type 2 diabetes mellitus: a systematic review. Arch Surg. 2011 Jun;146(6):744-50. PMID 21690453.

292. Meneghini CVFLF. Obesity, bariatric surgery and type 2 diabetes - a systematic review. Diabetes/Metabolism Research and Reviews. 2004;20(6):438-45.

293. Meshcheriakova VAP, O. A. Sharafetdinov, KhKh Iatsyshina, T. A. [The use of the combined food products with soy protein in diet therapy for patients with diabetes mellitus type 2]. Vopr Pitan. 2002;71(5):19-24. PMID 12599994.

294. Meyer LR, S. Becker, J. Pradignac, A. Meyer, C. Schlienger, J. L. Simon, C. Retrospective study of laparoscopic adjustable silicone gastric banding for the treatment of morbid obesity: results and complications in 127 patients. Diabetes Metab. 2004 Feb;30(1):53-60. PMID 15029098.

295. Mijailovic VM, D. Mijailovic, M. [Effects of a one-year weight reduction program and physical activity on obesity and comorbid conditions]. Med Pregl. 2004 Jan-Feb;57(1-2):55-9. PMID 15327191.

296. Miles JML, L. Hollander, P. Wadden, T. Anderson, J. W. Doyle, M. Foreyt, J. Aronne, L. Klein, S. Effect of orlistat in overweight and obese patients with type 2 diabetes treated with metformin. Diabetes Care. 2002 Jul;25(7):1123-8. PMID 12087008.

297. Miller KM, E. Pichler, M. Hell, E. . Quality-of-life outcomes of patients with the Lap-Band registered versus non-operative treatment of obesity. Preliminary results of an ongoing long-term follow-up study. Obes Surg 1997;7:280.

298. Miller YDD, D. W. The effectiveness of physical activity interventions for the treatment of overweight and obesity and type 2 diabetes. J Sci Med Sport. 2004 Apr;7(1 Suppl):52-9. PMID 15214602.

299. Mingrone G, DeGaetano A, Greco AV, et al. Reversibility of insulin resistance in obese diabetic patients: role of plasma lipids. Diabetologia. 1997 May;40(5):599-605. PMID 9165230.

300. Mittermair RPW, H. Nehoda, H. Kirchmayr, W. Aigner, F. Laparoscopic Swedish adjustable gastric banding: 6-year follow-up and comparison to other laparoscopic bariatric procedures. Obes Surg. 2003 Jun;13(3):412-7. PMID 12841903.

301. Mohos E, Schmaldienst E, Prager M. Quality of life parameters, weight change and improvement of co-morbidities after laparoscopic Roux Y gastric bypass and laparoscopic gastric sleeve resection-- comparative study. Obes Surg. 2011 Mar;21(3):288-94. PMID 20628831.

302. Moo TAR, F. Gastrointestinal surgery as treatment for type 2 diabetes. Curr Opin Endocrinol Diabetes Obes. 2008 Apr;15(2):153-8. PMID 18316951.

303. Morinigo RC, R. Delgado, S. Lacy, A. Deulofeu, R. Conget, I. Barcelo-Batllori, S. Gomis, R. Vidal, J. Insulin resistance, inflammation, and the metabolic syndrome following Roux-en-Y gastric bypass surgery in severely obese subjects. Diabetes Care. 2007 Jul;30(7):1906-8. PMID 17468354.

304. Morinigo RV, J. Lacy, A. M. Delgado, S. Casamitjana, R. Gomis, R. Circulating peptide YY, weight loss, and glucose homeostasis after gastric bypass surgery in morbidly obese subjects. Ann Surg. 2008 Feb;247(2):270-5. PMID 18216532.

305. Morino MT, M. Forestieri, P. Angrisani, L. Allaix, M. E. Scopinaro, N. Mortality after bariatric surgery: analysis of 13,871 morbidly obese patients from a national registry. Ann Surg. 2007 Dec;246(6):1002-7; discussion 7-9. PMID 18043102.

306. Morris JHW, D. A. Bolinger, R. E. Effect of Oral Sulfonylurea on Plasma Triglycerides in Diabetics. Diabetes. 1964 Jan-Feb;13:87-9. PMID 14104182.

307. Morris M, Jackson S, Johnson AB. Reality bites! Experiences of one year Post-Laparoscopic Gastric Banding (LAGB) for people with and without type 2 diabetes. Diabetic Medicine. 2010;27(2):2-3.

308. Mumme DE, Mathiason MA, Kallies KJ, et al. Effect of laparoscopic Roux-en-Y gastric bypass surgery on hemoglobin A1c levels in diabetic patients: a matched-cohort analysis. Surg Obes Relat Dis. 2009 Jan-Feb;5(1):4-10. PMID 19161932.

309. Murr MMS, M. R. Sarr, M. G. Results of Bariatric Surgery for Morbid Obesity in Patients Older than 50 Years. Obes Surg. 1995 Nov;5(4):399-402. PMID 10733835.

310. Muscelli EM, G. Camastra, S. Manco, M. Pereira, J. A. Pareja, J. C. Ferrannini, E. Differential effect of weight loss on insulin resistance in surgically treated obese patients. Am J Med. 2005 Jan;118(1):51-7. PMID 15639210.

311. Nain P, Virk S, Ahuja A, et al. To compare the weight and metabolic parameters before and after laparoscopic sleeve gastrectomy in 74 bariatric patients. Surgical Endoscopy and Other Interventional Techniques. 2011;25:S243.

312. Navarrete SA, Leyba JL, Llopis SN. Laparoscopic sleeve gastrectomy with duodenojejunal bypass for the treatment of type 2 diabetes in non-obese patients: technique and preliminary results. Obes Surg. 2011 May;21(5):663-7. PMID 21336559.

313. Nehoda HH, K. Sauper, T. Mittermair, R. Lanthaler, M. Aigner, F. Weiss, H. Laparoscopic gastric banding in older patients. Arch Surg. 2001 Oct;136(10):1171-6. PMID 11585511.

314. Nelson RHM, J. M. The use of orlistat in the treatment of obesity, dyslipidaemia and Type 2 diabetes. Expert Opin Pharmacother. 2005 Nov;6(14):2483-91. PMID 16259579.

315. Nguyen DA, Kim GJ, Liu CD. Diabetic patients have less lean body mass which is correlated with less excess weight loss in laparoscopic adjustable gastric banding (LAGB) over three years, N=601. Gastroenterology. 2011;140(5):S1058.

316. Nguyen NT, Masoomi H, Magno CP, et al. Trends in use of bariatric surgery, 2003-2008. Journal of the American College of Surgeons. 2011;213(2):261-6.

317. Nguyen NTH, M. Fayad, C. Varela, E. Wilson, S. E. Use and outcomes of laparoscopic versus open gastric bypass at academic medical centers. J Am Coll Surg. 2007 Aug;205(2):248-55. PMID 17660071.

318. Nguyen NTV, E. Sabio, A. Tran, C. L. Stamos, M. Wilson, S. E. Resolution of hyperlipidemia after laparoscopic Roux-en-Y gastric bypass. J Am Coll Surg. 2006 Jul;203(1):24-9. PMID 16798484.

319. Nield LM, H. J. Hooper, L. Cruickshank, J. K. Vyas, A. Whittaker, V. Summerbell, C. D. Dietary advice for treatment of type 2 diabetes mellitus in adults. Cochrane Database Syst Rev. 2007(3):CD004097. PMID 17636747.

320. Nielsen JVJ, E. Low-carbohydrate diet in type 2 diabetes. Stable improvement of bodyweight and glycemic control during 22 months follow-up. Nutr Metab (Lond). 2006;3:22. PMID 16774674.

321. Nielsen JVJ, E. A. Low-carbohydrate diet in type 2 diabetes: stable improvement of bodyweight and glycemic control during 44 months follow-up. Nutr Metab (Lond). 2008;5:14. PMID 18495047.

322. Nienhuijs SW, de Zoete JP, Berende CA, et al. Evaluation of laparoscopic sleeve gastrectomy on weight loss and co-morbidity. Int J Surg. 2010;8(4):302-4. PMID 20304112.

323. Nightengale MLS, M. G. Kelly, K. A. Jensen, M. D. Zinsmeister, A. R. Palumbo, P. J. Prospective evaluation of vertical banded gastroplasty as the primary operation for morbid obesity. Mayo Clin Proc. 1991 Aug;66(8):773-82. PMID 1861548.

324. Nijhawan S, Majid SF, Sedrak M, et al. First human NOTES(registered trademark) experience for sleeve gastrectomy at University of California at San Diego (UCSD). Gastrointestinal Endoscopy. 2011;73(4):AB147.

325. Nilsell KT, A. Sjostedt, S. Apelman, J. Pettersson, N. Prospective randomised comparison of adjustable gastric banding and vertical banded gastroplasty for morbid obesity. Eur J Surg. 2001 Jul;167(7):504-9. PMID 11560385.

326. Nugent CB, C. Elariny, H. Gopalakrishnan, P. Quigley, C. Garone, M., Jr. Afendy, M. Chan, O. Wheeler, A. Afendy, A. Younossi, Z. M. Metabolic syndrome after laparoscopic bariatric surgery. Obes Surg. 2008 Oct;18(10):1278-86. PMID 18401668.

327. Nuttall FQG, M. C. Saeed, A. Jordan, K. Hoover, H. The metabolic response of subjects with type 2 diabetes to a high-protein, weight-maintenance diet. J Clin Endocrinol Metab. 2003 Aug;88(8):3577-83. PMID 12915639.

328. Nwobu COJ, C. C. Targeting obesity to reduce the risk for type 2 diabetes and other co-morbidities in African American youth: a review of the literature and recommendations for prevention. Diab Vasc Dis Res. 2007 Dec;4(4):311-9. PMID 18158701.

329. O'Brien PED, J. B. Lap-band: outcomes and results. J Laparoendosc Adv Surg Tech A. 2003 Aug;13(4):265-70. PMID 14561255.

330. O'Brien PED, J. B. Laparoscopic adjustable gastric banding in the treatment of morbid obesity. Arch Surg. 2003 Apr;138(4):376-82. PMID 12686523.

331. O'Kane MW, P. G. Wales, J. K. Fluoxetine in the treatment of obese type 2 diabetic patients. Diabet Med. 1994 Jan-Feb;11(1):105-10. PMID 8181239.

332. Ohta M, Hirashita T, Iwashita Y, et al. Japanese experience in laparoscopic adjustable gastric banding: 5-year results. Surgical Endoscopy and Other Interventional Techniques. 2011;25:S244.

333. Olbers TB, S. Lindroos, A. Maleckas, A. Lonn, L. Sjostrom, L. Lonroth, H. Body composition, dietary intake, and energy expenditure after laparoscopic Roux-en-Y gastric bypass and laparoscopic vertical banded gastroplasty: a randomized clinical trial. Ann Surg. 2006 Nov;244(5):715-22. PMID 17060764.

334. Olbers TL, H. Dalenback, J. Haglind, E. Lundell, L. Laparoscopic vertical banded gastroplasty--an effective long-term therapy for morbidly obese patients? Obes Surg. 2001 Dec;11(6):726-30. PMID 11775570.

335. Olivan BMDT, Julio M. D. Bose, Mousumi PhD Bawa, Baani B. A. Chang, Tangel M. S. Summe, Heather M. S. Lee, Hongchan M. D. Laferrere, Blandine M. D. Effect of Weight Loss by Diet or Gastric Bypass Surgery on Peptide YY3-36 Levels. Ann Surg. 2009;249(6):948-53.

336. Omana JJ, Nguyen SQ, Herron D, et al. Comparison of comorbidity resolution and improvement between laparoscopic sleeve gastrectomy and laparoscopic adjustable gastric banding. Surg Endosc. 2010 Oct;24(10):2513-7. PMID 20339873.

337. Padwal RSM, S. R. Drug treatments for obesity: orlistat, sibutramine, and rimonabant. Lancet. 2007 Jan 6;369(9555):71-7. PMID 17208644.

338. Paisey RBF, J. Harvey, P. Paisey, A. Bower, L. Paisey, R. M. Taylor, P. Belka, I. Five year results of a prospective very low calorie diet or conventional weight loss programme in type 2 diabetes. J Hum Nutr Diet. 2002 Apr;15(2):121-7. PMID 11972741.

339. Paisey RBH, P. Rice, S. Belka, I. Bower, L. Dunn, M. Taylor, P. Paisey, R. M. Frost, J. Ash, I. An intensive weight loss programme in established type 2 diabetes and controls: effects on weight and atherosclerosis risk factors at 1 year. Diabet Med. 1998 Jan;15(1):73-9. PMID 9472867.

340. Paran HS, Liat Shwartz, Ivan Gutman, Mordechai. Long-term Follow-up on the Effect of Silastic Ring Vertical Gastroplasty on Weight and Co-Morbidities. Obesity Surgery. 2007;17(6):737-41.

341. Parikh ML, Helen Chang, Christopher Collings, Dinee Fielding, George Ren, Christine. Comparison of outcomes after laparoscopic adjustable gastric banding in African-Americans and whites. Surgery for Obesity and Related Diseases.2(6):607-10.

342. Pascale RWW, R. R. Butler, B. A. Mullen, M. Bononi, P. Effects of a behavioral weight loss program stressing calorie restriction versus calorie plus fat restriction in obese individuals with NIDDM or a family history of diabetes. Diabetes Care. 1995 Sep;18(9):1241-8. PMID 8612437.

343. Pasnik KK, J. Stanowski, E. Vertical banded gastroplasty: 6 years experience at a center in Poland. Obes Surg. 2005 Feb;15(2):223-7. PMID 15802065.

344. Patti ME, Goldfine AB. Hypoglycaemia following gastric bypass surgery--diabetes remission in the extreme? Diabetologia. 2010 Nov;53(11):2276-9. PMID 20730413.

345. Paxton JHM, J. B. The cost effectiveness of laparoscopic versus open gastric bypass surgery. Obes Surg. 2005 Jan;15(1):24-34. PMID 15760496.

346. Pedersen OG, P. Intensified multifactorial intervention and cardiovascular outcome in type 2 diabetes: the Steno-2 study. Metabolism. 2003 Aug;52(8 Suppl 1):19-23. PMID 12939735.

347. Pedersen SDK, J. Kline, G. A. Portion control plate for weight loss in obese patients with type 2 diabetes mellitus: a controlled clinical trial. Arch Intern Med. 2007 Jun 25;167(12):1277-83. PMID 17592101.

348. Penn LW, Martin Oldroyd, John Walker, Mark Alberti, K George Mathers, John. Prevention of type 2 diabetes in adults with impaired glucose tolerance: the European Diabetes Prevention RCT in Newcastle upon Tyne, UK. BMC Public Health. 2009;9(1):342. PMID doi:10.1186/1471-2458-9-342.

349. Peterli R, Beglinger C, Von Flue M, et al. Improved glucose metabolism 1 year after bariatric surgery: Comparison of laparoscopic Roux-en-Y gastric bypass (LRYGB) and laparoscopic sleeve gastrectomy (LSG)-a prospective randomized trial. Obesity Surgery. 2010;20(6):823.

350. Phelan SW, T. A. Berkowitz, R. I. Sarwer, D. B. Womble, L. G. Cato, R. K. Rothman, R. Impact of weight loss on the metabolic syndrome. Int J Obes (Lond). 2007 Sep;31(9):1442-8. PMID 17356528.

351. Pi-Sunyer FXA, L. J. Heshmati, H. M. Devin, J. Rosenstock, J. Effect of rimonabant, a cannabinoid-1 receptor blocker, on weight and cardiometabolic risk factors in overweight or obese patients: RIO-North America: a randomized controlled trial. JAMA. 2006 Feb 15;295(7):761-75. PMID 16478899.

352. Pi-Sunyer XB, G. Brancati, F. L. Bray, G. A. Bright, R. Clark, J. M. Curtis, J. M. Espeland, M. A. Foreyt, J. P. Graves, K. Haffner, S. M. Harrison, B. Hill, J. O. Horton, E. S. Jakicic, J. Jeffery, R. W. Johnson, K. C. Kahn, S. Kelley, D. E. Kitabchi, A. E. Knowler, W. C. Lewis, C. E. Maschak-Carey, B. J. Montgomery, B. Nathan, D. M. Patricio, J. Peters, A. Redmon, J. B. Reeves, R. S. Ryan, D. H. Safford, M. Van Dorsten, B. Wadden, T. A. Wagenknecht, L. Wesche-Thobaben, J. Wing, R. R. Yanovski, S. Z. Reduction in weight and cardiovascular disease risk factors in individuals with type 2 diabetes: one-year results of the look AHEAD trial. Diabetes Care. 2007 Jun;30(6):1374-83. PMID 17363746.

353. Pignone M. Bariatric surgery reduces the need for glycemic control medications and related health care costs. Clinical Diabetes. 2011;29(1):34-5.

354. Pinkey J. Bariatric surgery for diabetes: gastric banding is simple and safe. Br J Diabetes Vasc Dis. 2010;10:139-42.

355. Pinkney JHS, C. D. Gale, E. A. Should surgeons treat diabetes in severely obese people? Lancet. 2001 Apr 28;357(9265):1357-9. PMID 11343762.

356. Pinkney JK, D. Current status of bariatric surgery in the treatment of type 2 diabetes. Obes Rev. 2004 Feb;5(1):69-78. PMID 14969508.

357. Podnos YDJ, J. C. Wilson, S. E. Stevens, C. M. Nguyen, N. T. Complications after laparoscopic gastric bypass: a review of 3464 cases. Arch Surg. 2003 Sep;138(9):957-61. PMID 12963651.

358. Ponce JH, B. Paynter, S. Fromm, R. Lindsey, B. Shafer, A. Manahan, E. Sutterfield, C. Effect of Lap-Band-induced weight loss on type 2 diabetes mellitus and hypertension. Obes Surg. 2004 Nov-Dec;14(10):1335-42. PMID 15603648.

359. Pories WJM, K. G., Jr. Morgan, E. J. Sinha, M. K. Dohm, G. L. Swanson, M. S. Barakat, H. A. Khazanie, P. G. Leggett-Frazier, N. Long, S. D. et al.,. Surgical treatment of obesity and its effect on diabetes: 10-y follow-up. Am J Clin Nutr. 1992 Feb;55(2 Suppl):582S-5S. PMID 1733132.

360. Pories WJS, M. S. MacDonald, K. G. Long, S. B. Morris, P. G. Brown, B. M. Barakat, H. A. deRamon, R. A. Israel, G. Dolezal, J. M. et al.,. Who would have thought it? An operation proves to be the most effective therapy for adult-onset diabetes mellitus. Ann Surg. 1995 Sep;222(3):339-50; discussion 50-2. PMID 7677463.

361. Pournaras DJ, Osborne A, Hawkins SC, et al. Remission of type 2 diabetes after gastric bypass and banding: mechanisms and 2 year outcomes. Ann Surg. 2010 Dec;252(6):966-71. PMID 21107106.

362. Puzziferri NA-S, I. T. Wolfe, B. M. Wilson, S. E. Nguyen, N. T. Three-year follow-up of a prospective randomized trial comparing laparoscopic versus open gastric bypass. Ann Surg. 2006 Feb;243(2):181-8. PMID 16432350.

363. Rae AB, D. Evans, S. North, F. Roberman, B. Walters, B. A randomised controlled trial of dietary energy restriction in the management of obese women with gestational diabetes. Aust N Z J Obstet Gynaecol. 2000 Nov;40(4):416-22. PMID 11194427.

364. Raynor HAJ, R. W. Ruggiero, A. M. Clark, J. M. Delahanty, L. M. Weight loss strategies associated with BMI in overweight adults with type 2 diabetes at entry into the Look AHEAD (Action for Health in Diabetes) trial. Diabetes Care. 2008 Jul;31(7):1299-304. PMID 18375417.

365. Raz IH, M. Xu, L. Caria, C. Williams-Herman, D. Khatami, H. Efficacy and safety of the dipeptidyl peptidase-4 inhibitor sitagliptin as monotherapy in patients with type 2 diabetes mellitus. Diabetologia. 2006 Nov;49(11):2564-71. PMID 17001471.

366. Reaven GS, K. Hauptman, J. Boldrin, M. Lucas, C. Effect of orlistat-assisted weight loss in decreasing coronary heart disease risk in patients with syndrome X. Am J Cardiol. 2001 Apr 1;87(7):827-31. PMID 11274935.

367. Redmon JBB, A. G. Connelly, S. Fenney, P. A. Glasser, S. Glick, H. Greenway, F. Hesson, L. A. Lawlor, M. S. Montez, M. Montgomery, B. Effect of the Look AHEAD Study Intervention on Medication Use and Related Cost to Treat Cardiovascular Disease Risk Factors in Individuals with Type 2 Diabetes. Diabetes Care. 2010 Mar 23PMID 20332353.

368. Redmon JBR, S. K. Reck, K. P. Swanson, J. E. Kwong, C. A. Fan, Q. Thomas, W. Bantle, J. P. One-year outcome of a combination of weight loss therapies for subjects with type 2 diabetes: a randomized trial. Diabetes Care. 2003 Sep;26(9):2505-11. PMID 12941710.

369. Redmon JBR, S. K. Kwong, C. A. Swanson, J. E. Thomas, W. Bantle, J. P. Pharmacologic induction of weight loss to treat type 2 diabetes. Diabetes Care. 1999 Jun;22(6):896-903. PMID 10372238.

370. Redmon JBR, K. P. Raatz, S. K. Swanson, J. E. Kwong, C. A. Ji, H. Thomas, W. Bantle, J. P. Two-year outcome of a combination of weight loss therapies for type 2 diabetes. Diabetes Care. 2005 Jun;28(6):1311-5. PMID 15920044.

371. Reinhold RB. Late results of gastric bypass surgery for morbid obesity. J Am Coll Nutr. 1994 Aug;13(4):326-31. PMID 7963136.

372. Ricciardi RT, R. J. Kellogg, T. A. Ikramuddin, S. Baxter, N. N. Outcomes after open versus laparoscopic gastric bypass. Surg Laparosc Endosc Percutan Tech. 2006 Oct;16(5):317-20. PMID 17057571.

373. Richardson DW, Elizabeth Mason M, Vinik AI. Update: Metabolic and Cardiovascular Consequences of Bariatric Surgery. Endocrinology and Metabolism Clinics of North America. 2011;40(1):81-96.

374. Richelsen BT, S. Rossner, S. Toubro, S. Niskanen, L. Madsbad, S. Mustajoki, P. Rissanen, A. Effect of orlistat on weight regain and cardiovascular risk factors following a very-low-energy diet in abdominally obese patients: a 3-year randomized, placebo-controlled study. Diabetes Care. 2007 Jan;30(1):27-32. PMID 17192328.

375. Riddle MF, J. Zhang, B. Maier, H. Brown, C. Lutz, K. Kolterman, O. Pramlintide improved glycemic control and reduced weight in patients with type 2 diabetes using basal insulin. Diabetes Care. 2007 Nov;30(11):2794-9. PMID 17698615.

376. Rizzello M, Abbatini F, Casella G, et al. Early postoperative insulin-resistance changes after sleeve gastrectomy. Obes Surg. 2010 Jan;20(1):50-5. PMID 19916040.

377. Robinson JCF, A. R. Nabulsi, A. A. Watson, R. Brancati, F. L. Cai, J. Can postmenopausal hormone replacement improve plasma lipids in women with diabetes? The Atherosclerosis Risk in Communities Study Investigators. Diabetes Care. 1996 May;19(5):480-5. PMID 8732713.

378. Rodriguez LR, Eliana Fagalde, Pilar Oltra, Maria Soledad Saba, Jorge Aylwin, Carmen Gloria Prieto, Carolina Ramos, Almino Galvao, Manoel Gersin, Keith S. Sorli, Christopher. Pilot Clinical Study of an Endoscopic, Removable Duodenal-Jejunal Bypass Liner for the Treatment of Type 2 Diabetes. Diabetes Technology & Therapeutics. 2009;11(11):725-32. PMID 19905889.

379. Rosenstock JH, P. Gadde, K. M. Sun, X. Strauss, R. Leung, A. A randomized, double-blind, placebo-controlled, multicenter study to assess the efficacy and safety of topiramate controlled release in the treatment of obese type 2 diabetic patients. Diabetes Care. 2007 Jun;30(6):1480-6. PMID 17363756.

380. Roslin MSO, Jonathan H. Yatco, Edward Shah, Paresh C. PL-205: Abnormal glucose tolerance testing following gastric bypass. Surgery for Obesity and Related Diseases. 2009;5(3, Supplement 1):S10-S.

381. Ross R. Does exercise without weight loss improve insulin sensitivity? Diabetes Care. 2003 Mar;26(3):944-5. PMID 12610063.

382. Ross RF, J. A. Janssen, I. Exercise alone is an effective strategy for reducing obesity and related comorbidities. Exerc Sport Sci Rev. 2000 Oct;28(4):165-70. PMID 11064850.

383. Rubenstein RB. Laparoscopic adjustable gastric banding at a U.S. center with up to 3-year follow-up. Obes Surg. 2002 Jun;12(3):380-4. PMID 12082892.

384. Rutledge R. Subjective vs. objective resolution of diabetes mellitus following mini-gastric bypass: Patients' subjective assessment of resolution lags 1-3 years behind objective resolution. Obesity Surgery. 2010;20(8):1041-2.

385. Ryan DHE, M. A. Foster, G. D. Haffner, S. M. Hubbard, V. S. Johnson, K. C. Kahn, S. E. Knowler, W. C. Yanovski, S. Z. Look AHEAD (Action for Health in Diabetes): design and methods for a clinical trial of weight loss for the prevention of cardiovascular disease in type 2 diabetes. Control Clin Trials. 2003 Oct;24(5):610-28. PMID 14500058.

386. Saenz AF-E, I. Mataix, A. Ausejo, M. Roque, M. Moher, D. Metformin monotherapy for type 2 diabetes mellitus. Cochrane Database Syst Rev. 2005(3):CD002966. PMID 16034881.

387. Sahay BK. Yoga and diabetes. J Assoc Physicians India. 1986 Sep;34(9):645-8. PMID 3793701.

388. Salas MW, A. Caro, J. Health and economic effects of adding nateglinide to metformin to achieve dual control of glycosylated hemoglobin and postprandial glucose levels in a model of type 2 diabetes mellitus. Clin Ther. 2002 Oct;24(10):1690-705. PMID 12462297.

389. Salmela SP, M. Kasila, K. Vahasarja, K. Vanhala, M. Transtheoretical model-based dietary interventions in primary care: a review of the evidence in diabetes. Health Educ Res. 2009 Apr;24(2):237-52. PMID 18408218.

390. Salmon PA. The results of small intestine bypass operations for the treatment of obesity. Surg Gynecol Obstet. 1971 Jun;132(6):965-79. PMID 5578437.

391. Sampalis JSL, M. Auger, S. Christou, N. V. The impact of weight reduction surgery on health-care costs in morbidly obese patients. Obes Surg. 2004 Aug;14(7):939-47. PMID 15329183.

392. Sanchez-Pernaute A, Rubio MA, Martin E, et al. Metabolic results and weight loss outcome after single anastomosis duodeno-ileal bypass with sleeve gastrectomy (SADI-S). Threeyear results. Obesity Surgery. 2010;20(6):826.

393. Sartorelli DSS, E. C. Franco, L. J. Cardoso, M. A. Beneficial effects of short-term nutritional counselling at the primary health-care level among Brazilian adults. Public Health Nutr. 2005 Oct;8(7):820-5. PMID 16277797.

394. Schachter M. Metabolic effects of moxonidine and other centrally acting antihypertensives. Diabetes Obes Metab. 1999 Nov;1(6):317-22. PMID 11225647.

395. Schauer PRB, B. Ikramuddin, S. Cottam, D. Gourash, W. Hamad, G. Eid, G. M. Mattar, S. Ramanathan, R. Barinas-Mitchel, E. Rao, R. H. Kuller, L. Kelley, D. Effect of laparoscopic Roux-en Y gastric bypass on type 2 diabetes mellitus. Ann Surg. 2003 Oct;238(4):467-84; discussion 84-5. PMID 14530719.

396. Schauer PRI, S. Gourash, W. Ramanathan, R. Luketich, J. Outcomes after laparoscopic Roux-en-Y gastric bypass for morbid obesity. Ann Surg. 2000 Oct;232(4):515-29. PMID 10998650.

397. Scheen AJ. [Info-congress. Prevention of type 2 diabetes in obese patients: first results with orlistat in the XENDOS study]. Rev Med Liege. 2002 Sep;57(9):617-21. PMID 12440353.

398. Scheen AJE, P. New antiobesity agents in type 2 diabetes: overview of clinical trials with sibutramine and orlistat. Diabetes Metab. 2002 Dec;28(6 Pt 1):437-45. PMID 12522323.

399. Scheen AJVG, L. F. [Cardiometabolic effects of rimonabant in obese/overweight subjects with dyslipidaemia or type 2 diabetes]. Rev Med Liege. 2007 Feb;62(2):81-5. PMID 17461296.

400. Schindler KP, G. Ballaban, T. Kretschmer, S. Riener, R. Buranyi, B. Maier, C. Luger, A. Ludvik, B. Impact of laparoscopic adjustable gastric banding on plasma ghrelin, eating behaviour and body weight. Eur J Clin Invest. 2004 Aug;34(8):549-54. PMID 15305889.

401. Schok MG, R. van Antwerpen, T. de Wit, P. Brand, N. van Ramshorst, B. Quality of life after laparoscopic adjustable gastric banding for severe obesity: postoperative and retrospective preoperative evaluations. Obes Surg. 2000 Dec;10(6):502-8. PMID 11175956.

402. Schouten RMDR, Carianne S. M. D. Bouvy, Nicole D. M. D. PhD Hameeteman, Wim M. D. PhD Koek, Ger H. M. D. PhD Janssen, Ignace M. C. M. D. Greve, Jan-Willem M. M. D. PhD. A Multicenter, Randomized Efficacy Study of the EndoBarrier Gastrointestinal Liner for Presurgical Weight Loss Prior to Bariatric Surgery. [Miscellaneous Article]. Ann Surg. 2010;251(2):236-43.

403. Schouten RvD, F. M. Greve, J. W. Re-operation after laparoscopic adjustable gastric banding leads to a further decrease in BMI and obesity-related co-morbidities: results in 33 patients. Obes Surg. 2006 Jul;16(7):821-8. PMID 16839477.

404. Schouten RW, D. van Dielen, F. Greve, J. Laparoscopic adjustable gastric banding (LAGB) versus open vertical banded gastroplasty (VBG): long-term results of a prospective randomized trial. Obes Surg 2008;18:459.

405. Scopinaro NM, G. M. Camerini, G. B. Papadia, F. S. Adami, G. F. Specific effects of biliopancreatic diversion on the major components of metabolic syndrome: a long-term follow-up study. Diabetes Care. 2005 Oct;28(10):2406-11. PMID 16186271.

406. Scopinaro NP, F. Camerini, G. Marinari, G. Civalleri, D. Gian Franco, A. A comparison of a personal series of biliopancreatic diversion and literature data on gastric bypass help to explain the mechanisms of resolution of type 2 diabetes by the two operations. Obes Surg. 2008 Aug;18(8):1035-8. PMID 18463931.

407. Scott WR, Batterham RL. Roux-en-Y gastric bypass and laparoscopic sleeve gastrectomy: understanding weight loss and improvements in type 2 diabetes after bariatric surgery. Am J Physiol Regul Integr Comp Physiol. 2011 Jul;301(1):R15-27. PMID 21474429.

408. See CC, P. L. Elliott, D. Mullenix, P. Eggebroten, W. Porter, C. Watts, D. An institutional experience with laparoscopic gastric bypass complications seen in the first year compared with open gastric bypass complications during the same period. Am J Surg. 2002 May;183(5):533-8. PMID 12034387.

409. Segal JBC, J. M. Shore, A.D. Dominici, F. Magnuson, T. Richards, T.M. Weiner, J.P. Bass, E. B. Wu, A.W. Makary, M.A. Prompt Reducation in Use of Medications for Comorbid Conditions After Bariatric Surgery (Prepared by Johns Hopkins University DEcIDE Center under Contract No. HHSA29020050034-1TO2) Agency for Healthcare Research and Quality. Rockville, MD: June 2010. http://effectivehealthcare.ahrq.gov/reports/final.cfm.

410. Segal JBD, S.M. Millman, E.A. Herbert, R. Bass, E. B. Wu, A.W. Who Uses Exenatide for Glucose Control in Diabetes Mellitus? A Retrospective Cohort Study of a New Therapy (Prepared by Johns Hopkins University DEcIDE Center under Contract No. 290-2005-0034-1) Agency for Healthcare Research and Quality. Rockville, MD: July 2010. http://effectivehealthcare.ahrq.gov/reports/final.cfm.

411. Segato G, Busetto L, De Luca M, et al. Weight loss and changes in use of antidiabetic medication in obese type 2 diabetics after laparoscopic gastric banding. Surg Obes Relat Dis. 2010 Mar 4;6(2):132-7. PMID 19926528.

412. Selby JVE, B. Swain, B. E. Brown, J. B. First 20 months' experience with use of metformin for type 2 diabetes in a large health maintenance organization. Diabetes Care. 1999 Jan;22(1):38-44. PMID 10333901.

413. Serra-Majem LR, B. Estruch, R. Scientific evidence of interventions using the Mediterranean diet: a systematic review. Nutr Rev. 2006 Feb;64(2 Pt 2):S27-47. PMID 16532897.

414. Shah PS, Todkar JS, Shah SS. Effectiveness of laparoscopic sleeve gastrectomy on glycemic control in obese Indians with type 2 diabetes mellitus. Surg Obes Relat Dis. 2010 Mar 4;6(2):138-41. PMID 19733515.

415. Shah PST, Jayashree S. Shah, Shashank S. PL-214: Behavior of type 2 diabetes mellitus in obese Indian patients submitted to sleeve gastrectomy. Surgery for Obesity and Related Diseases. 2009;5(3, Supplement 1):S13-S4.

416. Shakeri-Manesch S, Ludvik B, Bohdjalian A, et al. Efficacy of bariatric surgery in the treatment of obesity-related type ii diabetes mellitus - 24 months follow up. Obesity Surgery. 2010;20(8):1038-9.

417. Singer DLH, D. Long-term experience with sulfonylureas and placebo. N Engl J Med. 1967 Aug 31;277(9):450-6. PMID 5340346.

418. Sjostrom CDP, M. Sjostrom, L. Blood pressure and pulse pressure during long-term weight loss in the obese: the Swedish Obese Subjects (SOS) Intervention Study. Obes Res. 2001 Mar;9(3):188-95. PMID 11323444.

419. Sjostrom L. Analysis of the XENDOS study (Xenical in the Prevention of Diabetes in Obese Subjects). Endocr Pract. 2006 Jan-Feb;12 Suppl 1:31-3. PMID 16627377.

420. Sjostrom LL, A. K. Peltonen, M. Torgerson, J. Bouchard, C. Carlsson, B. Dahlgren, S. Larsson, B. Narbro, K. Sjostrom, C. D. Sullivan, M. Wedel, H. Lifestyle, diabetes, and cardiovascular risk factors 10 years after bariatric surgery. N Engl J Med. 2004 Dec 23;351(26):2683-93. PMID 15616203.

421. Sjostrom LR, A. Andersen, T. Boldrin, M. Golay, A. Koppeschaar, H. P. Krempf, M. Randomised placebo-controlled trial of orlistat for weight loss and prevention of weight regain in obese patients. European Multicentre Orlistat Study Group. Lancet. 1998 Jul 18;352(9123):167-72. PMID 9683204.

422. Skroubis GA, S. Kehagias, I. Mead, N. Vagenas, K. Kalfarentzos, F. Roux-en-Y gastric bypass versus a variant of biliopancreatic diversion in a non-superobese population: prospective comparison of the efficacy and the incidence of metabolic deficiencies. Obes Surg. 2006 Apr;16(4):488-95. PMID 16608616.

423. Slim KB, J. Kwiatkowski, F. Lescure, G. Pezet, D. Chipponi, J. Quality of life before and after laparoscopic fundoplication. Am J Surg. 2000 Jul;180(1):41-5. PMID 11036138.

424. Smith DEW, R. R. Diminished weight loss and behavioral compliance during repeated diets in obese patients with type II diabetes. Health Psychol. 1991;10(6):378-83. PMID 1765032.

425. Smith SCE, C. B. Goodman, G. N. Changes in Diabetic Management After Roux-en-Y Gastric Bypass. Obes Surg. 1996 Aug;6(4):345-8. PMID 10729876.

426. Sosa JLP, H. Pallavicini, H. Ruiz-Rodriguez, M. Laparoscopic gastric bypass beyond age 60. Obes Surg. 2004 Nov-Dec;14(10):1398-401. PMID 15603658.

427. Souto SB, Souto EB, Braga DC, et al. Prevention and current onset delay approaches of type 2 diabetes mellitus (T2DM). European Journal of Clinical Pharmacology. 2011;67(7):653-61.

428. Sovik TT, Aasheim ET, Taha O, et al. Weight loss, cardiovascular risk factors, and quality of life after gastric bypass and duodenal switch: a randomized trial. Ann Intern Med. 2011 Sep 6;155(5):281-91. PMID 21893621.

429. Sovik TT, Irandoust B, Birkeland KI, et al. [Type 2 diabetes and metabolic syndrome before and after gastric bypass]. Tidsskr Nor Laegeforen. 2010 Jul 1;130(13):1347-50. PMID 20596116.

430. St Peter SDC, R. O. Tiede, J. L. Swain, J. M. Impact of advanced age on weight loss and health benefits after laparoscopic gastric bypass. Arch Surg. 2005 Feb;140(2):165-8. PMID 15723998.

431. Stenlof KR, S. Vercruysse, F. Kumar, A. Fitchet, M. Sjostrom, L. Topiramate in the treatment of obese subjects with drug-naive type 2 diabetes. Diabetes Obes Metab. 2007 May;9(3):360-8. PMID 17391164.

432. Stern LI, N. Seshadri, P. Chicano, K. L. Daily, D. A. McGrory, J. Williams, M. Gracely, E. J. Samaha, F. F. The effects of low-carbohydrate versus conventional weight loss diets in severely obese adults: one-year follow-up of a randomized trial. Ann Intern Med. 2004 May 18;140(10):778-85. PMID 15148064.

433. Stoeckli RC, R. Langer, I. Keller, U. Changes of body weight and plasma ghrelin levels after gastric banding and gastric bypass. Obes Res. 2004 Feb;12(2):346-50. PMID 14981228.

434. Stumvoll MN, N. Perriello, G. Dailey, G. Gerich, J. E. Metabolic effects of metformin in non-insulin-dependent diabetes mellitus. N Engl J Med. 1995 Aug 31;333(9):550-4. PMID 7623903.

435. Su Y, Su YH, Lee WJ, et al. C-peptide predicts the remission of type ii diabetes (T2DM) after sleeve gastrectomy. Obesity Surgery. 2010;20(8):979.

436. Sucharda P. [Metabolic surgery--the most effective diabetes treatment]. Vnitr Lek. 2011 Apr;57(4):396-401. PMID 21612067.

437. Sugerman HJK, J. M., Jr. DeMaria, E. J. Reines, H. D. Conversion of failed or complicated vertical banded gastroplasty to gastric bypass in morbid obesity. Am J Surg. 1996 Feb;171(2):263-9. PMID 8619465.

438. Sugerman HJL, G. L. Kellum, J. M. Wolf, L. Liszka, T. Engle, K. M. Birkenhauer, R. Starkey, J. V. Weight loss with vertical banded gastroplasty and Roux-Y gastric bypass for morbid obesity with selective versus random assignment. Am J Surg. 1989 Jan;157(1):93-102. PMID 2910132.

439. Sugerman HJW, L. G. Sica, D. A. Clore, J. N. Diabetes and hypertension in severe obesity and effects of gastric bypass-induced weight loss. Ann Surg. 2003 Jun;237(6):751-6; discussion 7-8. PMID 12796570.

440. Sultan S, Gupta D, Parikh M, et al. Five-year outcomes of patients with type 2 diabetes who underwent laparoscopic adjustable gastric banding. Surg Obes Relat Dis. 2010 Jul-Aug;6(4):373-6. PMID 20627708.

441. Summerbell CDW, C. Higgins, J. P. Garrow, J. S. Randomised controlled trial of novel, simple, and well supervised weight reducing diets in outpatients. BMJ. 1998 Nov 28;317(7171):1487-9. PMID 9831574.

442. Super P, Kitchen M, Krempic A, et al. Medium term metabolic outcomes of obese diabetic patients following laparoscopic adjustable gastric banding. Obesity Surgery. 2010;20(6):820.

443. Suter M, Donadini A, Romy S, et al. Laparoscopic Roux-En-Y gastric bypass: Significant long-term weight loss, improvement of obesity-related comorbidities and quality of life. Annals of Surgery. 2011;254(2):267-73.

444. Suter MG, V. Worreth, M. Heraief, E. Calmes, J. M. Laparoscopic gastric banding: a prospective, randomized study comparing the Lapband and the SAGB: early results. Ann Surg. 2005 Jan;241(1):55-62. PMID 15621991.

445. Tan JTK, S. Wijeratne, T. Chandraratna, H. S. Diagnosis and management of gastric leaks after laparoscopic sleeve gastrectomy for morbid obesity. Obes Surg. 2010 Apr;20(4):403-9. PMID 19936855.

446. Tarnoff MR, L. Escalona, A. Ramos, A. Neto, M. Alamo, M. Reyes, E. Pimentel, F. Ibanez, L. Open label, prospective, randomized controlled trial of an endoscopic duodenal-jejunal bypass sleeve versus low calorie diet for pre-operative weight loss in bariatric surgery. Surgical Endoscopy. 2009;23(3):650-6.

447. Taskin MZ, K. Apaydin, B. B. Unal, E. Laparoscopy in Turkish bariatric surgery: initial experience. Obes Surg. 2000 Jun;10(3):263-5. PMID 10932258.

448. Taylor CL, Laurent. Laparoscopic Adjustable Gastric Banding in Patients ≥60 Years Old: Is it Worthwhile? Obesity Surgery. 2006;16(12):1579-83.

449. Tayyem RM, Ali A. Short term outcome and health related quality of life of laparoscopic adjustable gastric band versus laparoscopic sleeve gastrectomy. Surgical Endoscopy and Other Interventional Techniques. 2011;25:S37.

450. Temple PCT, B. Sachs, L. Strasser, S. Choban, P. Flancbaum, L. Functioning and well-being of patients before and after elective surgical procedures. J Am Coll Surg. 1995 Jul;181(1):17-25. PMID 7599766.

451. The Danish Obesity Project. Randomised trial of jejunoileal bypass versus medical treatment in morbid obesity. . Lancet. 1979 Dec 15;2(8155):1255-8. PMID 93179.

452. The Diabetes Control and Complications Trial Research Group. Lifetime benefits and costs of intensive therapy as practiced in the diabetes control and complications trial. . JAMA. 1996 Nov 6;276(17):1409-15. PMID 8892716.

453. The Diabetes Prevention Program. Design and methods for a clinical trial in the prevention of type 2 diabetes. Diabetes Care. 1999 Apr;22(4):623-34. PMID 10189543.

454. Thomas DEE, E. J. Naughton, G. A. Exercise for type 2 diabetes mellitus. Cochrane Database Syst Rev. 2006;3:CD002968. PMID 16855995.

455. Tinker LFB, D. E. Margolis, K. L. Manson, J. E. Howard, B. V. Larson, J. Perri, M. G. Beresford, S. A. Robinson, J. G. Rodriguez, B. Safford, M. M. Wenger, N. K. Stevens, V. J. Parker, L. M. Low-fat dietary pattern and risk of treated diabetes mellitus in postmenopausal women: the Women's Health Initiative randomized controlled dietary modification trial. Arch Intern Med. 2008 Jul 28;168(14):1500-11. PMID 18663162.

456. Titi MJ, J. T. Modak, P. Galloway, D. J. Quality of life and alteration in comorbidity following laparoscopic adjustable gastric banding. Postgrad Med J. 2007 Jul;83(981):487-91. PMID 17621620.

457. Todkar JS, Shah SS, Shah PS, et al. Long-term effects of laparoscopic sleeve gastrectomy in morbidly obese subjects with type 2 diabetes mellitus. Surg Obes Relat Dis. 2010 Mar 4;6(2):142-5. PMID 19733513.

458. Toplak HH, A. Moore, R. Masson, E. Gorska, M. Vercruysse, F. Sun, X. Fitchet, M. Efficacy and safety of topiramate in combination with metformin in the treatment of obese subjects with type 2 diabetes: a randomized, double-blind, placebo-controlled study. Int J Obes (Lond). 2007 Jan;31(1):138-46. PMID 16703004.

459. Toplak HM, K. [Reduction of obesity and improvement in metabolic parameters by inhibition of intestinal lipases: current results with orlistat]. Acta Med Austriaca. 1998;25(4-5):142-5. PMID 9879390.

460. Toppino MM, M. Bonnet, G. Nigra, I. Siliquini, R. Laparoscopic surgery for morbid obesity: preliminary results from SICE registry (Italian Society of Endoscopic and Minimally Invasive Surgery). Obes Surg. 1999 Feb;9(1):62-5. PMID 10065587.

461. Torgerson JSH, J. Boldrin, M. N. Sjostrom, L. XENical in the prevention of diabetes in obese subjects (XENDOS) study: a randomized study of orlistat as an adjunct to lifestyle changes for the prevention of type 2 diabetes in obese patients. Diabetes Care. 2004 Jan;27(1):155-61. PMID 14693982.

462. Torquati AL, R. Abumrad, N. Richards, W. O. Is Roux-en-Y gastric bypass surgery the most effective treatment for type 2 diabetes mellitus in morbidly obese patients? J Gastrointest Surg. 2005 Nov;9(8):1112-6; discussion 7-8. PMID 16269382.

463. Torquati AW, K. Melvin, W. Richards, W. Effect of gastric bypass operation on Framingham and actual risk of cardiovascular events in class II to III obesity. J Am Coll Surg. 2007 May;204(5):776-82; discussion 82-3. PMID 17481482.

464. Trakhtenbroit MAL, J. G. Algahim, M. F. Miller, C. C., 3rd Moody, F. G. Lux, T. R. Taegtmeyer, H. Body weight, insulin resistance, and serum adipokine levels 2 years after 2 types of bariatric surgery. Am J Med. 2009 May;122(5):435-42. PMID 19375553.

465. Tsujiuchi TK, H. Yoshiuchi, K. He, D. Tsujiuchi, Y. Kuboki, T. Suematsu, H. Hirao, K. The effect of Qi-gong relaxation exercise on the control of type 2 diabetes mellitus: a randomized controlled trial. Diabetes Care. 2002 Jan;25(1):241-2. PMID 11772923.

466. Turnin MCB, O. Cathelineau, G. Leguerrier, A. M. Halimi, S. Sandre-Banon, D. Coliche, V. Breux, M. Verlet, E. Labrousse, F. Bensoussan, D. Grenier, J. L. Poncet, M. F. Tordjmann, F. Brun, J. M. Blickle, J. F. Mattei, C. Bolzonella, C. Buisson, J. C. Fabre, D. Tauber, J. P. Hanaire-Broutin, H. Multicenter randomized evaluation of a nutritional education software in obese patients. Diabetes Metab. 2001 Apr;27(2 Pt 1):139-47. PMID 11353880.

467. Tuthill AQ, A. McColgan, D. McKenna, M. O'Shea, D. McKenna, T. J. A prospective randomized controlled trial of lifestyle intervention on quality of life and cardiovascular risk score in patients with obesity and type 2 diabetes. Diabetes Obes Metab. 2007 Nov;9(6):917-9. PMID 17451423.

468. Umeda LM, Silva EA, Carneiro G, et al. Early Improvement in Glycemic Control After Bariatric Surgery and Its Relationships with Insulin, GLP-1, and Glucagon Secretion in Type 2 Diabetic Patients. Obes Surg. 2011 Jul;21(7):896-901. PMID 21559794.

469. Umpierrez GEC, W. S. Steen, M. T. Sulfonylurea treatment prevents recurrence of hyperglycemia in obese African-American patients with a history of hyperglycemic crises. Diabetes Care. 1997 Apr;20(4):479-83. PMID 9096964.

470. Valera-Mora MES, B. Gagliardi, L. Scarfone, A. Nanni, G. Castagneto, M. Manco, M. Mingrone, G. Ferrannini, E. Predictors of weight loss and reversal of comorbidities in malabsorptive bariatric surgery. Am J Clin Nutr. 2005 Jun;81(6):1292-7. PMID 15941878.

471. van Dam HAvdH, F. G. Knoops, L. Ryckman, R. M. Crebolder, H. F. van den Borne, B. H. Social support in diabetes: a systematic review of controlled intervention studies. Patient Educ Couns. 2005 Oct;59(1):1-12. PMID 16198213.

472. van Dielen FMS, P. B. de Brauw, L. M. Greve, J. W. Laparoscopic adjustable gastric banding versus open vertical banded gastroplasty: a prospective randomized trial. Obes Surg. 2005 Oct;15(9):1292-8. PMID 16259890.

473. Van Gaal LFR, A. M. Scheen, A. J. Ziegler, O. Rossner, S. Effects of the cannabinoid-1 receptor blocker rimonabant on weight reduction and cardiovascular risk factors in overweight patients: 1-year experience from the RIO-Europe study. Lancet. 2005 Apr 16-22;365(9468):1389-97. PMID 15836887.

474. van Gemert WGA, E. M. Kop, M. Vos, G. Greve, J. W. Soeters, P. B. A prospective cost-effectiveness analysis of vertical banded gastroplasty for the treatment of morbid obesity. Obes Surg. 1999 Oct;9(5):484-91. PMID 10605908.

475. van Gemert WGA, E. M. Greve, J. W. Soeters, P. B. Quality of life assessment of morbidly obese patients: effect of weight-reducing surgery. Am J Clin Nutr. 1998 Feb;67(2):197-201. PMID 9459366.

476. Vasudevan ARB, A. Fonseca, V. A. The effectiveness of intensive glycemic control for the prevention of vascular complications in diabetes mellitus. Treat Endocrinol. 2006;5(5):273-86. PMID 17002487.

477. Vertruyen M. Experience with Lap-band System up to 7 years. Obes Surg. 2002 Aug;12(4):569-72. PMID 12194553.

478. Vetter MLC, S. Rickels, M. R. Iqbal, N. Narrative review: effect of bariatric surgery on type 2 diabetes mellitus. Ann Intern Med. 2009 Jan 20;150(2):94-103. PMID 19153412.

479. Vidal JI, A. Nicolau, J. Vidov, M. Delgado, S. Martinez, G. Balust, J. Morinigo, R. Lacy, A. Short-term effects of sleeve gastrectomy on type 2 diabetes mellitus in severely obese subjects. Obes Surg. 2007 Aug;17(8):1069-74. PMID 17953241.

480. Vijgen SMH, M. Baan, C. A. de Wit, G. A. Limburg, W. Feenstra, T. L. Cost effectiveness of preventive interventions in type 2 diabetes mellitus: a systematic literature review. Pharmacoeconomics. 2006;24(5):425-41. PMID 16706569.

481. Vogel JAF, B. A. Zalesin, K. C. Trivax, J. E. Krause, K. R. Chengelis, D. L. McCullough, P. A. Reduction in predicted coronary heart disease risk after substantial weight reduction after bariatric surgery. Am J Cardiol. 2007 Jan 15;99(2):222-6. PMID 17223422.

482. Volokh MA, Gubochkin NG, Shapovalov VM, et al. [Surgical complications following operative treatment of abdominal obesity in type 2 diabetes mellitus patients]. Vestn Khir Im I I Grek. 2011;170(1):18-21. PMID 21506349.

483. Wadden TAW, D. S. Delahanty, L. Jakicic, J. Rejeski, J. Williamson, D. Berkowitz, R. I. Kelley, D. E. Tomchee, C. Hill, J. O. Kumanyika, S. The Look AHEAD study: a description of the lifestyle intervention and the evidence supporting it. Obesity (Silver Spring). 2006 May;14(5):737-52. PMID 16855180.

484. Walker EAM, M. Kramer, M. K. Kahn, S. Ma, Y. Edelstein, S. Smith, K. Johnson, M. K. Kitabchi, A. Crandall, J. Adherence to preventive medications: predictors and outcomes in the Diabetes Prevention Program. Diabetes Care. 2006 Sep;29(9):1997-2002. PMID 16936143.

485. Walton SJ, Date RS. Surgical cure for type II diabetes: Myth or reality? Annals of Surgery. 2011;254(1):180-1.

486. Weiner RAK, M. Matzig, E. Weiner, S. Karcz, W. K. Junginger, T. Early results with a new telemetrically adjustable gastric banding. Obes Surg. 2007 Jun;17(6):717-21. PMID 17879567.

487. Weinstock RSD, H. Wadden, T. A. Diet and exercise in the treatment of obesity: effects of 3 interventions on insulin resistance. Arch Intern Med. 1998 Dec 7-21;158(22):2477-83. PMID 9855386.

488. West DSD, V. Bursac, Z. Gore, S. A. Greene, P. G. Motivational interviewing improves weight loss in women with type 2 diabetes. Diabetes Care. 2007 May;30(5):1081-7. PMID 17337504.

489. White SB, E. Jurikova, L. Stubbs, R. S. Long-term outcomes after gastric bypass. Obes Surg. 2005 Feb;15(2):155-63. PMID 15802056.

490. Wilding JVG, L. Rissanen, A. Vercruysse, F. Fitchet, M. A randomized double-blind placebo-controlled study of the long-term efficacy and safety of topiramate in the treatment of obese subjects. Int J Obes Relat Metab Disord. 2004 Nov;28(11):1399-410. PMID 15486569.

491. Williams KVK, D. E. Metabolic consequences of weight loss on glucose metabolism and insulin action in type 2 diabetes. Diabetes Obes Metab. 2000 Jun;2(3):121-9. PMID 11220547.

492. Williamson DAR, Jack Lang, Wei Van Dorsten, Brent Fabricatore, Anthony N. Toledo, Katie for the Look AHEAD Research Group,. Impact of a Weight Management Program on Health-Related Quality of Life in Overweight Adults With Type 2 Diabetes. Arch Intern Med. 2009 January 26, 2009;169(2):163-71.

493. Wing RRA, K. Effectiveness of a behavioral weight control program for blacks and whites with NIDDM. Diabetes Care. 1996 May;19(5):409-13. PMID 8732700.

494. Wing RRB, E. H. Bononi, P. Marcus, M. D. Watanabe, R. Bergman, R. N. Caloric restriction per se is a significant factor in improvements in glycemic control and insulin sensitivity during weight loss in obese NIDDM patients. Diabetes Care. 1994 Jan;17(1):30-6. PMID 8112186.

495. Wing RRB, E. Marcus, M. Epstein, L. H. Harvey, J. Year-long weight loss treatment for obese patients with type II diabetes: does including an intermittent very-low-calorie diet improve outcome? Am J Med. 1994 Oct;97(4):354-62. PMID 7942937.

496. Wing RRE, L. H. Paternostro-Bayles, M. Kriska, A. Nowalk, M. P. Gooding, W. Exercise in a behavioural weight control programme for obese patients with Type 2 (non-insulin-dependent) diabetes. Diabetologia. 1988 Dec;31(12):902-9. PMID 3071485.

497. Wing RRM, M. D. Salata, R. Epstein, L. H. Miaskiewicz, S. Blair, E. H. Effects of a very-low-calorie diet on long-term glycemic control in obese type 2 diabetic subjects. Arch Intern Med. 1991 Jul;151(7):1334-40. PMID 2064484.

498. Wing RRM, M. D. Epstein, L. H. Jawad, A. A "family-based" approach to the treatment of obese type II diabetic patients. J Consult Clin Psychol. 1991 Feb;59(1):156-62. PMID 2002132.

499. Wing RRS, M. Marcus, M. D. McDermott, M. Gooding, W. Variables associated with weight loss and improvements in glycemic control in type II diabetic patients in behavioral weight control programs. Int J Obes. 1990 Jun;14(6):495-503. PMID 2401586.

500. Wing RRV, E. Jakicic, J. M. Polley, B. A. Lang, W. Lifestyle intervention in overweight individuals with a family history of diabetes. Diabetes Care. 1998 Mar;21(3):350-9. PMID 9540015.

501. Wittgrove ACC, G. W. Laparoscopic gastric bypass, Roux-en-Y- 500 patients: technique and results, with 3-60 month follow-up. Obes Surg. 2000 Jun;10(3):233-9. PMID 10929154.

502. Wittgrove ACC, G. W. Laparoscopic Gastric Bypass, Roux-en-Y: Experience of 27 Cases, with 3-18 Months Follow-up. Obes Surg. 1996 Feb;6(1):54-7. PMID 10731251.

503. Wittgrove ACC, G. W. Tremblay, L. J. Laparoscopic Gastric Bypass, Roux-en-Y: Preliminary Report of Five Cases. Obes Surg. 1994 Nov;4(4):353-7. PMID 10742801.

504. Wittgrove ACC, G. W. Schubert, K. R. Laparoscopic Gastric Bypass, Roux-en-Y: Technique and Results in 75 Patients With 3-30 Months Follow-up. Obes Surg. 1996 Dec;6(6):500-4. PMID 10729899.

505. Woelnerhanssen B, Peterli R, Steinert RE, et al. Effects of postbariatric surgery weight loss on adipokines and metabolic parameters: comparison of laparoscopic Roux-en-Y gastric bypass and

laparoscopic sleeve gastrectomy-a prospective randomized trial. Surg Obes Relat Dis. 2011 Mar 21PMID 21429816.

506. Wolf AMB, U. Kortner, B. Kuhlmann, H. W. Does gastric restriction surgery reduce the risks of metabolic diseases? Obes Surg. 1998 Feb;8(1):9-13. PMID 9562480.

507. Wolf AMC, M. R. Crowther, J. Q. Hazen, K. Y. L. Nadler J Oneida, B. Bovbjerg, V. E. Translating lifestyle intervention to practice in obese patients with type 2 diabetes: Improving Control with Activity and Nutrition (ICAN) study. Diabetes Care. 2004 Jul;27(7):1570-6. PMID 15220230.

508. Wolf AMK, H. W. Reoperation Due to Complications after Gastric Restriction Operation. Obes Surg. 1995 May;5(2):171-8. PMID 10733807.

509. Wolfe BM. Surgical treatment for diabetes mellitus type 2. Inflammation Research. 2010;59:s146.

510. Yang JG, Wang CC, Hu YZ, et al. [Treatment of obesity and type 2 diabetes mellitus by laparoscopic Roux-en-Y gastric bypass]. Zhonghua Wei Chang Wai Ke Za Zhi. 2010 Aug;13(8):594-7. PMID 20737312.

511. Yang K. A review of yoga programs for four leading risk factors of chronic diseases. Evid Based Complement Alternat Med. 2007 Dec;4(4):487-91. PMID 18227916.

512. Yates TK, K. Bull, F. Gorely, T. Davies, M. J. The role of physical activity in the management of impaired glucose tolerance: a systematic review. Diabetologia. 2007 Jun;50(6):1116-26. PMID 17415549.

513. Zehetner JH, F. Triaca, H. Klaiber, Ch. A 6-year experience with the Swedish adjustable gastric band Prospective long-term audit of laparoscopic gastric banding. Surg Endosc. 2005 Jan;19(1):21-8. PMID 15549627.

514. Zingmond DSM, M. L. Ko, C. Y. Hospitalization before and after gastric bypass surgery. JAMA. 2005 Oct 19;294(15):1918-24. PMID 16234498.

515. Zlabek JAG, M. S. Larson, C. J. Mathiason, M. A. Lambert, P. J. Kothari, S. N. The effect of laparoscopic gastric bypass surgery on dyslipidemia in severely obese patients. Surg Obes Relat Dis. 2005 Nov-Dec;1(6):537-42. PMID 16925287.

516. Zorrilla PGS, R. J. Salinas-Martinez, A. M. Vertical banded gastroplasty-gastric bypass with and without the interposition of jejunum: preliminary report. Obes Surg. 1999 Feb;9(1):29-32. PMID 10065577.

Reject Non Systematic Review:

1. Anvari M. Use of metabolic surgery for the treatment of type 2 diabetes. Canadian Journal of Diabetes. 2011;35(2):99-108.

2. Jackson L. Translating the Diabetes Prevention Program Into Practice: A Review of Community Interventions. The Diabetes Educator. 2009 March 1, 2009;35(2):309-20.

3. Kelley DEG, B. H. Effects of physical activity on insulin action and glucose tolerance in obesity. Med Sci Sports Exerc. 1999 Nov;31(11 Suppl):S619-23. PMID 10593537.

4. Pappachan JM, Chacko EC, Arunagirinathan G, et al. Management of hypertension and diabetes in obesity: non-pharmacological measures. Int J Hypertens. 2011;2011:398065. PMID 21629871.

5. Rubino F, Schauer PR, Kaplan LM, et al. Metabolic surgery to treat type 2 diabetes: clinical outcomes and mechanisms of action. Annu Rev Med. 2010;61:393-411. PMID 20059345.

6. Scheen AJVG, L. G. Despres, J. P. Pi-Sunyer, X. Golay, A. Hanotin, C. [Rimonabant improves cardiometabolic risk profile in obese or overweight subjects: overview of RIO studies]. Rev Med Suisse. 2006 Aug 23;2(76):1916-23. PMID 16972542.

7. Schernthaner G, Brix JM, Kopp HP, et al. Cure of type 2 diabetes by metabolic surgery? A critical analysis of the evidence in 2010. Diabetes Care. 2011 May;34 Suppl 2:S355-60. PMID 21525482.

8. Schulman APdG, F. Sinha, N. Rubino, F. "Metabolic" surgery for treatment of type 2 diabetes mellitus. Endocr Pract. 2009 Sep-Oct;15(6):624-31. PMID 19625245.

9. Sherwin RSA, R. M. Buse, J. B. Chin, M. H. Eddy, D. Fradkin, J. Ganiats, T. G. Ginsberg, H. N. Kahn, R. Nwankwo, R. Rewers, M. Schlessinger, L. Stern, M. Vinicor, F. Zinman, B. Prevention or delay of type 2 diabetes. Diabetes Care. 2004 Jan;27 Suppl 1:S47-54. PMID 14693925.

10. Varela JE. Bariatric surgery: a cure for diabetes? Curr Opin Clin Nutr Metab Care. 2011 Jul;14(4):396-401. PMID 21505331.

11. Villamizar N, Pryor AD. Safety, effectiveness, and cost effectiveness of metabolic surgery in the treatment of type 2 diabetes mellitus. J Obes. 2011;2011:790683. PMID 21113308.

Reject Non-Surgical Treatment with Follow-Up < 1 year:

1. Abbott WGB, V. L. Grundy, S. M. Howard, B. V. Effects of replacing saturated fat with complex carbohydrate in diets of subjects with NIDDM. Diabetes Care. 1989 Feb;12(2):102-7. PMID 2702893.

2. Abramson EA, R. A. Treatment of the obese diabetic. A comparative study of placebo, sulfonylurea and phenformin. Metabolism. 1967 Mar;16(3):204-12. PMID 5336062.

3. Albarracin CAF, B. C. Evans, J. L. Goldfine, I. D. Chromium picolinate and biotin combination improves glucose metabolism in treated, uncontrolled overweight to obese patients with type 2 diabetes. Diabetes Metab Res Rev. 2008 Jan-Feb;24(1):41-51. PMID 17506119.

4. Amano YS, M. Lee, J. S. Kawakubo, K. Mori, K. Tang, A. C. Akabayashi, A. Glycemic index-based nutritional education improves blood glucose control in Japanese adults: a randomized controlled trial. Diabetes Care. 2007 Jul;30(7):1874-6. PMID 17440171.

5. Andersen EH, P. Kindstedt, K. Hellstrom, K. Effects of a high-protein and low-fat diet vs a low-protein and high-fat diet on blood glucose, serum lipoproteins, and cholesterol metabolism in noninsulin-dependent diabetics. Am J Clin Nutr. 1987 Feb;45(2):406-13. PMID 3812340.

6. Anderson JWB-K, V. Hamilton, C. C. Logan, J. E. Collins, R. W. Gustafson, N. J. Food-containing hypocaloric diets are as effective as liquid-supplement diets for obese individuals with NIDDM. Diabetes Care. 1994 Jun;17(6):602-4. PMID 8082533.

7. Aro AU, M. Voutilainen, E. Hersio, K. Korhonen, T. Siitonen, O. Improved diabetic control and hypocholesterolaemic effect induced by long-term dietary supplementation with guar gum in type 2 (insulin-independent) diabetes. Diabetologia. 1981 Jul;21(1):29-33. PMID 6268475.

8. Baldi JCS, N. Resistance training improves glycaemic control in obese type 2 diabetic men. Int J Sports Med. 2003 Aug;24(6):419-23. PMID 12905089.

9. Barnard RJL, L. Holly, R. G. Cherny, S. Pritikin, N. Response of non-insulin-dependent diabetic patients to an intensive program of diet and exercise. Diabetes Care. 1982 Jul-Aug;5(4):370-4. PMID 7151652.

10. Barnes AJG, K. J. Crowley, M. F. Bloom, A. Effect of short and long term chlorpropamide treatment of insulin release and blood-glucose. Lancet. 1974 Jul 13;2(7872):69-72. PMID 4136696.

11. Barratt RF, G. Millward, D. J. Truby, H. A randomised controlled trial investigating the effect of an intensive lifestyle intervention v. standard care in adults with type 2 diabetes immediately after initiating insulin therapy. Br J Nutr. 2008 May;99(5):1025-31. PMID 18197995.

12. Bianchi RB, V. Bravenboer, B. Erkelens, D. W. Effects of benfluorex on insulin resistance and lipid metabolism in obese type II diabetic patients. Diabetes Care. 1993 Apr;16(4):557-9. PMID 8462377.

13. Bjorgaas MRV, J. T. Stolen, T. Lydersen, S. Grill, V. Regular use of pedometer does not enhance beneficial outcomes in a physical activity intervention study in type 2 diabetes mellitus. Metabolism. 2008 May;57(5):605-11. PMID 18442621.

14. Bogardus CR, E. Robbins, D. C. Wolfe, R. R. Horton, E. S. Sims, E. A. Effects of physical training and diet therapy on carbohydrate metabolism in patients with glucose intolerance and non-insulin-dependent diabetes mellitus. Diabetes. 1984 Apr;33(4):311-8. PMID 6368289.

15. Bonanome AV, A. Lusiani, L. Beltramello, G. Confortin, L. Biffanti, S. Sorgato, F. Costa, F. Pagnan, A. Carbohydrate and lipid metabolism in patients with non-insulin-dependent diabetes mellitus: effects of a low-fat, high-carbohydrate diet vs a diet high in monounsaturated fatty acids. Am J Clin Nutr. 1991 Sep;54(3):586-90. PMID 1877514.

16. Brand JCC, S. Crossman, S. Allen, A. Roberts, D. C. Truswell, A. S. Low-glycemic index foods improve long-term glycemic control in NIDDM. Diabetes Care. 1991 Feb;14(2):95-101. PMID 2060429.

17. Bratusch-Marrain PD, R. Waldhausl, W. [Weight reduction in obese diabetics: a double-blind study of diethylpropionate (author's transl)]. Wien Klin Wochenschr. 1979 Jun 22;91(13):455-8. PMID 380178.

18. Brunerova LS, V. Potockova, J. Andel, M. A comparison of the influence of a high-fat diet enriched in monounsaturated fatty acids and conventional diet on weight loss and metabolic parameters in obese non-diabetic and Type 2 diabetic patients. Diabet Med. 2007 May;24(5):533-40. PMID 17381504.

19. Brunzell JDL, R. L. Porte, D., Jr. Bierman, E. L. Effect of a fat free, high carbohydrate diet on diabetic subjects with fasting hyperglycemia. Diabetes. 1974 Feb;23(2):138-42. PMID 4811509.

20. Brunzell JDL, R. L. Hazzard, W. R. Porte, D., Jr. Bierman, E. L. Improved glucose tolerance with high carbohydrate feeding in mild diabetes. N Engl J Med. 1971 Mar 11;284(10):521-4. PMID 5100724.

21. Brussard HEGL, J.A. Frohlich, M. Kluft, C. Krans, H. M. Short-term oestrogen replacement improves insulin resistance, lipids and fibrinolysis in postmenopausal women with NIDDM. Diabetologia. 1997;40:843-9.

22. Buse JBH, R. R. Han, J. Kim, D. D. Fineman, M. S. Baron, A. D. Effects of exenatide (exendin-4) on glycemic control over 30 weeks in sulfonylurea-treated patients with type 2 diabetes. Diabetes Care. 2004 Nov;27(11):2628-35. PMID 15504997.

23. Cabrera-Pivaral CEG-P, G. Vega-Lopez, M. G. Centeno-Lopez, M. [Effects of an educational intervention on plasma levels of LDL cholesterol in type 2 diabetics]. Salud Publica Mex. 2001 Nov-Dec;43(6):556-62. PMID 11816230.

24. Cabrera-Pivaral CEG-P, G. Vega-Lopez, M. G. Arias-Merino, E. D. [Impact of participatory education on body mass index and blood glucose in obese type-2 diabetics]. Cad Saude Publica. 2004 Jan-Feb;20(1):275-81. PMID 15029330.

25. Campbell IWD, C. Patton, N. W. Broadhead, T. Tucker, G. T. Woods, H. F. The effect of metformin on glycaemic control, intermediary metabolism and blood pressure in non-insulin-dependent diabetes mellitus. Diabet Med. 1987 Jul-Aug;4(4):337-41. PMID 2956047.

26. Campbell LVB, R. Gosper, J. K. Jupp, J. J. Simons, L. A. Chisholm, D. J. Impact of intensive educational approach to dietary change in NIDDM. Diabetes Care. 1990 Aug;13(8):841-7. PMID 2209318.

27. Castaneda CL, J. E. Munoz-Orians, L. Gordon, P. L. Walsmith, J. Foldvari, M. Roubenoff, R. Tucker, K. L. Nelson, M. E. A randomized controlled trial of resistance exercise training to improve glycemic control in older adults with type 2 diabetes. Diabetes Care. 2002 Dec;25(12):2335-41. PMID 12453982.

28. Cederholm J. Short-term treatment of glucose intolerance in middle-aged subjects by diet, exercise and sulfonylurea. Ups J Med Sci. 1985;90(3):229-42. PMID 4095819.

29. Chapman IP, B. Doran, S. Feinle-Bisset, C. Wishart, J. Strobel, S. Wang, Y. Burns, C. Lush, C. Weyer, C. Horowitz, M. Effect of pramlintide on satiety and food intake in obese subjects and subjects with type 2 diabetes. Diabetologia. 2005 May;48(5):838-48. PMID 15843914.

30. Chazova IA, V. A. Shlyakhto, E. Moxonidine improves glycaemic control in mildly hypertensive, overweight patients: a comparison with metformin. Diabetes Obes Metab. 2006 Jul;8(4):456-65. PMID 16776753.

31. Chow CCK, G. T. Tsang, L. W. Yeung, V. T. Chan, J. C. Cockram, C. S. Dexfenfluramine in obese Chinese NIDDM patients. A placebo-controlled investigation of the effects on body weight, glycemic control, and cardiovascular risk factors. Diabetes Care. 1997 Jul;20(7):1122-7. PMID 9203448.

32. Christiansen ES, S. Palmvig, B. Tauber-Lassen, E. Pedersen, O. Intake of a diet high in trans monounsaturated fatty acids or saturated fatty acids. Effects on postprandial insulinemia and glycemia in obese patients with NIDDM. Diabetes Care. 1997 May;20(5):881-7. PMID 9135961.

33. Colman EK, L. I. Rogus, E. Coon, P. Muller, D. Goldberg, A. P. Weight loss reduces abdominal fat and improves insulin action in middle-aged and older men with impaired glucose tolerance. Metabolism. 1995 Nov;44(11):1502-8. PMID 7476341.

34. Coniff RFS, J. A. Seaton, T. B. Long-term efficacy and safety of acarbose in the treatment of obese subjects with non-insulin-dependent diabetes mellitus. Arch Intern Med. 1994 Nov 14;154(21):2442-8. PMID 7979840.

35. Connolly VMG, A. Kesson, C. M. A study of fluoxetine in obese elderly patients with type 2 diabetes. Diabet Med. 1995 May;12(5):416-8. PMID 7648804.

36. Coyle DP, A. J. Tam, R. Economic evaluation of pioglitazone hydrochloride in the management of type 2 diabetes mellitus in Canada. Pharmacoeconomics. 2002;20 Suppl 1:31-42. PMID 12036382.

37. Cuff DJM, G. S. Martin, A. Ignaszewski, A. Tildesley, H. D. Frohlich, J. J. Effective exercise modality to reduce insulin resistance in women with type 2 diabetes. Diabetes Care. 2003 Nov;26(11):2977-82. PMID 14578226.

38. Damsbo PH, L. S. Vaag, A. Hother-Nielsen, O. Beck-Nielsen, H. Irreversibility of the defect in glycogen synthase activity in skeletal muscle from obese patients with NIDDM treated with diet and metformin. Diabetes Care. 1998 Sep;21(9):1489-94. PMID 9727896.

39. Davey Smith GB, Y. Svendsen, K. H. Neaton, J. D. Haffner, S. M. Kuller, L. H. Incidence of type 2 diabetes in the randomized multiple risk factor intervention trial. Ann Intern Med. 2005 Mar 1;142(5):313-22. PMID 15738450.

40. Davidson JAM, S. O. Waterhouse, B. R. Cobitz, A. R. A 24-week, multicenter, randomized, double-blind, placebo-controlled, parallel-group study of the efficacy and tolerability of combination therapy with rosiglitazone and sulfonylurea in African American and Hispanic American patients with type 2 diabetes inadequately controlled with sulfonylurea monotherapy. Clin Ther. 2007 Sep;29(9):1900-14. PMID 18035190.

41. De Filippis EC, K. Ocampo, G. Berria, R. Buck, S. Consoli, A. Mandarino, L. J. Exercise-induced improvement in vasodilatory function accompanies increased insulin sensitivity in obesity and type 2 diabetes mellitus. J Clin Endocrinol Metab. 2006 Dec;91(12):4903-10. PMID 17018657.

42. De Jager JK, A. Lehert, P. Bets, D. Wulffele, M. G. Teerlink, T. Scheffer, P. G. Schalkwijk, C. G. Donker, A. J. Stehouwer, C. D. Effects of short-term treatment with metformin on markers of endothelial function and inflammatory activity in type 2 diabetes mellitus: a randomized, placebo-controlled trial. J Intern Med. 2005 Jan;257(1):100-9. PMID 15606381.

43. de Luis DAI, O. Aller, R. Cuellar, L. Terroba, M. C. Martin, T. Cabezas, G. Rojo, S. Domingo, M. A randomized clinical trial with two enteral diabetes-specific supplements in patients with diabetes mellitus type 2: metabolic effects. Eur Rev Med Pharmacol Sci. 2008 Jul-Aug;12(4):261-6. PMID 18727459.

44. Dejager SR, S. Foley, J. E. Schweizer, A. Vildagliptin in drug-naive patients with type 2 diabetes: a 24-week, double-blind, randomized, placebo-controlled, multiple-dose study. Horm Metab Res. 2007 Mar;39(3):218-23. PMID 17373638.

45. Dekker MJL, S. Hudson, R. Kilpatrick, K. Graham, T. E. Ross, R. Robinson, L. E. An exercise intervention without weight loss decreases circulating interleukin-6 in lean and obese men with and without type 2 diabetes mellitus. Metabolism. 2007 Mar;56(3):332-8. PMID 17292721.

46. Derosa GDA, A. Salvadeo, S. A. Ferrari, I. Gravina, A. Fogari, E. Maffioli, P. Cicero, A. F. Sibutramine effect on metabolic control of obese patients with type 2 diabetes mellitus treated with pioglitazone. Metabolism. 2008 Nov;57(11):1552-7. PMID 18940393.

47. Derosa GF, E. Cicero, A. F. D'Angelo, A. Ciccarelli, L. Piccinni, M. N. Pricolo, F. Salvadeo, S. A. Gravina, A. Ferrari, I. Fogari, R. Blood pressure control and inflammatory markers in type 2 diabetic patients treated with pioglitazone or rosiglitazone and metformin. Hypertens Res. 2007 May;30(5):387-94. PMID 17587750.

48. Didangelos TPT, A. K. Bousboulas, S. H. Sambanis, C. L. Athyros, V. G. Spanou, E. A. Dimitriou, K. C. Pappas, S. I. Karamanos, B. G. Karamitsos, D. T. The ORLIstat and CArdiovascular risk profile in patients with metabolic syndrome and type 2 DIAbetes (ORLICARDIA) Study. Curr Med Res Opin. 2004 Sep;20(9):1393-401. PMID 15383188.

49. Dornan TLH, S. R. Peck, G. M. Tattersall, R. B. Double-blind evaluation of efficacy and tolerability of metformin in NIDDM. Diabetes Care. 1991 Apr;14(4):342-4. PMID 2060439.

50. Dunstan DWD, R. M. Owen, N. Jolley, D. De Courten, M. Shaw, J. Zimmet, P. High-intensity resistance training improves glycemic control in older patients with type 2 diabetes. Diabetes Care. 2002 Oct;25(10):1729-36. PMID 12351469.

51. Dunstan DWD, R.M. Owen, N. et al. High resistance training improves glycemic control in older patients with type 2 diabetes. Diabetes Care. 2003;25:1729-36.

52. Einhorn DR, M. Rosenzweig, J. Egan, J. W. Mathisen, A. L. Schneider, R. L. Pioglitazone hydrochloride in combination with metformin in the treatment of type 2 diabetes mellitus: a randomized, placebo-controlled study. The Pioglitazone 027 Study Group. Clin Ther. 2000 Dec;22(12):1395-409. PMID 11192132.

53. Eliasson BG, S. Cederholm, J. Liang, Y. Vercruysse, F. Smith, U. Weight loss and metabolic effects of topiramate in overweight and obese type 2 diabetic patients: randomized double-blind placebo-controlled trial. Int J Obes (Lond). 2007 Jul;31(7):1140-7. PMID 17264849.

54. Fanghanel GS-R, L. Trujillo, C. Sotres, D. Espinosa-Campos, J. Metformin's effects on glucose and lipid metabolism in patients with secondary failure to sulfonylureas. Diabetes Care. 1996 Nov;19(11):1185-9. PMID 8908377.

55. Fanghanel GS, U. Sanchez-Reyes, L. Sisson, D. Sotres, D. Torres, E. M. Effects of metformin on fibrinogen levels in obese patients with type 2 diabetes. Rev Invest Clin. 1998 Sep-Oct;50(5):389-94. PMID 9949668.

56. Feinbock CL, A. Klingler, A. Egger, T. Bielesz, G. K. Winkler, F. Siebenhofer, A. Grossschadl, F. Frank, E. Irsigler, K. Prospective multicentre trial comparing the efficacy of, and compliance with, glimepiride or acarbose treatment in patients with type 2 diabetes not controlled with diet alone. Diabetes Nutr Metab. 2003 Aug;16(4):214-21. PMID 14768770.

57. Filippatos TDK, D. N. Liberopoulos, E. N. Georgoula, M. Mikhailidis, D. P. Elisaf, M. S. Effect of orlistat, micronised fenofibrate and their combination on metabolic parameters in overweight and obese patients with the metabolic syndrome: the FenOrli study. Curr Med Res Opin. 2005 Dec;21(12):1997-2006. PMID 16368051.

58. Fineman MSS, L. Z. Taylor, K. Kim, D. D. Baron, A. D. Effectiveness of progressive dose-escalation of exenatide (exendin-4) in reducing dose-limiting side effects in subjects with type 2 diabetes. Diabetes Metab Res Rev. 2004 Sep-Oct;20(5):411-7. PMID 15343588.

59. Finer NB, S. R. Frost, G. S. Banks, L. M. Griffiths, J. Sibutramine is effective for weight loss and diabetic control in obesity with type 2 diabetes: a randomised, double-blind, placebo-controlled study. Diabetes Obes Metab. 2000 Apr;2(2):105-12. PMID 11220522.

60. Fritsche AS, M. A. Haring, H. U. Glimepiride combined with morning insulin glargine, bedtime neutral protamine hagedorn insulin, or bedtime insulin glargine in patients with type 2 diabetes. A randomized, controlled trial. Ann Intern Med. 2003 Jun 17;138(12):952-9. PMID 12809451.

61. Fuh MML, M. M. Jeng, C. Y. Ma, F. Chen, Y. D. Reaven, G. M. Effect of low fat-high carbohydrate diets in hypertensive patients with non-insulin-dependent diabetes mellitus. Am J Hypertens. 1990 Jul;3(7):527-32. PMID 2194509.

62. Fujii SO, Y. Okada, K. Tanaka, S. Seki, J. Wada, M. Iseki, T. Effects of physical training on glucose tolerance and insulin response in diabetics. Osaka City Med J. 1982;28(1):1-8. PMID 6763179.

63. Fujioka KS, T. B. Rowe, E. Jelinek, C. A. Raskin, P. Lebovitz, H. E. Weinstein, S. P. Weight loss with sibutramine improves glycaemic control and other metabolic parameters in obese patients with type 2 diabetes mellitus. Diabetes Obes Metab. 2000 Jun;2(3):175-87. PMID 11220553.

64. Gannon MCN, F. Q. Effect of a high-protein, low-carbohydrate diet on blood glucose control in people with type 2 diabetes. Diabetes. 2004 Sep;53(9):2375-82. PMID 15331548.

65. Garg AB, A. Grundy, S. M. Zhang, Z. J. Unger, R. H. Comparison of a high-carbohydrate diet with a high-monounsaturated-fat diet in patients with non-insulin-dependent diabetes mellitus. N Engl J Med. 1988 Sep 29;319(13):829-34. PMID 3045553.

66. Garg AG, S. M. Unger, R. H. Comparison of effects of high and low carbohydrate diets on plasma lipoproteins and insulin sensitivity in patients with mild NIDDM. Diabetes. 1992 Oct;41(10):1278-85. PMID 1397701.

67. Glass LCQ, Y. Lenox, S. Kim, D. Gates, J. R. Brodows, R. Trautmann, M. Bergenstal, R. M. Effects of exenatide versus insulin analogues on weight change in subjects with type 2 diabetes: a pooled post-hoc analysis. Curr Med Res Opin. 2008 Mar;24(3):639-44. PMID 18218179.

68. Goldhaber-Fiebert JDG-F, S. N. Tristan, M. L. Nathan, D. M. Randomized controlled community-based nutrition and exercise intervention improves glycemia and cardiovascular risk factors in type 2 diabetic patients in rural Costa Rica. Diabetes Care. 2003 Jan;26(1):24-9. PMID 12502654.

69. Greco AVM, G. Capristo, E. De Gaetano, A. Ghirlanda, G. Castagneto, M. Effects of dexfenfluramine on free fatty acid turnover and oxidation in obese patients with type 2 diabetes mellitus. Metabolism. 1995 Feb;44(2 Suppl 2):57-61. PMID 7869940.

70. Gregorio FA, F. Angelici, F. Cristallini, S. Dini, F. L. Vespasiani, G. Santeusanio, F. Filipponi, P. [Body mass index, blood lactate and therapeutic effectiveness of metformin in type II diabetes mellitus]. Medicina (Firenze). 1989 Apr-Jun;9(2):200-4. PMID 2682123.

71. Gunton JEC, N. W. Hitchman, R. Hams, G. O'Sullivan, C. Foster-Powell, K. McElduff, A. Chromium supplementation does not improve glucose tolerance, insulin sensitivity, or lipid profile: a randomized, placebo-controlled, double-blind trial of supplementation in subjects with impaired glucose tolerance. Diabetes Care. 2005 Mar;28(3):712-3. PMID 15735214.

72. Gupta AG, R. Lal, B. Effect of Trigonella foenum-graecum (fenugreek) seeds on glycaemic control and insulin resistance in type 2 diabetes mellitus: a double blind placebo controlled study. J Assoc Physicians India. 2001 Nov;49:1057-61. PMID 11868855.

73. Guy-Grand BD, P. Eschwege, E. Gin, H. Joubert, J. M. Valensi, P. Effects of orlistat on obesity-related diseases - a six-month randomized trial. Diabetes Obes Metab. 2004 Sep;6(5):375-83. PMID 15287931.

74. Haisch JR, W. [Effectiveness and efficiency of ambulatory diabetes education programs. A comparison of specialty practice and general practice]. Dtsch Med Wochenschr. 2000 Feb 18;125(7):171-6. PMID 10719390.

75. Halimi SLB, M. A. Grange, V. Efficacy and safety of acarbose add-on therapy in the treatment of overweight patients with Type 2 diabetes inadequately controlled with metformin: a double-blind, placebo-controlled study. Diabetes Res Clin Pract. 2000 Sep;50(1):49-56. PMID 10936668.

76. Halpern AM, M. C. Suplicy, H. Zanella, M. T. Repetto, G. Gross, J. Jadzinsky, M. Barranco, J. Aschner, P. Ramirez, L. Matos, A. G. Latin-American trial of orlistat for weight loss and improvement in glycaemic profile in obese diabetic patients. Diabetes Obes Metab. 2003 May;5(3):180-8. PMID 12681025.

77. Han JRD, B. Sun, J. Chen, C. G. Corkey, B. E. Kirkland, J. L. Ma, J. Guo, W. Effects of dietary medium-chain triglyceride on weight loss and insulin sensitivity in a group of moderately overweight free-living type 2 diabetic Chinese subjects. Metabolism. 2007 Jul;56(7):985-91. PMID 17570262.

78. Heilbronn LKN, M. Clifton, P. M. The effect of high- and low-glycemic index energy restricted diets on plasma lipid and glucose profiles in type 2 diabetic subjects with varying glycemic control. J Am Coll Nutr. 2002 Apr;21(2):120-7. PMID 11999539.

79. Hermansen KK, M. Luo, E. Fanurik, D. Khatami, H. Stein, P. Efficacy and safety of the dipeptidyl peptidase-4 inhibitor, sitagliptin, in patients with type 2 diabetes mellitus inadequately controlled on

glimepiride alone or on glimepiride and metformin. Diabetes Obes Metab. 2007 Sep;9(5):733-45. PMID 17593236.

80. Hoffmann JS, M. Efficacy of 24-week monotherapy with acarbose, glibenclamide, or placebo in NIDDM patients. The Essen Study. Diabetes Care. 1994 Jun;17(6):561-6. PMID 8082525.

81. Holman RRT, R. C. Basal normoglycemia attained with chlorpropamide in mild diabetes. Metabolism. 1978 May;27(5):539-47. PMID 565457.

82. Horton ESC, C. Gatlin, M. Foley, J. Mallows, S. Shen, S. Nateglinide alone and in combination with metformin improves glycemic control by reducing mealtime glucose levels in type 2 diabetes. Diabetes Care. 2000 Nov;23(11):1660-5. PMID 11092289.

83. Howard BVA, W. G. Swinburn, B. A. Evaluation of metabolic effects of substitution of complex carbohydrates for saturated fat in individuals with obesity and NIDDM. Diabetes Care. 1991 Sep;14(9):786-95. PMID 1959472.

84. Hughes VAF, M. A. Fielding, R. A. Ferrara, C. M. Elahi, D. Evans, W. J. Long-term effects of a high-carbohydrate diet and exercise on insulin action in older subjects with impaired glucose tolerance. Am J Clin Nutr. 1995 Aug;62(2):426-33. PMID 7625352.

85. Hussain SA. Silymarin as an adjunct to glibenclamide therapy improves long-term and postprandial glycemic control and body mass index in type 2 diabetes. J Med Food. 2007 Sep;10(3):543-7. PMID 17887949.

86. Jenkins DJK, C. W. McKeown-Eyssen, G. Josse, R. G. Silverberg, J. Booth, G. L. Vidgen, E. Josse, A. R. Nguyen, T. H. Corrigan, S. Banach, M. S. Ares, S. Mitchell, S. Emam, A. Augustin, L. S. Parker, T. L. Leiter, L. A. Effect of a low-glycemic index or a high-cereal fiber diet on type 2 diabetes: a randomized trial. JAMA. 2008 Dec 17;300(23):2742-53. PMID 19088352.

87. Jimenez-Cruz AB-G, M. Turnbull, W. H. Rosales-Garay, P. Severino-Lugo, I. A flexible, low-glycemic index mexican-style diet in overweight and obese subjects with type 2 diabetes improves metabolic parameters during a 6-week treatment period. Diabetes Care. 2003 Jul;26(7):1967-70. PMID 12832297.

88. Josephkutty SP, J. M. Comparison of tolbutamide and metformin in elderly diabetic patients. Diabet Med. 1990 Jul;7(6):510-4. PMID 2142054.

89. Jun JKG, W. C. Mathur, R. Effects of pioglitazone on diabetes-related outcomes in Hispanic patients. Am J Health Syst Pharm. 2003 Mar 1;60(5):469-73. PMID 12635453.

90. Kadoglou NPI, F. Liapis, C. D. Perrea, D. Angelopoulou, N. Alevizos, M. Beneficial effects of combined treatment with rosiglitazone and exercise on cardiovascular risk factors in patients with type 2 diabetes. Diabetes Care. 2007 Sep;30(9):2242-4. PMID 17586747.

91. Kang JR, R. J. Hagberg, J. M. Kelley, D. E. Goss, F. L. DaSilva, S. G. Suminski, R. R. Utter, A. C. Effect of exercise intensity on glucose and insulin metabolism in obese individuals and obese NIDDM patients. Diabetes Care. 1996 Apr;19(4):341-9. PMID 8729157.

92. Karlander SA, I. Efendic, S. Metabolic effects and clinical value of beet fiber treatment in NIDDM patients. Diabetes Res Clin Pract. 1991 Feb;11(2):65-71. PMID 1850691.

93. Kattelmann KKC, K. Ren, C. The medicine wheel nutrition intervention: a diabetes education study with the Cheyenne River Sioux Tribe. J Am Diet Assoc. 2009 Sep;109(9):1532-9. PMID 19699832.

94. Keller UW, C. Messer, C. Riesen, W. [Comparison of a calorie-defined diet with the conventional exchange diet in Type 2 diabetes mellitus]. Schweiz Med Wochenschr. 1991 Jul 9;121(27-28):1014-9. PMID 1882212.

95. Kelley DEW, R. Buonocore, C. Sturis, J. Polonsky, K. Fitzsimmons, M. Relative effects of calorie restriction and weight loss in noninsulin-dependent diabetes mellitus. J Clin Endocrinol Metab. 1993 Nov;77(5):1287-93. PMID 8077323.

96. King ABA, D. U. Chinnapongse, S. Comparison of glycemic and lipid response to pioglitazone treatment in Mexican-Americans and non-Hispanic Caucasians with type 2 diabetes. Diabetes Care. 2003 Jan;26(1):245-6. PMID 12502690.

97. Kipnes MSK, A. Rendell, M. S. Egan, J. W. Mathisen, A. L. Schneider, R. L. Pioglitazone hydrochloride in combination with sulfonylurea therapy improves glycemic control in patients with type 2 diabetes mellitus: a randomized, placebo-controlled study. Am J Med. 2001 Jul;111(1):10-7. PMID 11448655.

98. Kuo CSP, D. Yao, C. Y. Hsieh, M. C. Kuo, S. W. Effect of orlistat in overweight poorly controlled Chinese female type 2 diabetic patients: a randomised, double-blind, placebo-controlled study. Int J Clin Pract. 2006 Aug;60(8):906-10. PMID 16893433.

99. Kutnowski MD, J. C. Friedman, H. Kolanowski, J. Krzentowski, G. Scheen, A. Van Gaal, L. Fluoxetine therapy in obese diabetic and glucose intolerant patients. Int J Obes Relat Metab Disord. 1992 Dec;16 Suppl 4:S63-6. PMID 1338388.

100. Lambers SVL, C. Van Acker, K. Calders, P. Influence of combined exercise training on indices of obesity, diabetes and cardiovascular risk in type 2 diabetes patients. Clin Rehabil. 2008 Jun;22(6):483-92. PMID 18511528.

101. Lamotte MA, L. Lefever, A. Nechelput, M. Masure, J. A health economic model to assess the long-term effects and cost-effectiveness of orlistat in obese type 2 diabetic patients. Diabetes Care. 2002 Feb;25(2):303-8. PMID 11815500.

102. Lee SK, J. L. Davidson, L. E. Hudson, R. Kilpatrick, K. Graham, T. E. Ross, R. Exercise without weight loss is an effective strategy for obesity reduction in obese individuals with and without Type 2 diabetes. J Appl Physiol. 2005 Sep;99(3):1220-5. PMID 15860689.

103. Lemon CCL, K. Lohse, B. Hubacher, D. O. Klawitter, B. Palta, M. Outcomes monitoring of health, behavior, and quality of life after nutrition intervention in adults with type 2 diabetes. J Am Diet Assoc. 2004 Dec;104(12):1805-15. PMID 15565074.

104. Leutenegger MB, B. Brun, J. M. Guillon-Metz, F. Martin, C. Nicolino-Peltier, C. Richard, J. L. Vannereau, D. Added benfluorex in obese insulin-requiring type 2 diabetes. Diabetes Metab. 1998 Feb;24(1):55-61. PMID 9534010.

105. Liu GCC, A. M. Lardinois, C. K. Hollenbeck, C. B. Moore, J. G. Reaven, G. M. Moderate weight loss and sulfonylurea treatment of non-insulin-dependent diabetes mellitus. Combined effects. Arch Intern Med. 1985 Apr;145(4):665-9. PMID 3885889.

106. Lousley SEJ, D. B. Slaughter, P. Carter, R. D. Jelfs, R. Mann, J. I. High carbohydrate-high fibre diets in poorly controlled diabetes. Diabet Med. 1984 May;1(1):21-5. PMID 6100938.

107. Lucas CPP, S. Stepke, T. Kinhal, V. Darga, L. L. Carroll-Michals, L. Spafford, T. R. Kasim, S. Achieving therapeutic goals in insulin-using diabetic patients with non-insulin-dependent diabetes mellitus. A weight reduction-exercise-oral agent approach. Am J Med. 1987 Sep 18;83(3A):3-9. PMID 3307404.

108. Ludvik BHM, K. Waldhaeusl, W. Hofer, A. Prager, R. Kautzky-Willer, A. Pacini, G. The effect of Ipomoea batatas (Caiapo) on glucose metabolism and serum cholesterol in patients with type 2 diabetes: a randomized study. Diabetes Care. 2002 Jan;25(1):239-40. PMID 11772921.

109. Ludvik BN, B. Pacini, G. Efficacy of Ipomoea batatas (Caiapo) on diabetes control in type 2 diabetic subjects treated with diet. Diabetes Care. 2004 Feb;27(2):436-40. PMID 14747225.

110. Luis Bautista JB, C. Dirnberger, G. Atherton, T. Efficacy and safety profile of glimepiride in Mexican American Patients with type 2 diabetes mellitus: a randomized, placebo-controlled study. Clin Ther. 2003 Jan;25(1):194-209. PMID 12637120.

111. Maeda HY, R. Hirao, K. Tochikubo, O. Effects of agar (kanten) diet on obese patients with impaired glucose tolerance and type 2 diabetes. Diabetes Obes Metab. 2005 Jan;7(1):40-6. PMID 15642074.

112. Maheux PD, F. Bourque, J. Garon, J. Chiasson, J. L. Fluoxetine improves insulin sensitivity in obese patients with non-insulin-dependent diabetes mellitus independently of weight loss. Int J Obes Relat Metab Disord. 1997 Feb;21(2):97-102. PMID 9043962.

113. Markovic TPC, L. V. Balasubramanian, S. Jenkins, A. B. Fleury, A. C. Simons, L. A. Chisholm, D. J. Beneficial effect on average lipid levels from energy restriction and fat loss in obese individuals with or without type 2 diabetes. Diabetes Care. 1998 May;21(5):695-700. PMID 9589226.

114. Markovic TPJ, A. B. Campbell, L. V. Furler, S. M. Kraegen, E. W. Chisholm, D. J. The determinants of glycemic responses to diet restriction and weight loss in obesity and NIDDM. Diabetes Care. 1998 May;21(5):687-94. PMID 9589225.

115. Mattoo VE, D. Widel, M. Duran, S. Fajardo, C. Strand, J. Knight, D. Grossman, L. Oakley, D. Tan, M. Metabolic effects of pioglitazone in combination with insulin in patients with type 2 diabetes mellitus whose disease is not adequately controlled with insulin therapy: results of a six-month, randomized, double-blind, prospective, multicenter, parallel-group study. Clin Ther. 2005 May;27(5):554-67. PMID 15978304.

116. McAuley KAW, S. M. Mann, J. I. Goulding, A. Chisholm, A. Wilson, N. Story, G. McLay, R. T. Harper, M. J. Jones, I. E. Intensive lifestyle changes are necessary to improve insulin sensitivity: a randomized controlled trial. Diabetes Care. 2002 Mar;25(3):445-52. PMID 11874928.

117. McKibbin CLP, T. L. Norman, G. Patrick, K. Jin, H. Roesch, S. Mudaliar, S. Barrio, C. O'Hanlon, K. Griver, K. Sirkin, A. Jeste, D. V. A lifestyle intervention for older schizophrenia patients with diabetes mellitus: a randomized controlled trial. Schizophr Res. 2006 Sep;86(1-3):36-44. PMID 16842977.

118. McLaughlin TC, S. Lamendola, C. Abbasi, F. Schaaf, P. Basina, M. Reaven, G. Clinical efficacy of two hypocaloric diets that vary in overweight patients with type 2 diabetes: comparison of moderate fat versus carbohydrate reductions. Diabetes Care. 2007 Jul;30(7):1877-9. PMID 17475941.

119. Meckling KAOS, C. Saari, D. Comparison of a low-fat diet to a low-carbohydrate diet on weight loss, body composition, and risk factors for diabetes and cardiovascular disease in free-living, overweight men and women. J Clin Endocrinol Metab. 2004 Jun;89(6):2717-23. PMID 15181047.

120. Meneilly GSG, N. Tildesley, H. Habener, J. F. Egan, J. M. Elahi, D. Effects of 3 months of continuous subcutaneous administration of glucagon-like peptide 1 in elderly patients with type 2 diabetes. Diabetes Care. 2003 Oct;26(10):2835-41. PMID 14514588.

121. Miller CKE, L. Kissling, G. Sanville, L. Evaluation of a theory-based nutrition intervention for older adults with diabetes mellitus. J Am Diet Assoc. 2002 Aug;102(8):1069-81. PMID 12171451.

122. Miyashita YK, N. Ohtsuka, M. Ozaki, H. Itoh, Y. Oyama, T. Uetake, T. Ariga, K. Shirai, K. Beneficial effect of low carbohydrate in low calorie diets on visceral fat reduction in type 2 diabetic patients with obesity. Diabetes Res Clin Pract. 2004 Sep;65(3):235-41. PMID 15331203.

123. Miyazaki YM, A. Matsuda, M. Glass, L. Mahankali, S. Ferrannini, E. Cusi, K. Mandarino, L. J. DeFronzo, R. A. Improved glycemic control and enhanced insulin sensitivity in type 2 diabetic subjects treated with pioglitazone. Diabetes Care. 2001 Apr;24(4):710-9. PMID 11315836.

124. Muchmore DBS, J. Miller, M. Self-monitoring of blood glucose in overweight type 2 diabetic patients. Acta Diabetol. 1994 Dec;31(4):215-9. PMID 7888692.

125. Nagulesparan MS, P. J. Bennion, L. J. Unger, R. H. Bennett, P. H. Diminished effect of caloric restriction on control of hyperglycemia with increasing known duration of type II diabetes mellitus. J Clin Endocrinol Metab. 1981 Sep;53(3):560-8. PMID 7021580.

126. Nam SYK, K. R. Cha, B. S. Song, Y. D. Lim, S. K. Lee, H. C. Huh, K. B. Low-dose growth hormone treatment combined with diet restriction decreases insulin resistance by reducing visceral fat and increasing muscle mass in obese type 2 diabetic patients. Int J Obes Relat Metab Disord. 2001 Aug;25(8):1101-7. PMID 11477493.

127. Nathan DMR, A. Godine, J. E. Glyburide or insulin for metabolic control in non-insulin-dependent diabetes mellitus. A randomized, double-blind study. Ann Intern Med. 1988 Mar;108(3):334-40. PMID 3124685.

128. Nolan JJJ, N. P. Patwardhan, R. Deacon, L. F. Rosiglitazone taken once daily provides effective glycaemic control in patients with Type 2 diabetes mellitus. Diabet Med. 2000 Apr;17(4):287-94. PMID 10821295.

129. Noury JN, A. Comparative three-month study of the efficacies of metformin and gliclazide in the treatment of NIDD. Diabete Metab. 1991 May;17(1 Pt 2):209-12. PMID 1936478.

130. Nuttall FQG, M. C. The metabolic response to a high-protein, low-carbohydrate diet in men with type 2 diabetes mellitus. Metabolism. 2006 Feb;55(2):243-51. PMID 16423633.

131. Osei KB, B. Dietary fructose as a natural sweetener in poorly controlled type 2 diabetes: a 12-month crossover study of effects on glucose, lipoprotein and apolipoprotein metabolism. Diabet Med. 1989 Aug;6(6):506-11. PMID 2527132.

132. Osei KF, J. Bossetti, B. M. Holland, G. C. Metabolic effects of fructose as a natural sweetener in the physiologic meals of ambulatory obese patients with type II diabetes. Am J Med. 1987 Aug;83(2):249-55. PMID 3618627.

133. Paniagua JAdlS, A. G. Sanchez, E. Romero, I. Vidal-Puig, A. Berral, F. J. Escribano, A. Moyano, M. J. Perez-Martinez, P. Lopez-Miranda, J. Perez-Jimenez, F. A MUFA-rich diet improves posprandial glucose, lipid and GLP-1 responses in insulin-resistant subjects. J Am Coll Nutr. 2007 Oct;26(5):434-44. PMID 17914131.

134. Parker BN, M. Luscombe, N. Clifton, P. Effect of a high-protein, high-monounsaturated fat weight loss diet on glycemic control and lipid levels in type 2 diabetes. Diabetes Care. 2002 Mar;25(3):425-30. PMID 11874925.

135. Pathan MFL, Z. A. Nazneen, N. E. Mili, S. U. Orlistat as an adjunct therapy in type 2 obese diabetic patients treated with sulphonylurea: a Bangladesh experience. Bangladesh Med Res Counc Bull. 2004 Apr;30(1):1-8. PMID 15376463.

136. Pereira MAJ, D. R., Jr. Pins, J. J. Raatz, S. K. Gross, M. D. Slavin, J. L. Seaquist, E. R. Effect of whole grains on insulin sensitivity in overweight hyperinsulinemic adults. Am J Clin Nutr. 2002 May;75(5):848-55. PMID 11976158.

137. Peters Harmel ALK, D. M. Buse, J. B. Boyle, P. J. Marchetti, A. Lau, H. Impact of adjunctive thiazolidinedione therapy on blood lipid levels and glycemic control in patients with type 2 diabetes. Curr Med Res Opin. 2004;20(2):215-23. PMID 15006017.

138. Petersen KFD, S. Befroy, D. Lehrke, M. Hendler, R. E. Shulman, G. I. Reversal of nonalcoholic hepatic steatosis, hepatic insulin resistance, and hyperglycemia by moderate weight reduction in patients with type 2 diabetes. Diabetes. 2005 Mar;54(3):603-8. PMID 15734833.

139. Phillips LSG, G. Miller, E. Patwardhan, R. Rappaport, E. B. Salzman, A. Once- and twice-daily dosing with rosiglitazone improves glycemic control in patients with type 2 diabetes. Diabetes Care. 2001 Feb;24(2):308-15. PMID 11213884.

140. Pi-Sunyer FXS, A. Mills, D. Dejager, S. Efficacy and tolerability of vildagliptin monotherapy in drug-naive patients with type 2 diabetes. Diabetes Res Clin Pract. 2007 Apr;76(1):132-8. PMID 17223217.

141. Pijl HO, S. Matsuda, M. Miyazaki, Y. Mahankali, A. Kumar, V. Pipek, R. Iozzo, P. Lancaster, J. L. Cincotta, A. H. DeFronzo, R. A. Bromocriptine: a novel approach to the treatment of type 2 diabetes. Diabetes Care. 2000 Aug;23(8):1154-61. PMID 10937514.

142. Pontiroli AEP, M. Piatti, P. M. Cassisa, C. Camisasca, R. Pozza, G. Benfluorex in obese noninsulin dependent diabetes mellitus patients poorly controlled by insulin: a double blind study versus placebo. J Clin Endocrinol Metab. 1996 Oct;81(10):3727-32. PMID 8855830.

143. Poon TN, P. Shen, L. Mihm, M. Taylor, K. Fineman, M. Kim, D. Exenatide improves glycemic control and reduces body weight in subjects with type 2 diabetes: a dose-ranging study. Diabetes Technol Ther. 2005 Jun;7(3):467-77. PMID 15929678.

144. Poppitt SDK, G. F. Prentice, A. M. Williams, D. E. Sonnemans, H. M. Valk, E. E. Robinson, E. Wareham, N. J. Long-term effects of ad libitum low-fat, high-carbohydrate diets on body weight and serum lipids in overweight subjects with metabolic syndrome. Am J Clin Nutr. 2002 Jan;75(1):11-20. PMID 11756055.

145. Pratley RER, J. Pi-Sunyer, F. X. Banerji, M. A. Schweizer, A. Couturier, A. Dejager, S. Management of type 2 diabetes in treatment-naive elderly patients: benefits and risks of vildagliptin monotherapy. Diabetes Care. 2007 Dec;30(12):3017-22. PMID 17878242.

146. Rabkin SWB, E. Wilson, A. Streja, D. A. A randomized clinical trial comparing behavior modification and individual counseling in the nutritional therapy of non-insulin-dependent diabetes mellitus: comparison of the effect on blood sugar, body weight, and serum lipids. Diabetes Care. 1983 Jan-Feb;6(1):50-6. PMID 6341015.

147. Rains SGW, G. A. Richmond, W. Elkeles, R. S. The effect of glibenclamide and metformin on serum lipoproteins in type 2 diabetes. Diabet Med. 1988 Oct;5(7):653-8. PMID 2975549.

148. Raskin PR, M. Riddle, M. C. Dole, J. F. Freed, M. I. Rosenstock, J. A randomized trial of rosiglitazone therapy in patients with inadequately controlled insulin-treated type 2 diabetes. Diabetes Care. 2001 Jul;24(7):1226-32. PMID 11423507.

149. Rasmussen OWT, C. Hansen, K. W. Vesterlund, M. Winther, E. Hermansen, K. Effects on blood pressure, glucose, and lipid levels of a high-monounsaturated fat diet compared with a high-carbohydrate diet in NIDDM subjects. Diabetes Care. 1993 Dec;16(12):1565-71. PMID 8117360.

150. Rave KR, K. Dellweg, S. Heise, T. tom Dieck, H. Improvement of insulin resistance after diet with a whole-grain based dietary product: results of a randomized, controlled cross-over study in obese subjects with elevated fasting blood glucose. Br J Nutr. 2007 Nov;98(5):929-36. PMID 17562226.

151. Reaven GM. Beneficial effect of moderate weight loss in older patients with non-insulin-dependent diabetes mellitus poorly controlled with insulin. J Am Geriatr Soc. 1985 Feb;33(2):93-5. PMID 3881506.

152. Reboussin DMG, D. C., Jr. Lipkin, E. W. Herrington, D. M. Summerson, J. Steffes, M. Crouse, R. J., 3rd Jovanovic, L. Feinglos, M. N. Probstfield, J. L. Banerji, M. A. Pettitt, D. J. Williamson, J. The combination oral and nutritional treatment of late-onset diabetes mellitus (CONTROL DM) trial results. Diabet Med. 2004 Oct;21(10):1082-9. PMID 15384954.

153. Richter HK, K. Kleinwechter, H. Demandt, N. Meincke, G. Dabelstein, A. Weisser, B. [Effects of a telephone intervention in patients with type 2 diabetes]. Dtsch Med Wochenschr. 2008 Oct;133(43):2203-8. PMID 18924053.

154. Riddle MCR, J. Gerich, J. The treat-to-target trial: randomized addition of glargine or human NPH insulin to oral therapy of type 2 diabetic patients. Diabetes Care. 2003 Nov;26(11):3080-6. PMID 14578243.

155. Rizkalla SWT, L. Laromiguiere, M. Huet, D. Boillot, J. Rigoir, A. Elgrably, F. Slama, G. Improved plasma glucose control, whole-body glucose utilization, and lipid profile on a low-glycemic index diet in type 2 diabetic men: a randomized controlled trial. Diabetes Care. 2004 Aug;27(8):1866-72. PMID 15277409.

156. Rodriguez-Villar CM, J. M. Casals, E. Perez-Heras, A. Zambon, D. Gomis, R. Ros, E. High-monounsaturated fat, olive oil-rich diet has effects similar to a high-carbohydrate diet on fasting and postprandial state and metabolic profiles of patients with type 2 diabetes. Metabolism. 2000 Dec;49(12):1511-7. PMID 11145109.

157. Roger PA, J. Drain, P. Addition of benfluorex to biguanide improves glycemic control in obese non-insulin-dependent diabetes: a double-blind study versus placebo. J Diabetes Complications. 1999 Mar-Apr;13(2):62-7. PMID 10432168.

158. Ronnemaa TM, J. Puukka, P. Kuusi, T. Effects of long-term physical exercise on serum lipids, lipoproteins and lipid metabolizing enzymes in type 2 (non-insulin-dependent) diabetic patients. Diabetes Res. 1988 Feb;7(2):79-84. PMID 3396267.

159. Rosenstock JE, D. Hershon, K. Glazer, N. B. Yu, S. Efficacy and safety of pioglitazone in type 2 diabetes: a randomised, placebo-controlled study in patients receiving stable insulin therapy. Int J Clin Pract. 2002 May;56(4):251-7. PMID 12074206.

160. Rosenstock JR, J. Bush, M. Yang, F. Stewart, M. Potential of albiglutide, a long-acting GLP-1 receptor agonist, in type 2 diabetes: a randomized controlled trial exploring weekly, biweekly, and monthly dosing. Diabetes Care. 2009 Oct;32(10):1880-6. PMID 19592625.

161. Ruderman NBG, O. P. Johansen, K. The effect of physical training on glucose tolerance and plasma lipids in maturity-onset diabetes. Diabetes. 1979 Jan;28 Suppl 1:89-92. PMID 761721.

162. Rudnick PAT, K. W. Effect of Prolonged Carbohydrate Restriction on Serum-Insulin Levels in Mild Diabetes. Br Med J. 1965 May 8;1(5444):1225-8. PMID 14275022.

163. Sahin MT, N. B. Ertugrul, D. Tanaci, N. Guvener, N. D. Effects of metformin or rosiglitazone on serum concentrations of homocysteine, folate, and vitamin B12 in patients with type 2 diabetes mellitus. J Diabetes Complications. 2007 Mar-Apr;21(2):118-23. PMID 17331860.

164. Saldalamacchia GM, P. Pacioni, D. Giordano, C. Tia, V. N. Pellegrino, S. Lilli, S. Riccardi, G. Rivellese, A. A. Weight loss in obese type 2 diabetic patients on an intensive therapeutic programme: Importance of an initial short hospitalization period. Nutr Metab Cardiovasc Dis. 2008 Feb;18(2):e1-2. PMID 18029160.

165. Salman SS, F. Satman, I. Yilmaz, Y. Ozer, E. Sengul, A. Demirel, H. O. Karsidag, K. Dinccag, N. Yilmaz, M. T. Comparison of acarbose and gliclazide as first-line agents in patients with type 2 diabetes. Curr Med Res Opin. 2001;16(4):296-306. PMID 11268714.

166. Sanchez-Tainta AE, R. Bullo, M. Corella, D. Gomez-Gracia, E. Fiol, M. Algorta, J. Covas, M. I. Lapetra, J. Zazpe, I. Ruiz-Gutierrez, V. Ros, E. Martinez-Gonzalez, M. A. Adherence to a Mediterranean-type diet and reduced prevalence of clustered cardiovascular risk factors in a cohort of 3,204 high-risk patients. Eur J Cardiovasc Prev Rehabil. 2008 Oct;15(5):589-93. PMID 18830087.

167. Sargrad KRH, C. Mozzoli, M. Boden, G. Effect of high protein vs high carbohydrate intake on insulin sensitivity, body weight, hemoglobin A1c, and blood pressure in patients with type 2 diabetes mellitus. J Am Diet Assoc. 2005 Apr;105(4):573-80. PMID 15800559.

168. Scarlett JAG, R. S. Griffin, J. Olefsky, J. M. Kolterman, O. G. Insulin treatment reverses the insulin resistance of type II diabetes mellitus. Diabetes Care. 1982 Jul-Aug;5(4):353-63. PMID 6759075.

169. Schnack CR, G. Luger, A. Schernthaner, G. Effects of the alpha-glucosidase inhibitor 1 desoxynojirimycin (Bay m 1099) on postprandial blood glucose, serum insulin and C-peptide levels in type II diabetic patients. Eur J Clin Pharmacol. 1986;30(4):417-9. PMID 3527720.

170. Scott RW, M. Sanchez, M. Stein, P. Efficacy and tolerability of the dipeptidyl peptidase-4 inhibitor sitagliptin as monotherapy over 12 weeks in patients with type 2 diabetes. Int J Clin Pract. 2007 Jan;61(1):171-80. PMID 17156104.

171. Segal KRE, A. Abalos, A. Albu, J. Blando, L. Tomas, M. B. Pi-Sunyer, F. X. Effect of exercise training on insulin sensitivity and glucose metabolism in lean, obese, and diabetic men. J Appl Physiol. 1991 Dec;71(6):2402-11. PMID 1778939.

172. Shahar DRA, R. Elhayany, A. Vardi, H. Fraser, D. Does dairy calcium intake enhance weight loss among overweight diabetic patients? Diabetes Care. 2007 Mar;30(3):485-9. PMID 17327309.

173. Shaw KMW, M. S. Campbell, D. B. Ward, J. D. Home blood glucose monitoring in non-insulin-dependent diabetics: the effect of gliclazide on blood glucose and weight control, a multicentre trial. Diabet Med. 1985 Nov;2(6):484-90. PMID 2951123.

174. Shi YFP, C. Y. Hill, J. Gao, Y. Orlistat in the treatment of overweight or obese Chinese patients with newly diagnosed Type 2 diabetes. Diabet Med. 2005 Dec;22(12):1737-43. PMID 16401321.

175. Simpson HCS, R. W. Lousley, S. Carter, R. D. Geekie, M. Hockaday, T. D. Mann, J. I. A high carbohydrate leguminous fibre diet improves all aspects of diabetic control. Lancet. 1981 Jan 3;1(8210):1-5. PMID 6109047.

176. Slama GS, A. Hautecouverture, M. Tchobroutsky, G. Double blind clinical trial of mazindol on weight loss blood glucose, plasma insulin and serum lipids in overweight diabetic patients. Diabete Metab. 1978 Sep;4(3):193-9. PMID 361463.

177. Smutok MAR, C. Kokkinos, P. F. Farmer, C. M. Dawson, P. K. DeVane, J. Patterson, J. Goldberg, A. P. Hurley, B. F. Effects of exercise training modality on glucose tolerance in men with abnormal glucose regulation. Int J Sports Med. 1994 Aug;15(6):283-9. PMID 7822064.

178. Solomon TPH, J. M. Kelly, K. R. Cook, M. D. Riccardi, M. Rocco, M. Kashyap, S. R. Barkoukis, H. Kirwan, J. P. Randomized trial on the effects of a 7-d low-glycemic diet and exercise intervention on insulin resistance in older obese humans. Am J Clin Nutr. 2009 Nov;90(5):1222-9. PMID 19793849.

179. Sun JW, Y. Chen, X. Chen, Y. Feng, Y. Zhang, X. Pan, Y. Hu, T. Xu, J. Du, L. Zhou, W. Zhao, H. Riley, R. E. Mustad, V. A. An integrated intervention program to control diabetes in overweight Chinese women and men with type 2 diabetes. Asia Pac J Clin Nutr. 2008;17(3):514-24. PMID 18818173.

180. Suter SLN, J. J. Wallace, P. Gumbiner, B. Olefsky, J. M. Metabolic effects of new oral hypoglycemic agent CS-045 in NIDDM subjects. Diabetes Care. 1992 Feb;15(2):193-203. PMID 1547676.

181. Takami KT, N. Nakashima, K. Takami, R. Hayashi, M. Ozeki, S. Yamada, A. Kokubo, Y. Sato, M. Kawachi, S. Sasaki, A. Yasuda, K. Effects of dietary treatment alone or diet with voglibose or glyburide on abdominal adipose tissue and metabolic abnormalities in patients with newly diagnosed type 2 diabetes. Diabetes Care. 2002 Apr;25(4):658-62. PMID 11919121.

182. Tankova TD, G. Lazarova, M. Dakovska, L. Kirilov, G. Koev, D. Sibutramine in the treatment of obesity in type 2 diabetic patients and in nondiabetic subjects. Acta Diabetol. 2004 Dec;41(4):146-53. PMID 15660196.

183. Tariq SHK, E. Thomas, D. R. Thomson, K. Philpot, C. Chapel, D. L. Morley, J. E. The use of a no-concentrated-sweets diet in the management of type 2 diabetes in nursing homes. J Am Diet Assoc. 2001 Dec;101(12):1463-6. PMID 11762744.

184. Trovati MC, Q. Cavalot, F. Vitali, S. Banaudi, C. Lucchina, P. G. Fiocchi, F. Emanuelli, G. Lenti, G. Influence of physical training on blood glucose control, glucose tolerance, insulin secretion, and insulin action in non-insulin-dependent diabetic patients. Diabetes Care. 1984 Sep-Oct;7(5):416-20. PMID 6389056.

185. Turner-McGrievy GMB, N. D. Cohen, J. Jenkins, D. J. Gloede, L. Green, A. A. Changes in nutrient intake and dietary quality among participants with type 2 diabetes following a low-fat vegan diet or a conventional diabetes diet for 22 weeks. J Am Diet Assoc. 2008 Oct;108(10):1636-45. PMID 18926128.

186. Uusitupa ML, M. Sarlund, H. Majander, H. Takala, J. Penttila, I. Long term effects of a very low calorie diet on metabolic control and cardiovascular risk factors in the treatment of obese non-insulin-dependent diabetics. Int J Obes. 1989;13 Suppl 2:163-4. PMID 2613415.

187. Valensi PM, I. Le Magoarou, M. Paries, J. Perret, G. Attali, J. R. Short-term effects of continuous subcutaneous insulin infusion treatment on insulin secretion in non-insulin-dependent overweight patients with poor glycaemic control despite maximal oral anti-diabetic treatment. Diabetes Metab. 1997 Feb;23(1):51-7. PMID 9059766.

188. Van Duyn MAL, T. A. McIvor, M. E. Behall, K. M. Michnowski, J. E. Mendeloff, A. I. Nutritional risk of high-carbohydrate, guar gum dietary supplementation in non-insulin-dependent diabetes mellitus. Diabetes Care. 1986 Sep-Oct;9(5):497-503. PMID 3021407.

189. Vancea DMMV, José Nelson Pires, Maria Izabel Fernandes Reis, Marco Antonio Moura, Rafael Brandão Dib, Sergio Atala. Effect of frequency of physical exercise on glycemic control and body composition in type 2 diabetic patients. Arquivos Brasileiros de Cardiologia. 2009;92:23-30.

190. Verdy MC, L. Verdy, I. Belanger, R. Bolte, E. Chiasson, J. L. Fenfluramine in the treatment of non-insulin-dependent diabetics: hypoglycemic versus anorectic effect. Int J Obes. 1983;7(4):289-97. PMID 6629637.

191. Vernon MCM, J. Transue, M. Yancy, W. S. Westman, E. C. Clinical experience of a carbohydrate-restricted diet: effect on diabetes mellitus. Metab Syndr Relat Disord. 2003 Sep;1(3):233-7. PMID 18370667.

192. Vukovic ML, M. Kalezic, N. Gvozdenovic, B. S. [The effect of metformin on fasting and postprandial insulin secretion in obese patients with diabetes mellitus type 2]. Srp Arh Celok Lek. 2007 Jul-Aug;135(7-8):447-52. PMID 17929538.

193. Vuksan VJ, D. J. Spadafora, P. Sievenpiper, J. L. Owen, R. Vidgen, E. Brighenti, F. Josse, R. Leiter, L. A. Bruce-Thompson, C. Konjac-mannan (glucomannan) improves glycemia and other associated risk factors for coronary heart disease in type 2 diabetes. A randomized controlled metabolic trial. Diabetes Care. 1999 Jun;22(6):913-9. PMID 10372241.

194. Wales JK. The effect of fenfluramine on obese, maturity-onset diabetic patients. Acta Endocrinol (Copenh). 1979 Apr;90(4):616-23. PMID 373358.

195. Wall JRP, D. A. Oakley, W. G. Effect of carbohydrate restriction in obese diabetics: relationship of control to weight loss. Br Med J. 1973 Mar 10;1(5853):577-8. PMID 4694404.

196. Wang TFP, D. Li, J. C. Tsai, W. C. Tsai, C. C. Yao, C. Y. Chang, E. T. Hsieh, M. C. Su, K. Y. Kuo, S. W. Effects of sibutramine in overweight, poorly controlled Chinese female type 2 diabetic patients: a randomised, double-blind, placebo-controlled study. Int J Clin Pract. 2005 Jul;59(7):746-50. PMID 15963197.

197. Watanabe MO, A. Shimamoto, K. Ueshima, H. Short-term effectiveness of an individual counseling program for impaired fasting glucose and mild type 2 diabetes in Japan: a multi-center randomized control trial. Asia Pac J Clin Nutr. 2007;16(3):489-97. PMID 17704031.

198. Weinsier RLS, A. Herrera, M. G. Assal, J. P. Soeldner, J. S. Gleason, R. E. High- and low-carbohydrate diets in diabetes mellitus. Study of effects on diabetic control, insulin secretion, and blood lipids. Ann Intern Med. 1974 Mar;80(3):332-41. PMID 4816173.

199. Willey KAM, L. M. Overland, J. E. Yue, D. K. The effects of dexfenfluramine on blood glucose control in patients with type 2 diabetes. Diabet Med. 1992 May;9(4):341-3. PMID 1600704.

200. Willms BR, D. Comparison of acarbose and metformin in patients with Type 2 diabetes mellitus insufficiently controlled with diet and sulphonylureas: a randomized, placebo-controlled study. Diabet Med. 1999 Sep;16(9):755-61. PMID 10510952.

201. Wing RRN, M. P. Epstein, L. H. Koeske, R. Calorie-counting compared to exchange system diets in the treatment of overweight patients with type II diabetes. Addict Behav. 1986;11(2):163-8. PMID 3739801.

202. Winnick JJG, T. Schuster, D. P. Resistance training differentially affects weight loss and glucose metabolism of White and African American patients with type 2 diabetes mellitus. Ethn Dis. 2008 Spring;18(2):152-6. PMID 18507266.

203. Winnick JJS, W. M. Habash, D. L. Stout, M. B. Failla, M. L. Belury, M. A. Schuster, D. P. Short-term aerobic exercise training in obese humans with type 2 diabetes mellitus improves whole-body insulin sensitivity through gains in peripheral, not hepatic insulin sensitivity. J Clin Endocrinol Metab. 2008 Mar;93(3):771-8. PMID 18073312.

204. Wolffenbuttel BHW, R. F. Van Koetsveld, P. M. Verschoor, L. Limitations of diet therapy in patients with non-insulin-dependent diabetes mellitus. Int J Obes. 1989;13(2):173-82. PMID 2744929.

205. Woo JS, M. M. Tong, P. Ko, G. T. Lee, Z. Chan, J. Chow, F. C. Effectiveness of a lifestyle modification programme in weight maintenance in obese subjects after cessation of treatment with Orlistat. J Eval Clin Pract. 2007 Dec;13(6):853-9. PMID 18070255.

206. Wycherley TPB, G. D. Noakes, M. Buckley, J. D. Clifton, P. M. Effect of caloric restriction with and without exercise training on oxidative stress and endothelial function in obese subjects with type 2 diabetes. Diabetes Obes Metab. 2008 Nov;10(11):1062-73. PMID 18435772.

207. Yamanouchi KS, T. Chikada, K. Nishikawa, T. Ito, K. Shimizu, S. Ozawa, N. Suzuki, Y. Maeno, H. Kato, K. et al.,. Daily walking combined with diet therapy is a useful means for obese NIDDM patients not only to reduce body weight but also to improve insulin sensitivity. Diabetes Care. 1995 Jun;18(6):775-8. PMID 7555502.

208. Yancy WS, Jr. Olsen, M. K. Guyton, J. R. Bakst, R. P. Westman, E. C. A low-carbohydrate, ketogenic diet versus a low-fat diet to treat obesity and hyperlipidemia: a randomized, controlled trial. Ann Intern Med. 2004 May 18;140(10):769-77. PMID 15148063.

209. Yip IG, V. L. DeShields, S. Saltsman, P. Bellman, M. Thames, G. Murray, S. Wang, H. J. Elashoff, R. Heber, D. Liquid meal replacements and glycemic control in obese type 2 diabetes patients. Obes Res. 2001 Nov;9 Suppl 4:341S-7S. PMID 11707563.

210. Ziemer DCB, K. J. Panayioto, R. M. El-Kebbi, I. M. Musey, V. C. Anderson, L. A. Wanko, N. S. Fowke, M. L. Brazier, C. W. Dunbar, V. G. Slocum, W. Bacha, G. M. Gallina, D. L. Cook, C. B. Phillips, L. S. A simple meal plan emphasizing healthy food choices is as effective as an exchange-based meal plan for urban African Americans with type 2 diabetes. Diabetes Care. 2003 Jun;26(6):1719-24. PMID 12766100.

Reject Published Before 1990:

1. Ackerman NB. Observations on the improvements in carbohydrate metabolism in diabetic and other morbidly obese patients after jejunoileal bypass. Surg Gynecol Obstet. 1981 May;152(5):581-6. PMID 7013122.

2. Bendezu RW, R. G. Green, S. G. Hallberg, M. C. Marsters, R. W. Certain metabolic consequences of jejunoileal bypass. Am J Clin Nutr. 1976 Apr;29(4):366-70. PMID 1266786.

3. Buchwald H. Ileal bypass in the treatment of the hyperlipidemias. J Atheroscler Res. 1969 Jul-Aug;10(1):1-4. PMID 5380901.

4. Buchwald H. Lowering of Cholesterol Absorption and Blood Levels by Ileal Exclusion. Experimental Basis and Preliminary Clinical Report. Circulation. 1964 May;29:713-20. PMID 14156865.

5. Buchwald HM, R. B. Frantz, I. D., Jr. Varco, R. L. Cholesterol reduction by partial ileal bypass in a pediatric population. Surgery. 1970 Dec;68(6):1101-11. PMID 5483243.

6. Buchwald HV, R. L. Partial ileal bypass for hypercholesterolemia and atherosclerosis. Surg Gynecol Obstet. 1967 Jun;124(6):1231-8. PMID 6024201.

7. Dobrea GMW, R. G. Johnson, M. W. The effect of rapid weight loss due to jejunoileal bypass on total cholesterol and high-density lipoprotein. Am J Clin Nutr. 1981 Oct;34(10):1994-6. PMID 7293931.

8. Flickinger EGP, W. J. Meelheim, H. D. Sinar, D. R. Blose, I. L. Thomas, F. T. The Greenville gastric bypass. Progress report at 3 years. Ann Surg. 1984 May;199(5):555-62. PMID 6721605.

9. Gleysteen JJB, J. J. Improvement in heart disease risk factors after gastric bypass. Arch Surg. 1983 Jun;118(6):681-4. PMID 6847361.

10. Goldberg RBW, R. B. Landau, R. L. Changes in plasma apolipoproteins A-I, A-II, and B, and lipoprotein cholesterol after jejunoileal bypass. Gastroenterology. 1983 Apr;84(4):732-6. PMID 6402411.

11. Gomez CA. Gastroplasty in the surgical treatment of morbid obesity. Am J Clin Nutr. 1980 Feb;33(2 Suppl):406-15. PMID 7355812.

12. Gonen BH, J. D. Schonfeld, G. Lipoprotein levels in morbidly obese patients with massive, surgically-induced weight loss. Metabolism. 1983 May;32(5):492-6. PMID 6843360.

13. Halverson JDK, J. Cave, A. Permutt, A. Santiago, J. Altered glucose tolerance, insulin response, and insulin sensitivity after massive weight reduction subsequent to gastric bypass. Surgery. 1982 Aug;92(2):235-40. PMID 7048596.

14. Hardie GHS, G. CoBabe, T. Gastric bypass: a safe, effective procedure? Wis Med J. 1979 Nov;78(11):34-8. PMID 516786.

15. Herbst CAH, T. A. Gwynne, J. T. Buckwalter, J. A. Gastric bariatric operation in insulin-treated adults. Surgery. 1984 Feb;95(2):209-14. PMID 6364435.

16. Hocking MPD, M. C. O'Leary, J. P. Woodward, E. R. Jejunoileal bypass for morbid obesity. Late follow-up in 100 cases. N Engl J Med. 1983 Apr 28;308(17):995-9. PMID 6835318.

17. Holt JBC, C. L. Trowbridge, P. E. Immediate and long-term results of vertical banded gastroplasty for morbid obesity. Conn Med. 1987 Oct;51(10):638-42. PMID 3677666.

18. Hughes TAG, J. T. Switzer, B. R. Herbst, C. White, G. Effects of caloric restriction and weight loss on glycemic control, insulin release and resistance, and atherosclerotic risk in obese patients with type II diabetes mellitus. Am J Med. 1984 Jul;77(1):7-17. PMID 6377892.

19. Lewis LAT, R. B., Jr. Page, I. H. Effects of jejunocolic shunt on obesity, serum lipoproteins, lipids, and electrolytes. Arch Intern Med. 1966 Jan;117(1):4-16. PMID 5900488.

20. Mason EEI, C. Gastric bypass in obesity. Surg Clin North Am. 1967 Dec;47(6):1345-51. PMID 6073761.

21. Moore RBB, H. Varco, R. L. The effect of partial ileal bypass on plasma lipoproteins. Circulation. 1980 Sep;62(3):469-76. PMID 7398005.

22. Naslund I. Gastric bypass versus gastroplasty. A prospective study of differences in two surgical procedures for morbid obesity. Acta Chir Scand Suppl. 1987;536:1-60. PMID 3475886.

23. Naslund IW, G. Christoffersson, E. Agren, G. A prospective randomized comparison of gastric bypass and gastroplasty. Complications and early results. Acta Chir Scand. 1986 Nov;152:681-9. PMID 3551425.

24. Olsson SAP, B. G. Sorbris, R. Nilsson-Ehle, P. Effects of weight reduction after gastroplasty on glucose and lipid metabolism. Am J Clin Nutr. 1984 Dec;40(6):1273-80. PMID 6391138.

25. Payne JHD, L. T. Surgical treatment of obesity. Am J Surg. 1969 Aug;118(2):141-7. PMID 5798387.

26. Pories WJC, J. F. Flickinger, E. G. Meelheim, H. D. Swanson, M. S. The control of diabetes mellitus (NIDDM) in the morbidly obese with the Greenville Gastric Bypass. Ann Surg. 1987 Sep;206(3):316-23. PMID 3632094.

27. Pories WJF, E. G. Meelheim, D. Van Rij, A. M. Thomas, F. T. The effectiveness of gastric bypass over gastric partition in morbid obesity: consequence of distal gastric and duodenal exclusion. Ann Surg. 1982 Oct;196(4):389-99. PMID 7125726.

28. Quaade FB, O. Stokholm, K. H. Andersen, T. The Copenhagen PLAFA project: a randomized trial of gastroplasty versus very-low-calorie diet in the treatment of severe obesity (preliminary results). Int J Obes. 1981;5(3):257-61. PMID 7024154.

29. Ranlov PJ. Serum lipid changes after gastroplasty for morbid obesity. Acta Med Scand. 1984;216(5):503-8. PMID 6524454.

30. Rossner SH, D. Serum lipoproteins in massive obesity. A study and after jejunoileal shunt operation. Acta Med Scand. 1978;204(1-2):103-10. PMID 210633.

31. Rucker RD, Jr. Goldenberg, F. Varco, R. L. Buchwald, H. Lipid effects of obesity operations. J Surg Res. 1981 Mar;30(3):229-35. PMID 7230770.

32. Sanderson ID, M. Bojm, M. A. The handling of glucose and insulin response before and after weight loss with jejuno-ileal bypass: a preliminary report. JPEN J Parenter Enteral Nutr. 1983 May-Jun;7(3):274-6. PMID 6345839.

33. Schrumpf EB, A. Djoseland, O. Fausa, O. Flaten, O. Skagen, D. W. Tronier, B. The effect of gastric bypass operation on glucose tolerance in obesity. Scand J Gastroenterol Suppl. 1985;107:24-31. PMID 3885381.

34. Schwartz RWS, W. E. Simpson, W. S. Griffen, W. O., Jr. Gastric bypass revision: lessons learned from 920 cases. Surgery. 1988 Oct;104(4):806-12. PMID 3051478.

35. Scott HW, Jr. Dean, R. H. Younger, R. K. Butts, W. H. Changes in hyperlipidemia and hyperlipoproteinemia in morbidly obese patients treated by jejunoileal bypass. Surg Gynecol Obstet. 1974 Mar;138(3):353-8. PMID 4811320.

36. Scott HW, Jr. Dean, R. H. Shull, H. J. Gluck, F. Results of jejunoileal bypass in two hundred patients with morbid obesity. Surg Gynecol Obstet. 1977 Nov;145(5):661-73. PMID 910208.

37. Sherman CD, Jr. May, A. G. Nye, W. Waterhouse, C. Clinical and metabolic studies following bowel by-passing for obesity. Ann N Y Acad Sci. 1965 Oct 8;131(1):614-22. PMID 5216995.

38. Shibata HRM, J. R. Long, R. C. Metabolic effects of controlled jejunocolic bypass. Arch Surg. 1967 Sep;95(3):413-28. PMID 6035465.

39. Solhaug JHG, I. Metabolic changes after jejuno-ileal bypass for obesity. Scand J Gastroenterol. 1978;13(2):169-75. PMID 635457.

40. Sugerman HJS, J. V. Birkenhauer, R. A randomized prospective trial of gastric bypass versus vertical banded gastroplasty for morbid obesity and their effects on sweets versus non-sweets eaters. Ann Surg. 1987 Jun;205(6):613-24. PMID 3296971.

41. Vessby BB, M. Lindahl, B. Lithell, H. Thoren, L. Werner, I. Serum lipoprotein lipid and apolipoprotein concentrations in grossly obese patients before and after jejuno-ileal shunt operation. Eur J Clin Invest. 1981 Feb;11(1):49-54. PMID 6783429.

42. Yale CE. Gastric surgery for morbid obesity. Complications and long-term weight control. Arch Surg. 1989 Aug;124(8):941-6. PMID 2757508.

Reject Treatment Not of Interest:

1. Ahn SM, Pomp A, Rubino F. Metabolic surgery for type 2 diabetes. Ann N Y Acad Sci. 2010 Nov;1212(1):E37-45. PMID 21732953.

2. Babio NB, M. Basora, J. Martinez-Gonzalez, M. A. Fernandez-Ballart, J. Marquez-Sandoval, F. Molina, C. Salas-Salvado, J. Adherence to the Mediterranean diet and risk of metabolic syndrome and its components. Nutr Metab Cardiovasc Dis. 2009 Oct;19(8):563-70. PMID 19176282.

3. Belcher GL, C. Goh, K. L. Edwards, G. Valbuena, M. Cardiovascular effects of treatment of type 2 diabetes with pioglitazone, metformin and gliclazide. Int J Clin Pract. 2004 Sep;58(9):833-7. PMID 15529516.

4. Berne C. A randomized study of orlistat in combination with a weight management programme in obese patients with Type 2 diabetes treated with metformin. Diabet Med. 2005 May;22(5):612-8. PMID 15842517.

5. Berry M. Metabolic surgery in non obese type 2 diabetic patients. Obesity Surgery. 2010;20(8):981.

6. Birkeland KIR, U. Hanssen, K. F. Vaaler, S. NIDDM: a rapid progressive disease. Results from a long-term, randomised, comparative study of insulin or sulphonylurea treatment. Diabetologia. 1996 Dec;39(12):1629-33. PMID 8960854.

7. Bravard A, Lefai E, Meugnier E, et al. FTO is increased in muscle during type 2 diabetes, and its overexpression in myotubes alters insulin signaling, enhances lipogenesis and ROS production, and induces mitochondrial dysfunction. Diabetes. 2011 Jan;60(1):258-68. PMID 20943749.

8. Buse JBK, D. C. Nielsen, L. L. Guan, X. Bowlus, C. L. Holcombe, J. H. Maggs, D. G. Wintle, M. E. Metabolic effects of two years of exenatide treatment on diabetes, obesity, and hepatic biomarkers in patients with type 2 diabetes: an interim analysis of data from the open-label, uncontrolled extension of three double-blind, placebo-controlled trials. Clin Ther. 2007 Jan;29(1):139-53. PMID 17379054.

9. Campbell IWM, D. G. Chalmers, J. McBain, A. M. Brown, I. R. One year comparative trial of metformin and glipizide in type 2 diabetes mellitus. Diabete Metab. 1994 Jul-Aug;20(4):394-400. PMID 7843470.

10. Castagneto MDG, A. Mingrone, G. Tacchino, R. Nanni, G. Capristo, E. Benedetti, G. Tataranni, P. A. Greco, A. V. Normalization of Insulin Sensitivity in the Obese Patient after Stable Weight Reduction with Biliopancreatic Diversion. Obes Surg. 1994 May;4(2):161-8. PMID 10742775.

11. Chiasson JLJ, R. G. Hunt, J. A. Palmason, C. Rodger, N. W. Ross, S. A. Ryan, E. A. Tan, M. H. Wolever, T. M. The efficacy of acarbose in the treatment of patients with non-insulin-dependent diabetes mellitus. A multicenter controlled clinical trial. Ann Intern Med. 1994 Dec 15;121(12):928-35. PMID 7734015.

12. Clark MH, S. E. Implementing a psychological intervention to improve lifestyle self-management in patients with type 2 diabetes. Patient Educ Couns. 2001 Mar;42(3):247-56. PMID 11164324.

13. Clarke BFD, L. J. Comparison of chlorpropamide and metformin treatment on weight and blood-glucose response of uncontrolled obese diabetics. Lancet. 1968 Jan 20;1(7534):123-6. PMID 4169605.

14. Dansinger MLG, J. A. Griffith, J. L. Selker, H. P. Schaefer, E. J. Comparison of the Atkins, Ornish, Weight Watchers, and Zone diets for weight loss and heart disease risk reduction: a randomized trial. JAMA. 2005 Jan 5;293(1):43-53. PMID 15632335.

15. de Fine Olivarius NA, A. H. Siersma, V. Richelsen, B. Beck-Nielsen, H. Changes in patient weight and the impact of antidiabetic therapy during the first 5 years after diagnosis of diabetes mellitus. Diabetologia. 2006 Sep;49(9):2058-67. PMID 16841232.

16. De Paula ALS, A. R. Macedo, A. Ribamar, J. Mancini, M. Halpern, A. Vencio, S. Prospective randomized controlled trial comparing 2 versions of laparoscopic ileal interposition associated with sleeve gastrectomy for patients with type 2 diabetes with BMI 21-34 kg/m(2). Surg Obes Relat Dis. 2010 May-Jun;6(3):296-304. PMID 20096647.

17. DePaula ALM, A. L. Schraibman, V. Mota, B. R. Vencio, S. Hormonal evaluation following laparoscopic treatment of type 2 diabetes mellitus patients with BMI 20-34. Surg Endosc. 2009 Aug;23(8):1724-32. PMID 18830747.

18. DePaula ALM, A. L. Mota, B. R. Schraibman, V. Laparoscopic ileal interposition associated to a diverted sleeve gastrectomy is an effective operation for the treatment of type 2 diabetes mellitus patients with BMI 21-29. Surg Endosc. 2009 Jun;23(6):1313-20. PMID 18830750.

19. DePaula ALM, A. L. Rassi, N. Vencio, S. Machado, C. A. Mota, B. R. Silva, L. Q. Halpern, A. Schraibman, V. Laparoscopic treatment of metabolic syndrome in patients with type 2 diabetes mellitus. Surg Endosc. 2008 Dec;22(12):2670-8. PMID 18347866.

20. DePaula ALM, A. L. Rassi, N. Machado, C. A. Schraibman, V. Silva, L. Q. Halpern, A. Laparoscopic treatment of type 2 diabetes mellitus for patients with a body mass index less than 35. Surg Endosc. 2008 Mar;22(3):706-16. PMID 17704886.

21. DePaula ALS, A. R. DePaula, C. C. Halpern, A. Vencio, S. Impact on dyslipidemia of the laparoscopic ileal interposition associated to sleeve gastrectomy in type 2 diabetic patients. J Gastrointest Surg. 2010 Aug;14(8):1319-25. PMID 20556664.

22. Depaula ALS, A. Halpern, A. Vencio, S. Thirty-Day Morbidity and Mortality of the Laparoscopic Ileal Interposition Associated with Sleeve Gastrectomy for the Treatment of Type 2 Diabetic Patients with BMI <35: An Analysis of 454 Consecutive Patients. World J Surg. 2010 Nov 3PMID 21052999.

23. Derosa GC, A. F. Murdolo, G. Ciccarelli, L. Fogari, R. Comparison of metabolic effects of orlistat and sibutramine treatment in Type 2 diabetic obese patients. Diabetes Nutr Metab. 2004 Aug;17(4):222-9. PMID 15575343.

24. Derosa GC, A. F. Gaddi, A. Ragonesi, P. D. Fogari, E. Bertone, G. Ciccarelli, L. Piccinni, M. N. Metabolic effects of pioglitazone and rosiglitazone in patients with diabetes and metabolic syndrome treated with glimepiride: a twelve-month, multicenter, double-blind, randomized, controlled, parallel-group trial. Clin Ther. 2004 May;26(5):744-54. PMID 15220018.

25. Derosa GDA, A. Ragonesi, P. D. Ciccarelli, L. Piccinni, M. N. Pricolo, F. Salvadeo, S. A. Montagna, L. Gravina, A. Ferrari, I. Paniga, S. Cicero, A. F. Metabolic effects of pioglitazone and rosiglitazone in patients with diabetes and metabolic syndrome treated with metformin. Intern Med J. 2007 Feb;37(2):79-86. PMID 17229249.

26. Ferzli GSD, E. Ciaglia, M. Bluth, M. H. Gonzalez, A. Fingerhut, A. Clinical improvement after duodenojejunal bypass for nonobese type 2 diabetes despite minimal improvement in glycemic homeostasis. World J Surg. 2009 May;33(5):972-9. PMID 19288284.

27. Draeger KEW-P, K. Lomp, H. J. Schuler, E. Rosskamp, R. Long-term treatment of type 2 diabetic patients with the new oral antidiabetic agent glimepiride (Amaryl): a double-blind comparison with glibenclamide. Horm Metab Res. 1996 Sep;28(9):419-25. PMID 8911976.

28. Gerstein HCM, M. E. Byington, R. P. Goff, D. C., Jr. Bigger, J. T. Buse, J. B. Cushman, W. C. Genuth, S. Ismail-Beigi, F. Grimm, R. H., Jr. Probstfield, J. L. Simons-Morton, D. G. Friedewald, W. T. Effects of intensive glucose lowering in type 2 diabetes. N Engl J Med. 2008 Jun 12;358(24):2545-59. PMID 18539917.

29. Goel R, Amin P, Goel M, et al. Early resolution of type 2 diabetes mellitus by laparoscopic ileal transposition with sleeve gastrectomy surgery in 23 - 35 BMI patients. Obesity Reviews. 2010;11:254.

30. Goke BH, K. Kerr, D. Calle Pascual, A. Schweizer, A. Foley, J. Shao, Q. Dejager, S. Efficacy and safety of vildagliptin monotherapy during 2-year treatment of drug-naive patients with type 2 diabetes: comparison with metformin. Horm Metab Res. 2008 Dec;40(12):892-5. PMID 18726829.

31. Harrower AD. Comparison of diabetic control in type 2 (non-insulin dependent) diabetic patients treated with different sulphonylureas. Curr Med Res Opin. 1985;9(10):676-80. PMID 3935376.

32. Hollander PAL, P. Fineman, M. S. Maggs, D. G. Shen, L. Z. Strobel, S. A. Weyer, C. Kolterman, O. G. Pramlintide as an adjunct to insulin therapy improves long-term glycemic and weight control in patients with type 2 diabetes: a 1-year randomized controlled trial. Diabetes Care. 2003 Mar;26(3):784-90. PMID 12610038.

33. Holman RRT, K. I. Farmer, A. J. Davies, M. J. Keenan, J. F. Paul, S. Levy, J. C. Addition of biphasic, prandial, or basal insulin to oral therapy in type 2 diabetes. N Engl J Med. 2007 Oct 25;357(17):1716-30. PMID 17890232.

34. Horton ESW, F. Ghazzi, M. N. Venable, T. C. Whitcomb, R. W. Troglitazone in combination with sulfonylurea restores glycemic control in patients with type 2 diabetes. The Troglitazone Study Group. Diabetes Care. 1998 Sep;21(9):1462-9. PMID 9727892.

35. James SAJ, L. Raghunathan, T. E. Strogatz, D. S. Furth, E. D. Khazanie, P. G. Physical activity and NIDDM in African-Americans. The Pitt County Study. Diabetes Care. 1998 Apr;21(4):555-62. PMID 9571342.

36. Josse RG. Acarbose for the treatment of type II diabetes: the results of a Canadian multi-centre trial. Diabetes Res Clin Pract. 1995 Aug;28 Suppl:S167-72. PMID 8529510.

37. Kahn SEH, S. M. Heise, M. A. Herman, W. H. Holman, R. R. Jones, N. P. Kravitz, B. G. Lachin, J. M. O'Neill, M. C. Zinman, B. Viberti, G. Glycemic durability of rosiglitazone, metformin, or glyburide monotherapy. N Engl J Med. 2006 Dec 7;355(23):2427-43. PMID 17145742.

38. Keyserling TCA, A. S. Samuel-Hodge, C. D. Ingram, A. F. Skelly, A. H. Elasy, T. A. Johnston, L. F. Cole, A. S. Henriquez-Roldan, C. F. A diabetes management program for African American women with type 2 diabetes. Diabetes Educ. 2000 Sep-Oct;26(5):796-805. PMID 11140007.

39. Knowler WCH, R. F. Edelstein, S. L. Barrett-Connor, E. Ehrmann, D. A. Walker, E. A. Fowler, S. E. Nathan, D. M. Kahn, S. E. Prevention of type 2 diabetes with troglitazone in the Diabetes Prevention Program. Diabetes. 2005 Apr;54(4):1150-6. PMID 15793255.

40. Kumar KVU, S. Gupta, N. Naik, V. Kumar, P. Bhaskar, P. Modi, K. D. Ileal interposition with sleeve gastrectomy for control of type 2 diabetes. Diabetes Technol Ther. 2009 Dec;11(12):785-9. PMID 20001679.

41. Laaksonen MK, Paul Rissanen, Harri Härkänen, Tommi Virtala, Esa Marniemi, Jukka Aromaa, Arpo Heliövaara, Markku Reunanen, Antti. The relative importance of modifiable potential risk factors of type 2 diabetes: a meta-analysis of two cohorts. European Journal of Epidemiology. 2010;25(2):115-24.

42. Manson JEN, D. M. Krolewski, A. S. Stampfer, M. J. Willett, W. C. Hennekens, C. H. A prospective study of exercise and incidence of diabetes among US male physicians. JAMA. 1992 Jul 1;268(1):63-7. PMID 1608115.

43. Merriam PAT, T. L. Rosal, M. C. Olendzki, B. C. Ma, Y. Pagoto, S. L. Ockene, I. S. Methodology of a diabetes prevention translational research project utilizing a community-academic partnership for implementation in an underserved Latino community. BMC Med Res Methodol. 2009;9:20. PMID 19284663.

44. Mertes G. Safety and efficacy of acarbose in the treatment of Type 2 diabetes: data from a 5-year surveillance study. Diabetes Res Clin Pract. 2001 Jun;52(3):193-204. PMID 11323089.

45. Ong CRM, L. M. Constantino, M. I. Twigg, S. M. Yue, D. K. Long-term efficacy of metformin therapy in nonobese individuals with type 2 diabetes. Diabetes Care. 2006 Nov;29(11):2361-4. PMID 17065668.

46. Paajanen H, Suuronen S, Nordstrom P, et al. Laparoscopic versus open cholecystectomy in diabetic patients and postoperative outcome. Surg Endosc. 2011 Mar;25(3):764-70. PMID 20661751.

47. Paisey RE, R. S. Hambley, J. Magill, P. The effects of chlorpropamide and insulin on serum lipids, lipoproteins and fractional triglyceride removal. Diabetologia. 1978 Aug;15(2):81-5. PMID 700275.

48. Ramos ACGN, M. P. de Souza, Y. M. Galvao, M. Murakami, A. H. Silva, A. C. Canseco, E. G. Santamaria, R. Zambrano, T. A. Laparoscopic duodenal-jejunal exclusion in the treatment of type 2 diabetes mellitus in patients with BMI<30 kg/m2 (LBMI). Obes Surg. 2009 Mar;19(3):307-12. PMID 18987919.

49. Ratner REM, D. Nielsen, L. L. Stonehouse, A. H. Poon, T. Zhang, B. Bicsak, T. A. Brodows, R. G. Kim, D. D. Long-term effects of exenatide therapy over 82 weeks on glycaemic control and weight in over-weight metformin-treated patients with type 2 diabetes mellitus. Diabetes Obes Metab. 2006 Jul;8(4):419-28. PMID 16776749.

50. Raz IS, V. Stein, P. Influence of small-group education sessions on glucose homeostasis in NIDDM. Diabetes Care. 1988 Jan;11(1):67-71. PMID 3338379.

51. Ribisl PML, W. Jaramillo, S. A. Jakicic, J. M. Stewart, K. J. Bahnson, J. Bright, R. Curtis, J. F. Crow, R. S. Soberman, J. E. Exercise capacity and cardiovascular/metabolic characteristics of overweight and obese individuals with type 2 diabetes: the Look AHEAD clinical trial. Diabetes Care. 2007 Oct;30(10):2679-84. PMID 17644623.

52. Riddle MCH, R. R. Poon, T. H. Zhang, B. Mac, S. M. Holcombe, J. H. Kim, D. D. Maggs, D. G. Exenatide elicits sustained glycaemic control and progressive reduction of body weight in patients with type 2 diabetes inadequately controlled by sulphonylureas with or without metformin. Diabetes Metab Res Rev. 2006 Nov-Dec;22(6):483-91. PMID 16634116.

53. Schernthaner GM, D. R. Charbonnel, B. Hanefeld, M. Brunetti, P. Efficacy and safety of pioglitazone versus metformin in patients with type 2 diabetes mellitus: a double-blind, randomized trial. J Clin Endocrinol Metab. 2004 Dec;89(12):6068-76. PMID 15579760.

54. Schouten RvD, F. M. van Gemert, W. G. Greve, J. W. Conversion of vertical banded gastroplasty to Roux-en-Y gastric bypass results in restoration of the positive effect on weight loss and co-morbidities: evaluation of 101 patients. Obes Surg. 2007 May;17(5):622-30. PMID 17658021.

55. Schrier RWE, R. O. Mehler, P. S. Hiatt, W. R. Appropriate blood pressure control in hypertensive and normotensive type 2 diabetes mellitus: a summary of the ABCD trial. Nat Clin Pract Nephrol. 2007 Aug;3(8):428-38. PMID 17653121.

56. Suter MG, V. Heraief, E. Zysset, F. Calmes, J. M. Laparoscopic gastric banding. Surg Endosc. 2003 Sep;17(9):1418-25. PMID 12802666.

57. Tan MJ, D. Gonzalez Galvez, G. Antunez, O. Fabian, G. Flores-Lozano, F. Zuniga Guajardo, S. Garza, E. Morales, H. Konkoy, C. Herz, M. Effects of pioglitazone and glimepiride on glycemic control and insulin sensitivity in Mexican patients with type 2 diabetes mellitus: A multicenter, randomized, double-blind, parallel-group trial. Clin Ther. 2004 May;26(5):680-93. PMID 15220012.

58. Taylor KGJ, W. G. Matthews, K. A. Wright, A. D. A prospective study of the effect of 12 months treatment on serum lipids and apolipoproteins A-I and B in Type 2 (non-insulin-dependent) diabetes. Diabetologia. 1982 Dec;23(6):507-10. PMID 6818080.

59. Tinoco A, El-Kadre L, Aquiar L, et al. Short-Term and Mid-Term Control of Type 2 Diabetes Mellitus by Laparoscopic Sleeve Gastrectomy with Ileal Interposition. World J Surg. 2011 Jul 9PMID 21744166.

60. UK Prospective Diabetes Study (UKPDS) Group. Effect of intensive blood-glucose control with metformin on complications in overweight patients with type 2 diabetes (UKPDS 34). The Lancet. 1998;352(9131):854-65.

61. Vencio SAC, Stival AR, De Paula AL. Assessment of insulin secretion and insulin sensitivity with the hyperglycaemic clamp in type 2 diabetic patients with BMI below 35 Kg/m2 submitted to ileal interposition associated to sleeve gastrectomy. Diabetologia. 2010;53:S43.

62. Wake NH, A. Katayama, T. Kishikawa, H. Ohkubo, Y. Sakai, M. Araki, E. Shichiri, M. Cost-effectiveness of intensive insulin therapy for type 2 diabetes: a 10-year follow-up of the Kumamoto study. Diabetes Res Clin Pract. 2000 Jun;48(3):201-10. PMID 10802159.

63. Yates TD, M. Gorely, T. Bull, F. Khunti, K. Rationale, design and baseline data from the Pre-diabetes Risk Education and Physical Activity Recommendation and Encouragement (PREPARE) programme study: a randomized controlled trial. Patient Educ Couns. 2008 Nov;73(2):264-71. PMID 18653305.

64. Zinman BH, S. B. Neuman, J. Gerstein, H. C. Retnakaran, R. R. Raboud, J. Qi, Y. Hanley, A. J. Low-dose combination therapy with rosiglitazone and metformin to prevent type 2 diabetes mellitus (CANOE trial): a double-blind randomised controlled study. Lancet. 2010 Jul 10;376(9735):103-11. PMID 20605202.

Reject Non-Surgical Already Included in Systematic Reviews:

1. Absetz PV, R. Oldenburg, B. Heinonen, H. Nissinen, A. Fogelholm, M. Ilvesmaki, V. Talja, M. Uutela, A. Type 2 diabetes prevention in the "real world": one-year results of the GOAL Implementation Trial. Diabetes Care. 2007 Oct;30(10):2465-70. PMID 17586741.

2. Ackermann RTF, E. A. Brizendine, E. Zhou, H. Marrero, D. G. Translating the Diabetes Prevention Program into the community. The DEPLOY Pilot Study. Am J Prev Med. 2008 Oct;35(4):357-63. PMID 18779029.

3. Aldana SGB, M. Smith, R. Yanowitz, F. G. Adams, T. Loveday, L. Arbuckle, J. LaMonte, M. J. The diabetes prevention program: a worksite experience. AAOHN J. 2005 Nov;53(11):499-505; quiz 6-7. PMID 16309012.

4. Anderson JWW, K. Long-term effects of high-carbohydrate, high-fiber diets on glucose and lipid metabolism: a preliminary report on patients with diabetes. Diabetes Care. 1978 Mar-Apr;1(2):77-82. PMID 729433.

5. Anderssen SAH, I. Urdal, P. Torjesen, P. A. Holme, I. Improved carbohydrate metabolism after physical training and dietary intervention in individuals with the "atherothrombogenic syndrome'. Oslo Diet and Exercise Study (ODES). A randomized trial. J Intern Med. 1996 Oct;240(4):203-9. PMID 8918511.

6. Ash SR, M. M. Yeo, S. Morrison, G. Carey, D. Capra, S. Effect of intensive dietetic interventions on weight and glycaemic control in overweight men with Type II diabetes: a randomised trial. Int J Obes Relat Metab Disord. 2003 Jul;27(7):797-802. PMID 12821964.

7. Balducci SL, F. Di Mario, U. Fallucca, F. Is a long-term aerobic plus resistance training program feasible for and effective on metabolic profiles in type 2 diabetic patients? Diabetes Care. 2004 Mar;27(3):841-2. PMID 14988317.

8. Banerji MAC, R. L. Lebovitz, H. E. Prolongation of near-normoglycemic remission in black NIDDM subjects with chronic low-dose sulfonylurea treatment. Diabetes. 1995 Apr;44(4):466-70. PMID 7698517.

9. Barnard NDC, Joshua Jenkins, David JA Turner-McGrievy, Gabrielle Gloede, Lise Green, Amber Ferdowsian, Hope. A low-fat vegan diet and a conventional diabetes diet in the treatment of type 2 diabetes: a randomized, controlled, 74-wk clinical trial. Am J Clin Nutr. 2009 May 1, 2009;89(5):1588S-96.

10. Ben-Avraham SH-B, Ilana Schwarzfuchs, Dan Shai, Iris. Dietary strategies for patients with type 2 diabetes in the era of multi-approaches; review and results from the Dietary Intervention Randomized Controlled Trial (DIRECT). Diabetes Research and Clinical Practice. 2009;86(Supplement 1):S41-S8.

11. Blonde LK, E. J. Han, J. Zhang, B. Mac, S. M. Poon, T. H. Taylor, K. L. Trautmann, M. E. Kim, D. D. Kendall, D. M. Interim analysis of the effects of exenatide treatment on A1C, weight and cardiovascular risk factors over 82 weeks in 314 overweight patients with type 2 diabetes. Diabetes Obes Metab. 2006 Jul;8(4):436-47. PMID 16776751.

12. Blonk MCJ, M. A. Biesheuvel, E. H. Weeda-Mannak, W. L. Heine, R. J. Influences on weight loss in type 2 diabetic patients: little long-term benefit from group behaviour therapy and exercise training. Diabet Med. 1994 Jun;11(5):449-57. PMID 8088122.

13. Bloomgarden ZTK, W. Metzger, M. J. Brothers, M. Nechemias, C. Bookman, J. Faierman, D. Ginsberg-Fellner, F. Rayfield, E. Brown, W. V. Randomized, controlled trial of diabetic patient education: improved knowledge without improved metabolic status. Diabetes Care. 1987 May-Jun;10(3):263-72. PMID 3297575.

14. Bo SC, G. Baldi, C. Benini, L. Dusio, F. Forastiere, G. Lucia, C. Nuti, C. Durazzo, M. Cassader, M. Gentile, L. Pagano, G. Effectiveness of a lifestyle intervention on metabolic syndrome. A randomized controlled trial. J Gen Intern Med. 2007 Dec;22(12):1695-703. PMID 17922167.

15. Boltri JMD-S, Y. M. Seale, J. P. Shellenberger, S. Okosun, I. S. Cornelius, M. E. Diabetes prevention in a faith-based setting: results of translational research. J Public Health Manag Pract. 2008 Jan-Feb;14(1):29-32. PMID 18091037.

16. Bosch JL, E. Pogue, J. Arnold, J. M. Dagenais, G. R. Yusuf, S. Long-term effects of ramipril on cardiovascular events and on diabetes: results of the HOPE study extension. Circulation. 2005 Aug 30;112(9):1339-46. PMID 16129815.

17. Bourn DMM, J. I. McSkimming, B. J. Waldron, M. A. Wishart, J. D. Impaired glucose tolerance and NIDDM: does a lifestyle intervention program have an effect? Diabetes Care. 1994 Nov;17(11):1311-9. PMID 7821173.

18. Brinkworth GDN, M. Keogh, J. B. Luscombe, N. D. Wittert, G. A. Clifton, P. M. Long-term effects of a high-protein, low-carbohydrate diet on weight control and cardiovascular risk markers in obese hyperinsulinemic subjects. Int J Obes Relat Metab Disord. 2004 May;28(5):661-70. PMID 15007396.

19. Brinkworth GDN, M. Buckley, J. D. Keogh, J. B. Clifton, P. M. Long-term effects of a very-low-carbohydrate weight loss diet compared with an isocaloric low-fat diet after 12 mo. Am J Clin Nutr. 2009 Jul;90(1):23-32. PMID 19439458.

20. Brinkworth GDN, M. Parker, B. Foster, P. Clifton, P. M. Long-term effects of advice to consume a high-protein, low-fat diet, rather than a conventional weight-loss diet, in obese adults with type 2 diabetes: one-year follow-up of a randomised trial. Diabetologia. 2004 Oct;47(10):1677-86. PMID 15480538.

21. Brown SAB, S. A. Kouzekanani, K. Garcia, A. A. Winchell, M. Hanis, C. L. Dosage effects of diabetes self-management education for Mexican Americans: the Starr County Border Health Initiative. Diabetes Care. 2005 Mar;28(3):527-32. PMID 15735182.

22. Bruce DGC, E. M. Campbell, L. V. Chisholm, D. J. Insulin therapy in patients with poorly controlled non-insulin dependent diabetes mellitus. Med J Aust. 1987 Mar 2;146(5):240-2. PMID 3547052.

23. Brun JFB, S. Mercier, J. Jaussent, A. Picot, M. C. Prefaut, C. Cost-sparing effect of twice-weekly targeted endurance training in type 2 diabetics: a one-year controlled randomized trial. Diabetes Metab. 2008 Jun;34(3):258-65. PMID 18468933.

24. Buchanan TAX, A. H. Peters, R. K. Kjos, S. L. Marroquin, A. Goico, J. Ochoa, C. Tan, S. Berkowitz, K. Hodis, H. N. Azen, S. P. Preservation of pancreatic beta-cell function and prevention of type 2 diabetes by pharmacological treatment of insulin resistance in high-risk hispanic women. Diabetes. 2002 Sep;51(9):2796-803. PMID 12196473.

25. Buse JBG, B. Mathias, N. P. Nelson, D. M. Faja, B. W. Whitcomb, R. W. Troglitazone use in insulin-treated type 2 diabetic patients. The Troglitazone Insulin Study Group. Diabetes Care. 1998 Sep;21(9):1455-61. PMID 9727891.

26. Calle-Pascual ALR, C. Camacho, F. Sanchez, R. Martin-Alvarez, P. J. Yuste, E. Hidalgo, I. Diaz, R. J. Calle, J. R. Charro, A. L. Behaviour modification in obese subjects with type 2 diabetes mellitus. Diabetes Res Clin Pract. 1992 Feb;15(2):157-62. PMID 1563332.

27. Campbell EMR, S. Moffitt, P. S. Sanson-Fisher, R. W. The relative effectiveness of educational and behavioral instruction programs for patients with NIDDM: a randomized trial. Diabetes Educ. 1996 Jul-Aug;22(4):379-86. PMID 8846745.

28. Carr DBU, K. M. Boyko, E. J. Asberry, P. J. Hull, R. L. Kodama, K. Callahan, H. S. Matthys, C. C. Leonetti, D. L. Schwartz, R. S. Kahn, S. E. Fujimoto, W. Y. A reduced-fat diet and aerobic exercise in Japanese Americans with impaired glucose tolerance decreases intra-abdominal fat and improves insulin sensitivity but not beta-cell function. Diabetes. 2005 Feb;54(2):340-7. PMID 15677490.

29. Chiasson J-LJ, Robert G. Gomis, Ramon Hanefeld, Markolf Karasik, Avraham Laakso, Markku. Acarbose for prevention of type 2 diabetes mellitus: the STOP-NIDDM randomised trial. The Lancet. 2002;359(9323):2072-7.

30. Chiasson JLJ, R. G. Gomis, R. Hanefeld, M. Karasik, A. Laakso, M. Acarbose for the prevention of Type 2 diabetes, hypertension and cardiovascular disease in subjects with impaired glucose tolerance: facts and interpretations concerning the critical analysis of the STOP-NIDDM Trial data. Diabetologia. 2004 Jun;47(6):969-75; discussion 76-7. PMID 15164169.

31. Chiasson JLJ, R. G. Gomis, R. Hanefeld, M. Karasik, A. Laakso, M. Acarbose treatment and the risk of cardiovascular disease and hypertension in patients with impaired glucose tolerance: the STOP-NIDDM trial. JAMA. 2003 Jul 23;290(4):486-94. PMID 12876091.

32. Christian JGB, D. H. Byers, T. E. Christian, K. K. Goldstein, M. G. Bock, B. C. Clinic-based support to help overweight patients with type 2 diabetes increase physical activity and lose weight. Arch Intern Med. 2008 Jan 28;168(2):141-6. PMID 18227359.

33. Clark MH, S. E. Avery, L. Simpson, R. Effects of a tailored lifestyle self-management intervention in patients with type 2 diabetes. Br J Health Psychol. 2004 Sep;9(Pt 3):365-79. PMID 15296683.

34. Clarke PG, A. Adler, A. Stevens, R. Raikou, M. Cull, C. Stratton, I. Holman, R. Cost-effectiveness analysis of intensive blood-glucose control with metformin in overweight patients with type II diabetes (UKPDS No. 51). Diabetologia. 2001 Mar;44(3):298-304. PMID 11317659.

35. Collins RA, J. Parish, S. Sleigh, P. Peto, R. MRC/BHF Heart Protection Study of cholesterol-lowering with simvastatin in 5963 people with diabetes: a randomised placebo-controlled trial. Lancet. 2003 Jun 14;361(9374):2005-16. PMID 12814710.

36. Corpeleijn EF, E. J. Jansen, E. H. Mensink, M. Saris, W. H. de Bruin, T. W. Blaak, E. E. Improvements in glucose tolerance and insulin sensitivity after lifestyle intervention are related to changes in serum fatty acid profile and desaturase activities: the SLIM study. Diabetologia. 2006 Oct;49(10):2392-401. PMID 16896932.

37. Crandall JS, D. Ma, Y. Fujimoto, W. Y. Barrett-Connor, E. Fowler, S. Dagogo-Jack, S. Andres, R. The influence of age on the effects of lifestyle modification and metformin in prevention of diabetes. J Gerontol A Biol Sci Med Sci. 2006 Oct;61(10):1075-81. PMID 17077202.

38. Daly RMD, D. W. Owen, N. Jolley, D. Shaw, J. E. Zimmet, P. Z. Does high-intensity resistance training maintain bone mass during moderate weight loss in older overweight adults with type 2 diabetes? Osteoporos Int. 2005 Dec;16(12):1703-12. PMID 15937634.

39. Davis TMC, C. A. Holman, R. R. Relationship between ethnicity and glycemic control, lipid profiles, and blood pressure during the first 9 years of type 2 diabetes: U.K. Prospective Diabetes Study (UKPDS 55). Diabetes Care. 2001 Jul;24(7):1167-74. PMID 11423497.

40. Deakin TAC, J. E. Williams, R. Greenwood, D. C. Structured patient education: the diabetes X-PERT Programme makes a difference. Diabet Med. 2006 Sep;23(9):944-54. PMID 16922700.

41. Despres JPG, A. Sjostrom, L. Effects of rimonabant on metabolic risk factors in overweight patients with dyslipidemia. N Engl J Med. 2005 Nov 17;353(20):2121-34. PMID 16291982.

42. Di Loreto CF, C. Lucidi, P. Murdolo, G. De Cicco, A. Parlanti, N. Ranchelli, A. Fatone, C. Taglioni, C. Santeusanio, F. De Feo, P. Make your diabetic patients walk: long-term impact of different amounts of physical activity on type 2 diabetes. Diabetes Care. 2005 Jun;28(6):1295-302. PMID 15920042.

43. Diabetes Prevention Program Research Group. Effects of Withdrawal From Metformin on the Development of Diabetes in the Diabetes Prevention Program. Diabetes Care. 2003 April 2003;26(4):977-80.

44. Diabetes Prevention Program Research Group. Reduction in the Incidence of Type 2 Diabetes with Lifestyle Intervention or Metformin. N Engl J Med. 2002 February 7, 2002;346(6):393-403.

45. Dixon ANV, G. Hanif, M. W. Field, A. Boutsiadis, A. Harte, A. McTernan, P. G. Barnett, A. H. Kumar, S. Effect of the orlistat on serum endotoxin lipopolysaccharide and adipocytokines in South Asian individuals with impaired glucose tolerance. Int J Clin Pract. 2008 Jul;62(7):1124-9. PMID 18564278.

46. DREAM. Effect of ramipril on the incidence of diabetes. N Engl J Med. 2006;355:1608-10.

47. Dunstan DWD, R. M. Owen, N. Jolley, D. Vulikh, E. Shaw, J. Zimmet, P. Home-based resistance training is not sufficient to maintain improved glycemic control following supervised training in older individuals with type 2 diabetes. Diabetes Care. 2005 Jan;28(1):3-9. PMID 15616225.

48. Ebbeling CBL, M. M. Sinclair, K. B. Seger-Shippee, L. G. Feldman, H. A. Ludwig, D. S. Effects of an ad libitum low-glycemic load diet on cardiovascular disease risk factors in obese young adults. Am J Clin Nutr. 2005 May;81(5):976-82. PMID 15883418.

49. Eeley EAS, I. M. Hadden, D. R. Turner, R. C. Holman, R. R. UKPDS 18: estimated dietary intake in type 2 diabetic patients randomly allocated to diet, sulphonylurea or insulin therapy. UK Prospective Diabetes Study Group. Diabet Med. 1996 Jul;13(7):656-62. PMID 8840101.

50. Eriksson JL, J. Valle, T. Aunola, S. Hamalainen, H. Ilanne-Parikka, P. Keinanen-Kiukaanniemi, S. Laakso, M. Lauhkonen, M. Lehto, P. Lehtonen, A. Louheranta, A. Mannelin, M. Martikkala, V. Rastas, M. Sundvall, J. Turpeinen, A. Viljanen, T. Uusitupa, M. Tuomilehto, J. Prevention of Type II diabetes in subjects with impaired glucose tolerance: the Diabetes Prevention Study (DPS) in Finland. Study design and 1-year interim report on the feasibility of the lifestyle intervention programme. Diabetologia. 1999 Jul;42(7):793-801. PMID 10440120.

51. Eriksson KFL, F. No excess 12-year mortality in men with impaired glucose tolerance who participated in the Malmo Preventive Trial with diet and exercise. Diabetologia. 1998 Sep;41(9):1010-6. PMID 9754818.

52. Eriksson KFL, F. Prevention of type 2 (non-insulin-dependent) diabetes mellitus by diet and physical exercise. The 6-year Malmo feasibility study. Diabetologia. 1991 Dec;34(12):891-8. PMID 1778354.

53. Esposito KM, M. I. Ciotola, M. Di Palo, C. Scognamiglio, P. Gicchino, M. Petrizzo, M. Saccomanno, F. Beneduce, F. Ceriello, A. Giugliano, D. Effects of a Mediterranean-style diet on the need for antihyperglycemic drug therapy in patients with newly diagnosed type 2 diabetes: a randomized trial. Ann Intern Med. 2009 Sep 1;151(5):306-14. PMID 19721018.

54. Fitz JDS, E. M. Fein, H. G. A hypocaloric high-protein diet as primary therapy for adults with obesity-related diabetes: effective long-term use in a community hospital. Diabetes Care. 1983 Jul-Aug;6(4):328-33. PMID 6617408.

55. Fontbonne AD, I. Baccara-Dinet, M. Eschwege, E. Charles, M. A. Effects of 1-year treatment with metformin on metabolic and cardiovascular risk factors in non-diabetic upper-body obese subjects with mild glucose anomalies: a post-hoc analysis of the BIGPRO1 trial. Diabetes Metab. 2009 Nov;35(5):385-91. PMID 19665415.

56. Forlani GL, C. Moscatiello, S. Ridolfi, V. Melchionda, N. Di Domizio, S. Marchesini, G. Are behavioural approaches feasible and effective in the treatment of type 2 diabetes? A propensity score analysis vs. prescriptive diet. Nutrition, Metabolism and Cardiovascular Diseases. 2009;19(5):313-20.

57. Fraser AA, R. Lawlor, D. A. Fraser, D. Elhayany, A. A modified Mediterranean diet is associated with the greatest reduction in alanine aminotransferase levels in obese type 2 diabetes patients: results of a quasi-randomised controlled trial. Diabetologia. 2008 Sep;51(9):1616-22. PMID 18597068.

58. Freeman DJN, J. Sattar, N. Neely, R. D. Cobbe, S. M. Ford, I. Isles, C. Lorimer, A. R. Macfarlane, P. W. McKillop, J. H. Packard, C. J. Shepherd, J. Gaw, A. Pravastatin and the development of diabetes mellitus: evidence for a protective treatment effect in the West of Scotland Coronary Prevention Study. Circulation. 2001 Jan 23;103(3):357-62. PMID 11157685.

59. Fujimoto WYJ, K. A. Bray, G. A. Kriska, A. Barrett-Connor, E. Haffner, S. Hanson, R. Hill, J. O. Hubbard, V. Stamm, E. Pi-Sunyer, F. X. Body size and shape changes and the risk of diabetes in the diabetes prevention program. Diabetes. 2007 Jun;56(6):1680-5. PMID 17363740.

60. Gaede PL-A, H. Parving, H. H. Pedersen, O. Effect of a multifactorial intervention on mortality in type 2 diabetes. N Engl J Med. 2008 Feb 7;358(6):580-91. PMID 18256393.

61. Gallagher AH, W. Abraira, C. Dietary patterns and metabolic control in diabetic diets: a prospective study of 51 outpatient men on unmeasured and exchange diets. J Am Coll Nutr. 1987 Dec;6(6):525-32. PMID 3693756.

62. Gerstein HCY, S. Bosch, J. Pogue, J. Sheridan, P. Dinccag, N. Hanefeld, M. Hoogwerf, B. Laakso, M. Mohan, V. Shaw, J. Zinman, B. Holman, R. R. Effect of rosiglitazone on the frequency of diabetes in patients with impaired glucose tolerance or impaired fasting glucose: a randomised controlled trial. Lancet. 2006 Sep 23;368(9541):1096-105. PMID 16997664.

63. Gilliland SSA, S. P. Perez, G. E. Carter, J. S. Strong in body and spirit: lifestyle intervention for Native American adults with diabetes in New Mexico. Diabetes Care. 2002 Jan;25(1):78-83. PMID 11772905.

64. Group TDPPR. Effect of weight loss with lifestyle intervention on risk of diabetes. . Diabetes Care. 2006;29:2192-07.

65. Gruesser MB, U. Ellermann, P. Kronsbein, P. Joergens, V. Evaluation of a structured treatment and teaching program for non-insulin-treated type II diabetic outpatients in Germany after the nationwide introduction of reimbursement policy for physicians. Diabetes Care. 1993 Sep;16(9):1268-75. PMID 8404431.

66. Guare JCW, R. R. Grant, A. Comparison of obese NIDDM and nondiabetic women: short- and long-term weight loss. Obes Res. 1995 Jul;3(4):329-35. PMID 8521149.

67. Gurka MJW, A. M. Conaway, M. R. Crowther, J. Q. Nadler, J. L. Bovbjerg, V. E. Lifestyle intervention in obese patients with type 2 diabetes: impact of the patient's educational background. Obesity (Silver Spring). 2006 Jun;14(6):1085-92. PMID 16861614.

68. Gurlek AE, T. Gedik, O. Frequency of severe hypoglycaemia in type 1 and type 2 diabetes during conventional insulin therapy. Exp Clin Endocrinol Diabetes. 1999;107(3):220-4. PMID 10376450.

69. Haffner ST, M. Crandall, J. Fowler, S. Goldberg, R. Horton, E. Marcovina, S. Mather, K. Orchard, T. Ratner, R. Barrett-Connor, E. Intensive lifestyle intervention or metformin on inflammation and coagulation in participants with impaired glucose tolerance. Diabetes. 2005 May;54(5):1566-72. PMID 15855347.

70. Haimoto HI, M. Wakai, K. Umegaki, H. Long-term effects of a diet loosely restricting carbohydrates on HbA1c levels, BMI and tapering of sulfonylureas in type 2 diabetes: a 2-year follow-up study. Res Clin Pract. 2008;79:350-6.

71. Hamalainen HR, T. Virtanen, A. Lindstrom, J. Eriksson, J. G. Valle, T. T. Ilanne-Parikka, P. Keinanen-Kiukaanniemi, S. Rastas, M. Aunola, S. Uusitupa, M. Tuomilehto, J. Improved fibrinolysis by an intensive lifestyle intervention in subjects with impaired glucose tolerance. The Finnish Diabetes Prevention Study. Diabetologia. 2005 Nov;48(11):2248-53. PMID 16205886.

72. Hamman RFW, R. R. Edelstein, S. L. Lachin, J. M. Bray, G. A. Delahanty, L. Hoskin, M. Kriska, A. M. Mayer-Davis, E. J. Pi-Sunyer, X. Regensteiner, J. Venditti, B. Wylie-Rosett, J. Effect of weight loss with lifestyle intervention on risk of diabetes. Diabetes Care. 2006 Sep;29(9):2102-7. PMID 16936160.

73. Hanefeld MF, S. Schmechel, H. Rothe, G. Schulze, J. Dude, H. Schwanebeck, U. Julius, U. Diabetes Intervention Study. Multi-intervention trial in newly diagnosed NIDDM. Diabetes Care. 1991 Apr;14(4):308-17. PMID 2060433.

74. Hanefeld MS, G. The effects of orlistat on body weight and glycaemic control in overweight patients with type 2 diabetes: a randomized, placebo-controlled trial. Diabetes Obes Metab. 2002 Nov;4(6):415-23. PMID 12406041.

75. Heart Outcomes Prevention Evaluation Study Investigators. Effects of ramipril on cardiovascular and microvascular outcomes in people with diabetes mellitus: results of the HOPE study and MICRO-HOPE substudy. . Lancet. 2000 Jan 22;355(9200):253-9. PMID 10675071.

76. Heath GWW, R. H. Smith, J. Leonard, B. E. Community-based exercise and weight control: diabetes risk reduction and glycemic control in Zuni Indians. Am J Clin Nutr. 1991 Jun;53(6 Suppl):1642S-6S. PMID 2031500.

77. Heitzmann CAK, R. M. Wilson, D. K. Sandler, J. Sex differences in weight loss among adults with type II diabetes mellitus. J Behav Med. 1987 Apr;10(2):197-211. PMID 3612778.

78. Heller SRC, P. Daly, H. Davis, I. McCulloch, D. K. Allison, S. P. Tattersall, R. B. Group education for obese patients with type 2 diabetes: greater success at less cost. Diabet Med. 1988 Sep;5(6):552-6. PMID 2974778.

79. Herder CP, M. Koenig, W. Kraft, I. Muller-Scholze, S. Martin, S. Lakka, T. Ilanne-Parikka, P. Eriksson, J. G. Hamalainen, H. Keinanen-Kiukaanniemi, S. Valle, T. T. Uusitupa, M. Lindstrom, J. Kolb, H. Tuomilehto, J. Systemic immune mediators and lifestyle changes in the prevention of type 2 diabetes: results from the Finnish Diabetes Prevention Study. Diabetes. 2006 Aug;55(8):2340-6. PMID 16873699.

80. Hockaday TDH, J. M. Mann, J. I. Turner, R. C. Prospective comparison of modified fat-high-carbohydrate with standard low-carbohydrate dietary advice in the treatment of diabetes: one year follow-up study. Br J Nutr. 1978 Mar;39(2):357-62. PMID 629924.

81. Hollander P. Endocannabinoid blockade for improving glycemic control and lipids in patients with type 2 diabetes mellitus. Am J Med. 2007 Feb;120(2 Suppl 1):S18-28; discussion S9-32. PMID 17296341.

82. Hollander PAE, S. C. Hirsch, I. B. Kelley, D. McGill, J. Taylor, T. Weiss, S. R. Crockett, S. E. Kaplan, R. A. Comstock, J. Lucas, C. P. Lodewick, P. A. Canovatchel, W. Chung, J. Hauptman, J. Role of orlistat in the treatment of obese patients with type 2 diabetes. A 1-year randomized double-blind study. Diabetes Care. 1998 Aug;21(8):1288-94. PMID 9702435.

83. Holloszy JOS, J. Kusnierkiewicz, J. Hagberg, J. M. Ehsani, A. A. Effects of exercise on glucose tolerance and insulin resistance. Brief review and some preliminary results. Acta Med Scand Suppl. 1986;711:55-65. PMID 3535414.

84. Holman RRC, C. A. Turner, R. C. A randomized double-blind trial of acarbose in type 2 diabetes shows improved glycemic control over 3 years (U.K. Prospective Diabetes Study 44). Diabetes Care. 1999 Jun;22(6):960-4. PMID 10372249.

85. Horrocks PMB, R. Wright, A. D. A long-term follow-up of dietary advice in maturity onset diabetes: the experience of one centre in the UK prospective study. Diabet Med. 1987 May-Jun;4(3):241-4. PMID 2956027.

86. Hughes TAK, J. O. Segrest, J. P. Effects of glyburide therapy on lipoproteins in non-insulin-dependent diabetes mellitus. Am J Med. 1985 Sep 20;79(3B):86-91. PMID 3931466.

87. Hypertension in Diabetes Study III. Prospective study of therapy of hypertension in type 2 diabetic patients: efficacy of ACE inhibition and beta-blockade. Diabet Med. 1994 Oct;11(8):773-82. PMID 7851072.

88. Jarrett RJK, H. Fuller, J. H. McCartney, M. Worsening to diabetes in men with impaired glucose tolerance ("borderline diabetes"). Diabetologia. 1979 Jan;16(1):25-30. PMID 761734.

89. Johnston PSL, H. E. Coniff, R. F. Simonson, D. C. Raskin, P. Munera, C. L. Advantages of alpha-glucosidase inhibition as monotherapy in elderly type 2 diabetic patients. J Clin Endocrinol Metab. 1998 May;83(5):1515-22. PMID 9589648.

90. Jonsson BC, J. R. Pedersen, T. R. The cost-effectiveness of lipid lowering in patients with diabetes: results from the 4S trial. Diabetologia. 1999 Nov;42(11):1293-301. PMID 10550412.

91. Kaplan RMH, S. L. Wilson, D. K. Wallace, J. P. Effects of diet and exercise interventions on control and quality of life in non-insulin-dependent diabetes mellitus. J Gen Intern Med. 1987 Jul-Aug;2(4):220-8. PMID 3302144.

92. Karlstrom BN, M. Vessby, B. Dietary habits and effects of dietary advice in patients with type 2 diabetes. Results from a one-year intervention study. Eur J Clin Nutr. 1989 Jan;43(1):59-68. PMID 2543554.

93. Kawamori RT, N. Iwamoto, Y. Kashiwagi, A. Shimamoto, K. Kaku, K. [Alpha-glucosidase inhibitor for the prevention of type 2 diabetes mellitus: a randomised, double-blind trial in Japanese subjects with impaired glucose tolerance]. Nippon Rinsho. 2009 Sep;67(9):1821-5. PMID 19768922.

94. Kawamori RT, N. Iwamoto, Y. Kashiwagi, A. Shimamoto, K. Kaku, K. Voglibose for prevention of type 2 diabetes mellitus: a randomised, double-blind trial in Japanese individuals with impaired glucose tolerance. Lancet. 2009 May 9;373(9675):1607-14. PMID 19395079.

95. Keech AS, R. J. Barter, P. Best, J. Scott, R. Taskinen, M. R. Forder, P. Pillai, A. Davis, T. Glasziou, P. Drury, P. Kesaniemi, Y. A. Sullivan, D. Hunt, D. Colman, P. d'Emden, M. Whiting, M. Ehnholm, C. Laakso, M. Effects of long-term fenofibrate therapy on cardiovascular events in 9795 people with type 2 diabetes mellitus (the FIELD study): randomised controlled trial. Lancet. 2005 Nov 26;366(9500):1849-61. PMID 16310551.

96. Keen HJ, R. J. Ward, J. D. Fuller, J. H. Borderline diabetics and their response to tolbutamide. Adv Metab Disord. 1973;2:Suppl 2:521-31. PMID 4720382.

97. Keen HJ, R. J. McCartney, P. The ten-year follow-up of the Bedford survey (1962-1972): glucose tolerance and diabetes. Diabetologia. 1982 Feb;22(2):73-8. PMID 7060852.

98. Kilo CD, J. Kalb, E. Evaluation of saftey and efficacy of gliclazide in non-insulin-dependent diabetic patients. Diabetes Res Clin Pract. 1991(14):79S-82S.

99. Kirk AM, N. MacIntyre, P. Fisher, M. Effects of a 12-month physical activity counselling intervention on glycaemic control and on the status of cardiovascular risk factors in people with Type 2 diabetes. Diabetologia. 2004 May;47(5):821-32. PMID 15138687.

100. Kirkman MSW, M. Landsman, P. B. Samsa, G. P. Shortliffe, E. A. Simel, D. L. Feussner, J. R. A telephone-delivered intervention for patients with NIDDM. Effect on coronary risk factors. Diabetes Care. 1994 Aug;17(8):840-6. PMID 7956628.

101. Kitabchi AET, M. Knowler, W. C. Kahn, S. E. Fowler, S. E. Haffner, S. M. Andres, R. Saudek, C. Edelstein, S. L. Arakaki, R. Murphy, M. B. Shamoon, H. Role of insulin secretion and sensitivity in the

evolution of type 2 diabetes in the diabetes prevention program: effects of lifestyle intervention and metformin. Diabetes. 2005 Aug;54(8):2404-14. PMID 16046308.

102. Klonoff DCB, J. B. Nielsen, L. L. Guan, X. Bowlus, C. L. Holcombe, J. H. Wintle, M. E. Maggs, D. G. Exenatide effects on diabetes, obesity, cardiovascular risk factors and hepatic biomarkers in patients with type 2 diabetes treated for at least 3 years. Curr Med Res Opin. 2008 Jan;24(1):275-86. PMID 18053320.

103. Knowler WCB-C, E. Fowler, S. E. Hamman, R. F. Lachin, J. M. Walker, E. A. Nathan, D. M. Reduction in the incidence of type 2 diabetes with lifestyle intervention or metformin. N Engl J Med. 2002 Feb 7;346(6):393-403. PMID 11832527.

104. Korhonen TU, M. Aro, A. Kumpulainen, T. Siitonen, O. Voutilainen, E. Pyorala, K. Efficacy of dietary instructions in newly diagnosed non-insulin-dependent diabetic patients. Comparison of two different patient education regimens. Acta Med Scand. 1987;222(4):323-31. PMID 3425385.

105. Kosaka KN, M. Kuzuya, T. Prevention of type 2 diabetes by lifestyle intervention: a Japanese trial in IGT males. Diabetes Res Clin Pract. 2005 Feb;67(2):152-62. PMID 15649575.

106. Kramer MKK, A. M. Venditti, E. M. Miller, R. G. Brooks, M. M. Burke, L. E. Siminerio, L. M. Solano, F. X. Orchard, T. J. Translating the Diabetes Prevention Program: a comprehensive model for prevention training and program delivery. Am J Prev Med. 2009 Dec;37(6):505-11. PMID 19944916.

107. Kudlacek SS, G. The effect of insulin treatment on HbA1c, body weight and lipids in type 2 diabetic patients with secondary-failure to sulfonylureas. A five year follow-up study. Horm Metab Res. 1992 Oct;24(10):478-83. PMID 1464414.

108. Kulzer BH, Norbert Gorges, Daniela Schwarz, Peter Haak, Thomas. Prevention of Diabetes Self-Management Program (PREDIAS): Effects on Weight, Metabolic Risk Factors, and Behavioral Outcomes. Diabetes Care. 2009 July 2009;32(7):1143-6.

109. Laaksonen DEL, J. Lakka, T. A. Eriksson, J. G. Niskanen, L. Wikstrom, K. Aunola, S. Keinanen-Kiukaanniemi, S. Laakso, M. Valle, T. T. Ilanne-Parikka, P. Louheranta, A. Hamalainen, H. Rastas, M. Salminen, V. Cepaitis, Z. Hakumaki, M. Kaikkonen, H. Harkonen, P. Sundvall, J. Tuomilehto, J. Uusitupa, M. Physical activity in the prevention of type 2 diabetes: the Finnish diabetes prevention study. Diabetes. 2005 Jan;54(1):158-65. PMID 15616024.

110. Lachin JMC, C. A. Edelstein, S. L. Ehrmann, D. A. Hamman, R. F. Kahn, S. E. Knowler, W. C. Nathan, D. M. Factors associated with diabetes onset during metformin versus placebo therapy in the diabetes prevention program. Diabetes. 2007 Apr;56(4):1153-9. PMID 17395752.

111. Laitinen JHA, I. E. Sarkkinen, E. S. Winberg, R. L. Harmaakorpi-Iivonen, P. A. Uusitupa, M. I. Impact of intensified dietary therapy on energy and nutrient intakes and fatty acid composition of serum lipids in patients with recently diagnosed non-insulin-dependent diabetes mellitus. J Am Diet Assoc. 1993 Mar;93(3):276-83. PMID 8382712.

112. Lehtovirta MF, B. Gullstrom, M. Haggblom, M. Eriksson, J. G. Taskinen, M. R. Groop, L. Metabolic effects of metformin in patients with impaired glucose tolerance. Diabet Med. 2001 Jul;18(7):578-83. PMID 11553189.

113. Lewis EJH, L. G. Clarke, W. R. Berl, T. Pohl, M. A. Lewis, J. B. Ritz, E. Atkins, R. C. Rohde, R. Raz, I. Renoprotective effect of the angiotensin-receptor antagonist irbesartan in patients with nephropathy due to type 2 diabetes. N Engl J Med. 2001 Sep 20;345(12):851-60. PMID 11565517.

114. Ley SJM, P. A. Scragg, R. K. Swinburn, B. A. Long-term effects of a reduced fat diet intervention on cardiovascular disease risk factors in individuals with glucose intolerance. Diabetes Res Clin Pract. 2004 Feb;63(2):103-12. PMID 14739050.

115. Li CLP, C. Y. Lu, J. M. Zhu, Y. Wang, J. H. Deng, X. X. Xia, F. C. Wang, H. Z. Wang, H. Y. Effect of metformin on patients with impaired glucose tolerance. Diabet Med. 1999 Jun;16(6):477-81. PMID 10391395.

116. Li ZH, K. Saltsman, P. DeShields, S. Bellman, M. Thames, G. Liu, Y. Wang, H. J. Elashoff, R. Heber, D. Long-term efficacy of soy-based meal replacements vs an individualized diet plan in obese type II DM patients: relative effects on weight loss, metabolic parameters, and C-reactive protein. Eur J Clin Nutr. 2005 Mar;59(3):411-8. PMID 15674301.

117. Liao DA, P. J. Shofer, J. B. Callahan, H. Matthys, C. Boyko, E. J. Leonetti, D. Kahn, S. E. Austin, M. Newell, L. Schwartz, R. S. Fujimoto, W. Y. Improvement of BMI, body composition, and body fat distribution with lifestyle modification in Japanese Americans with impaired glucose tolerance. Diabetes Care. 2002 Sep;25(9):1504-10. PMID 12196418.

118. Lindahl BN, T. K. Jansson, J. H. Asplund, K. Hallmans, G. Improved fibrinolysis by intense lifestyle intervention. A randomized trial in subjects with impaired glucose tolerance. J Intern Med. 1999 Jul;246(1):105-12. PMID 10447232.

119. Lindgarde F. The effect of orlistat on body weight and coronary heart disease risk profile in obese patients: the Swedish Multimorbidity Study. J Intern Med. 2000 Sep;248(3):245-54. PMID 10971792.

120. Lindstrom JE, J. G. Valle, T. T. Aunola, S. Cepaitis, Z. Hakumaki, M. Hamalainen, H. Ilanne-Parikka, P. Keinanen-Kiukaanniemi, S. Laakso, M. Louheranta, A. Mannelin, M. Martikkala, V. Moltchanov, V. Rastas, M. Salminen, V. Sundvall, J. Uusitupa, M. Tuomilehto, J. Prevention of diabetes mellitus in subjects with impaired glucose tolerance in the Finnish Diabetes Prevention Study: results from a randomized clinical trial. J Am Soc Nephrol. 2003 Jul;14(7 Suppl 2):S108-13. PMID 12819313.

121. Lindstrom JI-P, P. Peltonen, M. Aunola, S. Eriksson, J. G. Hemio, K. Hamalainen, H. Harkonen, P. Keinanen-Kiukaanniemi, S. Laakso, M. Louheranta, A. Mannelin, M. Paturi, M. Sundvall, J. Valle, T. T. Uusitupa, M. Tuomilehto, J. Sustained reduction in the incidence of type 2 diabetes by lifestyle intervention: follow-up of the Finnish Diabetes Prevention Study. Lancet. 2006 Nov 11;368(9548):1673-9. PMID 17098085.

122. Lindstrom JL, A. Mannelin, M. Rastas, M. Salminen, V. Eriksson, J. Uusitupa, M. Tuomilehto, J. The Finnish Diabetes Prevention Study (DPS): Lifestyle intervention and 3-year results on diet and physical activity. Diabetes Care. 2003 Dec;26(12):3230-6. PMID 14633807.

123. Lindstrom JP, M. Eriksson, J. G. Aunola, S. Hamalainen, H. Ilanne-Parikka, P. Keinanen-Kiukaanniemi, S. Uusitupa, M. Tuomilehto, J. Determinants for the effectiveness of lifestyle intervention in the Finnish Diabetes Prevention Study. Diabetes Care. 2008 May;31(5):857-62. PMID 18252900.

124. Lindstrom JP, M. Eriksson, J. G. Louheranta, A. Fogelholm, M. Uusitupa, M. Tuomilehto, J. High-fibre, low-fat diet predicts long-term weight loss and decreased type 2 diabetes risk: the Finnish Diabetes Prevention Study. Diabetologia. 2006 May;49(5):912-20. PMID 16541277.

125. Lindstrom JP, M. Tuomilehto, J. Lifestyle strategies for weight control: experience from the Finnish Diabetes Prevention Study. Proc Nutr Soc. 2005 Feb;64(1):81-8. PMID 15877926.

126. Manning RMJ, R. T. Leese, G. P. Newton, R. W. The comparison of four weight reduction strategies aimed at overweight diabetic patients. Diabet Med. 1995 May;12(5):409-15. PMID 7648803.

127. Manning RMJ, R. T. Leese, G. P. Newton, R. W. The comparison of four weight reduction strategies aimed at overweight patients with diabetes mellitus: four-year follow-up. Diabet Med. 1998 Jun;15(6):497-502. PMID 9632125.

128. Mazzuca SAM, N. H. Wheeler, M. L. Norton, J. A. Fineberg, N. S. Vinicor, F. Cohen, S. J. Clark, C. M., Jr. The diabetes education study: a controlled trial of the effects of diabetes patient education. Diabetes Care. 1986 Jan-Feb;9(1):1-10. PMID 3948638.

129. McAuley KAS, K. J. Taylor, R. W. McLay, R. T. Williams, S. M. Mann, J. I. Long-term effects of popular dietary approaches on weight loss and features of insulin resistance. Int J Obes (Lond). 2006 Feb;30(2):342-9. PMID 16158081.

130. McBride PEE, J. A. Grant, H. Sargent, C. Underbakke, G. Vitcenda, M. Zeller, L. Stein, J. H. Putting the Diabetes Prevention Program into practice: a program for weight loss and cardiovascular risk reduction for patients with metabolic syndrome or type 2 diabetes mellitus. J Nutr Health Aging. 2008 Dec;12(10):745S-9S. PMID 19043651.

131. McCarron DAR, M. E. Reducing cardiovascular disease risk with diet. Obes Res. 2001 Nov;9 Suppl 4:335S-40S. PMID 11707562.

132. Mensink MB, E. E. Corpeleijn, E. Saris, W. H. de Bruin, T. W. Feskens, E. J. Lifestyle intervention according to general recommendations improves glucose tolerance. Obes Res. 2003 Dec;11(12):1588-96. PMID 14694225.

133. Mensink MB, E. E. Wagenmakers, A. J. Saris, W. H. Lifestyle intervention and fatty acid metabolism in glucose-intolerant subjects. Obes Res. 2005 Aug;13(8):1354-62. PMID 16129717.

134. Mensink MF, E. J. Saris, W. H. De Bruin, T. W. Blaak, E. E. Study on Lifestyle Intervention and Impaired Glucose Tolerance Maastricht (SLIM): preliminary results after one year. Int J Obes Relat Metab Disord. 2003 Mar;27(3):377-84. PMID 12629566.

135. Mertes G. Efficacy and safety of acarbose in the treatment of type 2 diabetes: data from a 2-year surveillance study. Diabetes Res Clin Pract. 1998 Apr;40(1):63-70. PMID 9699092.

136. Metz JAS, J. S. Kris-Etherton, P. Reusser, M. E. Morris, C. D. Hatton, D. C. Oparil, S. Haynes, R. B. Resnick, L. M. Pi-Sunyer, F. X. Clark, S. Chester, L. McMahon, M. Snyder, G. W. McCarron, D. A. A randomized trial of improved weight loss with a prepared meal plan in overweight and obese patients: impact on cardiovascular risk reduction. Arch Intern Med. 2000 Jul 24;160(14):2150-8. PMID 10904458.

137. Molitch MEF, W. Hamman, R. F. Knowler, W. C. The diabetes prevention program and its global implications. J Am Soc Nephrol. 2003 Jul;14(7 Suppl 2):S103-7. PMID 12819312.

138. New JPM, J. M. Freemantle, N. Teasdale, S. Wong, L. M. Bruce, N. J. Burns, J. A. Gibson, J. M. Specialist nurse-led intervention to treat and control hypertension and hyperlipidemia in diabetes (SPLINT): a randomized controlled trial. Diabetes Care. 2003 Aug;26(8):2250-5. PMID 12882844.

139. Nielsen JVJ, E. Nilsson, A. K. Lasting improvement of hyperglycaemia and bodyweight: low-carbohydrate diet in type 2 diabetes. A brief report. Ups J Med Sci. 2005;110(2):179-83. PMID 16075898.

140. Nijpels GB, W. Dekker, J. M. Kostense, P. J. Bouter, L. M. Heine, R. J. A study of the effects of acarbose on glucose metabolism in patients predisposed to developing diabetes: the Dutch acarbose intervention study in persons with impaired glucose tolerance (DAISI). Diabetes Metab Res Rev. 2008 Nov-Dec;24(8):611-6. PMID 18756586.

141. Nissen SEW, K. Topol, E. J. Effect of muraglitazar on death and major adverse cardiovascular events in patients with type 2 diabetes mellitus. JAMA. 2005 Nov 23;294(20):2581-6. PMID 16239637.

142. Oldroyd JCU, N. C. White, M. Mathers, J. C. Alberti, K. G. Randomised controlled trial evaluating lifestyle interventions in people with impaired glucose tolerance. Diabetes Res Clin Pract. 2006 May;72(2):117-27. PMID 16297488.

143. Orchard TJT, M. Goldberg, R. Haffner, S. Ratner, R. Marcovina, S. Fowler, S. The effect of metformin and intensive lifestyle intervention on the metabolic syndrome: the Diabetes Prevention Program randomized trial. Ann Intern Med. 2005 Apr 19;142(8):611-9. PMID 15838067.

144. Page RCH, K. E. Cook, J. T. Turner, R. C. Can life-styles of subjects with impaired glucose tolerance be changed? A feasibility study. Diabet Med. 1992 Jul;9(6):562-6. PMID 1643806.

145. Pan XL, G. Hu, Y. [Effect of dietary and/or exercise intervention on incidence of diabetes in 530 subjects with impaired glucose tolerance from 1986-1992]. Zhonghua Nei Ke Za Zhi. 1995 Feb;34(2):108-12. PMID 7796655.

146. Pan XRL, G. W. Hu, Y. H. Wang, J. X. Yang, W. Y. An, Z. X. Hu, Z. X. Lin, J. Xiao, J. Z. Cao, H. B. Liu, P. A. Jiang, X. G. Jiang, Y. Y. Wang, J. P. Zheng, H. Zhang, H. Bennett, P. H. Howard, B. V. Effects of diet and exercise in preventing NIDDM in people with impaired glucose tolerance. The Da Qing IGT and Diabetes Study. Diabetes Care. 1997 Apr;20(4):537-44. PMID 9096977.

147. Perreault LK, Steven E. Christophi, Costas A. Knowler, William C. Hamman, Richard F. Regression From Pre-Diabetes to Normal Glucose Regulation in the Diabetes Prevention Program. Diabetes Care. 2009 September 2009;32(9):1583-8.

148. Pritchard DAH, J. Taba, F. Nutritional counselling in general practice: a cost effective analysis. J Epidemiol Community Health. 1999 May;53(5):311-6. PMID 10396539.

149. Ratner RG, R. Haffner, S. Marcovina, S. Orchard, T. Fowler, S. Temprosa, M. Impact of intensive lifestyle and metformin therapy on cardiovascular disease risk factors in the diabetes prevention program. Diabetes Care. 2005 Apr;28(4):888-94. PMID 15793191.

150. Ratzmann KPW, S. Schulz, B. The effect of long-term glibenclamide treatment on glucose tolerance, insulin secretion and serum lipids in subjects with impaired glucose tolerance. Diabete Metab. 1983 May-Jun;9(2):87-93. PMID 6413265.

151. Ratzmann KPZ, E. Witt, S. Schulz, B. [Effect of a combined diet-training program on the insulin sensitivity of obese persons with normal or disordered glucose tolerance]. Z Gesamte Inn Med. 1982 May 15;37(10):304-8. PMID 7048770.

152. Ridgeway NAH, D. R. Harvill, L. M. Falin, T. M. Forester, G. M. Gose, O. D. Improved control of type 2 diabetes mellitus: a practical education/behavior modification program in a primary care clinic. South Med J. 1999 Jul;92(7):667-72. PMID 10414474.

153. Rossner SS, L. Noack, R. Meinders, A. E. Noseda, G. Weight loss, weight maintenance, and improved cardiovascular risk factors after 2 years treatment with orlistat for obesity. European Orlistat Obesity Study Group. Obes Res. 2000 Jan;8(1):49-61. PMID 10678259.

154. Roumen CC, E. Feskens, E. J. Mensink, M. Saris, W. H. Blaak, E. E. Impact of 3-year lifestyle intervention on postprandial glucose metabolism: the SLIM study. Diabet Med. 2008 May;25(5):597-605. PMID 18445174.

155. Rowley KGD, M. Skinner, K. Skinner, M. White, G. A. O'Dea, K. Effectiveness of a community-directed 'healthy lifestyle' program in a remote Australian aboriginal community. Aust N Z J Public Health. 2000 Apr;24(2):136-44. PMID 10790932.

156. Samaras KH, C. S. Sullivan, D. Kelly, R. P. Campbell, L. V. Effects of postmenopausal hormone replacement therapy on central abdominal fat, glycemic control, lipid metabolism, and vascular factors in type 2 diabetes: a prospective study. Diabetes Care. 1999 Sep;22(9):1401-7. PMID 10480500.

157. Sanchez-Reyes LF, G. Yamamoto, J. Martinez-Rivas, L. Campos-Franco, E. Berber, A. Use of sibutramine in overweight adult hispanic patients with type 2 diabetes mellitus: a 12-month, randomized, double-blind, placebo-controlled clinical trial. Clin Ther. 2004 Sep;26(9):1427-35. PMID 15531005.

158. Sarkadi AR, U. Field test of a group education program for type 2 diabetes: measures and predictors of success on individual and group levels. Patient Educ Couns. 2001 Aug;44(2):129-39. PMID 11479053.

159. Sartor GS, B. Carlstrom, S. Melander, A. Norden, A. Persson, G. Ten-year follow-up of subjects with impaired glucose tolerance: prevention of diabetes by tolbutamide and diet regulation. Diabetes. 1980 Jan;29(1):41-9. PMID 7380107.

160. Scheen AJF, N. Hollander, P. Jensen, M. D. Van Gaal, L. F. Efficacy and tolerability of rimonabant in overweight or obese patients with type 2 diabetes: a randomised controlled study. Lancet. 2006 Nov 11;368(9548):1660-72. PMID 17098084.

161. Scheen AJP, N. Lefebvre, P. J. [United Kingdom Prospective Diabetes Study (UKPDS): 10 years later]. Rev Med Liege. 2008 Oct;63(10):624-9. PMID 19009971.

162. Scherbaum WAS, A. Mari, A. Nilsson, P. M. Lalanne, G. Jauffret, S. Foley, J. E. Efficacy and tolerability of vildagliptin in drug-naive patients with type 2 diabetes and mild hyperglycaemia*. Diabetes Obes Metab. 2008 Aug;10(8):675-82. PMID 18248490.

163. Sever PSD, B. Poulter, N. R. Wedel, H. Beevers, G. Caulfield, M. Collins, R. Kjeldsen, S. E. Kristinsson, A. McInnes, G. T. Mehlsen, J. Nieminen, M. O'Brien, E. Ostergren, J. Prevention of coronary and stroke events with atorvastatin in hypertensive patients who have average or lower-than-average cholesterol concentrations, in the Anglo-Scandinavian Cardiac Outcomes Trial--Lipid Lowering Arm (ASCOT-LLA): a multicentre randomised controlled trial. Drugs. 2004;64 Suppl 2:43-60. PMID 15765890.

164. Sever PSP, N. R. Dahlof, B. Wedel, H. Collins, R. Beevers, G. Caulfield, M. Kjeldsen, S. E. Kristinsson, A. McInnes, G. T. Mehlsen, J. Nieminen, M. O'Brien, E. Ostergren, J. Reduction in cardiovascular events with atorvastatin in 2,532 patients with type 2 diabetes: Anglo-Scandinavian Cardiac Outcomes Trial--lipid-lowering arm (ASCOT-LLA). Diabetes Care. 2005 May;28(5):1151-7. PMID 15855581.

165. Simmons DF, C. Voyle, J. Fou, F. Feo, S. Gatland, B. A pilot urban church-based programme to reduce risk factors for diabetes among Western Samoans in New Zealand. Diabet Med. 1998 Feb;15(2):136-42. PMID 9507914.

166. Simmons DV, J. A. Fou, F. Feo, S. Leakehe, L. Tale of two churches: differential impact of a church-based diabetes control programme among Pacific Islands people in New Zealand. Diabet Med. 2004 Feb;21(2):122-8. PMID 14984446.

167. Sirtori CRC, G. Manzato, E. Mancini, M. Rivellese, A. Paoletti, R. Pazzucconi, F. Pamparana, F. Stragliotto, E. One-year treatment with ethyl esters of n-3 fatty acids in patients with hypertriglyceridemia and glucose intolerance: reduced triglyceridemia, total cholesterol and increased HDL-C without glycemic alterations. Atherosclerosis. 1998 Apr;137(2):419-27. PMID 9622285.

168. Skarfors ETW, T. A. Lithell, H. Selinus, I. Physical training as treatment for type 2 (non-insulin-dependent) diabetes in elderly men. A feasibility study over 2 years. Diabetologia. 1987 Dec;30(12):930-3. PMID 3436489.

169. Sol BGvdG, Y. van der Bijl, J. J. Goessens, B. M. Visseren, F. L. The role of self-efficacy in vascular risk factor management: a randomized controlled trial. Patient Educ Couns. 2008 May;71(2):191-7. PMID 18242934.

170. Sone HK, A. Ishibashi, S. Abe, R. Saito, Y. Murase, T. Yamashita, H. Yajima, Y. Ito, H. Ohashi, Y. Akanuma, Y. Yamada, N. Effects of lifestyle modifications on patients with type 2 diabetes: the Japan Diabetes Complications Study (JDCS) study design, baseline analysis and three year-interim report. Horm Metab Res. 2002 Sep;34(9):509-15. PMID 12384828.

171. Stone DBC, W. E. The prolonged effects of a low cholesterol, high carbohydrate diet upon the serum lipids in diabetic patients. Diabetes. 1963 Mar-Apr;12:127-32. PMID 13984377.

172. Swinburn BAM, P. A. Ley, S. J. Long-term (5-year) effects of a reduced-fat diet intervention in individuals with glucose intolerance. Diabetes Care. 2001 Apr;24(4):619-24. PMID 11315819.

173. Takekoshi HM, K. Suzuki, Y. Atsumi, Y. Kubo, A. Hayashi, K. Horiuchi, A. A ten year follow up study in NIDDM with or without exercise. J Med Assoc Thai. 1987 Mar;70 Suppl 2:149-52. PMID 3598424.

174. Tapsell LCB, M. J. Teuss, G. Tan, S. Y. Dalton, S. Quick, C. J. Gillen, L. J. Charlton, K. E. Long-term effects of increased dietary polyunsaturated fat from walnuts on metabolic parameters in type II diabetes. Eur J Clin Nutr. 2009 Aug;63(8):1008-15. PMID 19352378.

175. Tate DFJ, E. H. Wing, R. R. Effects of Internet behavioral counseling on weight loss in adults at risk for type 2 diabetes: a randomized trial. JAMA. 2003 Apr 9;289(14):1833-6. PMID 12684363.

176. Taylor CBM, N. H. Reilly, K. R. Greenwald, G. Cunning, D. Deeter, A. Abascal, L. Evaluation of a nurse-care management system to improve outcomes in patients with complicated diabetes. Diabetes Care. 2003 Apr;26(4):1058-63. PMID 12663573.

177. Tenkanen LM, M. Manninen, V. Some coronary risk factors related to the insulin resistance syndrome and treatment with gemfibrozil. Experience from the Helsinki Heart Study. Circulation. 1995 Oct 1;92(7):1779-85. PMID 7671361.

178. Torgerson JSH, J. Boldrin, M. N. Sjostrom, L. XENical in the prevention of diabetes in obese subjects (XENDOS) study: a randomized study of orlistat as an adjunct to lifestyle changes for the prevention of type 2 diabetes in obese patients. Diabetes Care. 2004 Jan;27(1):155-61. PMID 14693982.

179. Torjesen PAB, K. I. Anderssen, S. A. Hjermann, I. Holme, I. Urdal, P. Lifestyle changes may reverse development of the insulin resistance syndrome. The Oslo Diet and Exercise Study: a randomized trial. Diabetes Care. 1997 Jan;20(1):26-31. PMID 9028689.

180. Trento MP, P. Borgo, E. Tomalino, M. Bajardi, M. Cavallo, F. Porta, M. A 5-year randomized controlled study of learning, problem solving ability, and quality of life modifications in people with type 2 diabetes managed by group care. Diabetes Care. 2004 Mar;27(3):670-5. PMID 14988283.

181. Trento MP, P. Tomalino, M. Bajardi, M. Pomero, F. Allione, A. Vaccari, P. Molinatti, G. M. Porta, M. Group visits improve metabolic control in type 2 diabetes: a 2-year follow-up. Diabetes Care. 2001 Jun;24(6):995-1000. PMID 11375359.

182. Trento MP, P. Bajardi, M. Tomalino, M. Grassi, G. Borgo, E. Donnola, C. Cavallo, F. Bondonio, P. Porta, M. Lifestyle intervention by group care prevents deterioration of Type II diabetes: a 4-year randomized controlled clinical trial. Diabetologia. 2002 Sep;45(9):1231-9. PMID 12242455.

183. Tuomilehto JL, J. Eriksson, J. G. Valle, T. T. Hamalainen, H. Ilanne-Parikka, P. Keinanen-Kiukaanniemi, S. Laakso, M. Louheranta, A. Rastas, M. Salminen, V. Uusitupa, M. Prevention of type 2

diabetes mellitus by changes in lifestyle among subjects with impaired glucose tolerance. N Engl J Med. 2001 May 3;344(18):1343-50. PMID 11333990.

184. Turner RC, C. Holman, R. United Kingdom Prospective Diabetes Study 17: a 9-year update of a randomized, controlled trial on the effect of improved metabolic control on complications in non-insulin-dependent diabetes mellitus. Ann Intern Med. 1996 Jan 1;124(1 Pt 2):136-45. PMID 8554206.

185. Turner RCC, C. A. Frighi, V. Holman, R. R. Glycemic control with diet, sulfonylurea, metformin, or insulin in patients with type 2 diabetes mellitus: progressive requirement for multiple therapies (UKPDS 49). UK Prospective Diabetes Study (UKPDS) Group. JAMA. 1999 Jun 2;281(21):2005-12. PMID 10359389.

186. U.K. Prospective Diabetes Study Group. Quality of life in type 2 diabetic patients is affected by complications but not by intensive policies to improve blood glucose or blood pressure control (UKPDS 37). Diabetes Care. 1999 Jul;22(7):1125-36. PMID 10388978.

187. UK Prospective Diabetes Study (UKPDS) Group. Intensive blood-glucose control with sulphonylureas or insulin compared with conventional treatment and risk of complications in patients with type 2 diabetes (UKPDS 33). Lancet. 1998 Sep 12;352(9131):837-53. PMID 9742976.

188. UK prospective study of therapies of maturity-onset diabetes I. Effect of diet, sulphonylurea, insulin or biguanide therapy on fasting plasma glucose and body weight over one year. Diabetologia. 1983 Jun;24(6):404-11. PMID 6350078.

189. U.K. prospective diabetes study II. Reduction in HbA1c with basal insulin supplement, sulfonylurea, or biguanide therapy in maturity-onset diabetes. A multicenter study. Diabetes. 1985 Aug;34(8):793-8. PMID 2862087.

190. UKPDS Group. UK Prospective Diabetes Study 7: response of fasting plasma glucose to diet therapy in newly presenting type II diabetic patients. Metabolism. 1990 Sep;39(9):905-12. PMID 2392060.

191. United Kingdom Prospective Diabetes Study 24. a 6-year, randomized, controlled trial comparing sulfonylurea, insulin, and metformin therapy in patients with newly diagnosed type 2 diabetes that could not be controlled with diet therapy. United Kingdom Prospective Diabetes Study Group. Ann Intern Med. 1998 Feb 1;128(3):165-75. PMID 9454524.

192. United Kingdom Prospective Diabetes Study (UKPDS). 13: Relative efficacy of randomly allocated diet, sulphonylurea, insulin, or metformin in patients with newly diagnosed non-insulin dependent diabetes followed for three years. BMJ. 1995 Jan 14;310(6972):83-8. PMID 7833731.

193. Uusitupa ML, V. Louheranta, A. Salopuro, T. Lindstrom, J. Tuomilehto, J. Long-term improvement in insulin sensitivity by changing lifestyles of people with impaired glucose tolerance: 4-year results from the Finnish Diabetes Prevention Study. Diabetes. 2003 Oct;52(10):2532-8. PMID 14514637.

194. Uusitupa MP, Markku Lindström, Jaana Aunola, Sirkka Ilanne-Parikka, Pirjo Keinänen-Kiukaanniemi, Sirkka Valle, Timo T. Eriksson, Johan G. Tuomilehto, Jaakko for the Finnish Diabetes Prevention Study, Group. Ten-Year Mortality and Cardiovascular Morbidity in the Finnish Diabetes Prevention Study—Secondary Analysis of the Randomized Trial. PLoS ONE. 2009;4(5):e5656.

195. van Sluijs EMvP, M. N. Twisk, J. W. Chin, A. Paw M. J. Calfas, K. J. van Mechelen, W. Effect of a tailored physical activity intervention delivered in general practice settings: results of a randomized controlled trial. Am J Public Health. 2005 Oct;95(10):1825-31. PMID 16186461.

196. Vanninen EU, M. Lansimies, E. Siitonen, O. Laitinen, J. Effect of metabolic control on autonomic function in obese patients with newly diagnosed type 2 diabetes. Diabet Med. 1993 Jan-Feb;10(1):66-73. PMID 8435991.

197. Vanninen EU, M. Siitonen, O. Laitinen, J. Lansimies, E. Habitual physical activity, aerobic capacity and metabolic control in patients with newly-diagnosed type 2 (non-insulin-dependent) diabetes mellitus: effect of 1-year diet and exercise intervention. Diabetologia. 1992 Apr;35(4):340-6. PMID 1516762.

198. Venojarvi MP, R. Hamalainen, H. Marniemi, J. Rastas, M. Rusko, H. Nuutila, P. Hanninen, O. Aunola, S. Role of skeletal muscle-fibre type in regulation of glucose metabolism in middle-aged subjects with impaired glucose tolerance during a long-term exercise and dietary intervention. Diabetes Obes Metab. 2005 Nov;7(6):745-54. PMID 16219019.

199. Wadden TAW, D. S. Neiberg, R. H. Wing, R. R. Ryan, D. H. Johnson, K. C. Foreyt, J. P. Hill, J. O. Trence, D. L. Vitolins, M. Z. One-year weight losses in the Look AHEAD study: factors associated with success. Obesity (Silver Spring). 2009 Apr;17(4):713-22. PMID 19180071.

200. Watanabe MY, K. Yokotsuka, M. Tango, T. Randomized controlled trial of a new dietary education program to prevent type 2 diabetes in a high-risk group of Japanese male workers. Diabetes Care. 2003 Dec;26(12):3209-14. PMID 14633803.

201. Wein PB, N. Harris, C. Permezel, M. A trial of simple versus intensified dietary modification for prevention of progression to diabetes mellitus in women with impaired glucose tolerance. Aust N Z J Obstet Gynaecol. 1999 May;39(2):162-6. PMID 10755770.

202. Weitgasser RL, M. Luger, A. Klingler, A. Effects of glimepiride on HbA(1c) and body weight in Type 2 diabetes: results of a 1.5-year follow-up study. Diabetes Res Clin Pract. 2003 Jul;61(1):13-9. PMID 12849919.

203. Wing RRK, R. Epstein, L. H. Nowalk, M. P. Gooding, W. Becker, D. Long-term effects of modest weight loss in type II diabetic patients. Arch Intern Med. 1987 Oct;147(10):1749-53. PMID 3310940.

204. Wolever TMG, A. L. Mehling, C. Chiasson, J. L. Connelly, P. W. Josse, R. G. Leiter, L. A. Maheux, P. Rabasa-Lhoret, R. Rodger, N. W. Ryan, E. A. The Canadian Trial of Carbohydrates in Diabetes (CCD), a 1-y controlled trial of low-glycemic-index dietary carbohydrate in type 2 diabetes: no effect on glycated hemoglobin but reduction in C-reactive protein. Am J Clin Nutr. 2008 Jan;87(1):114-25. PMID 18175744.

205. Woollard JB, V. Beilin, L. J. Verheijden, M. Bulsara, M. K. Effects of a general practice-based intervention on diet, body mass index and blood lipids in patients at cardiovascular risk. J Cardiovasc Risk. 2003 Feb;10(1):31-40. PMID 12569235.

206. Wright ADC, C. A. Macleod, K. M. Holman, R. R. Hypoglycemia in Type 2 diabetic patients randomized to and maintained on monotherapy with diet, sulfonylurea, metformin, or insulin for 6 years from diagnosis: UKPDS73. J Diabetes Complications. 2006 Nov-Dec;20(6):395-401. PMID 17070446.

207. Yamanouchi TS, T. Igarashi, K. Ichiyanagi, K. Watanabe, H. Kawasaki, T. Comparison of metabolic effects of pioglitazone, metformin, and glimepiride over 1 year in Japanese patients with newly diagnosed Type 2 diabetes. Diabet Med. 2005 Aug;22(8):980-5. PMID 16026361.

208. Yancy WS, Jr Westman, Eric C. McDuffie, Jennifer R. Grambow, Steven C. Jeffreys, Amy S. Bolton, Jamiyla Chalecki, Allison Oddone, Eugene Z. A Randomized Trial of a Low-Carbohydrate Diet vs Orlistat Plus a Low-Fat Diet for Weight Loss. Arch Intern Med. 2010 January 25, 2010;170(2):136-45.

209. Yates TD, Melanie Gorely, Trish Bull, Fiona Khunti, Kamlesh. Effectiveness of a Pragmatic Education Program Designed to Promote Walking Activity in Individuals With Impaired Glucose Tolerance. Diabetes Care. 2009 August 2009;32(8):1404-10.

210. Yusuf SG, H. Hoogwerf, B. Pogue, J. Bosch, J. Wolffenbuttel, B. H. Zinman, B. Ramipril and the development of diabetes. JAMA. 2001 Oct 17;286(15):1882-5. PMID 11597291.

Reject Wrong Population –Cancer Patients

1. Lanzarini E, Csendes A, Lembach H, et al. Evolution of type 2 diabetes mellitus in non morbid obese gastrectomized patients with Roux en-Y reconstruction: retrospective study. World J Surg. 2010 Sep;34(9):2098-102. PMID 20532768.

Reject N < 10, case reports / case series

1. Cohen RVS, C. A. Pinheiro, J. S. Correa, J. L. Rubino, F. Duodenal-jejunal bypass for the treatment of type 2 diabetes in patients with body mass index of 22-34 kg/m2: a report of 2 cases. Surg Obes Relat Dis. 2007 Mar-Apr;3(2):195-7. PMID 17386401.

2. Ikramuddin S, Leslie D, Swan T, et al. Outcomes of Roux-en Y gastric bypass for patients with BMI <35 Kg/M2. Obesity Surgery. 2010;20(8):998-9.

3. Lee HC, Kim MK, Kwon HS, et al. Early changes in incretin secretion after laparoscopic duodenal-jejunal bypass surgery in type 2 diabetic patients. Obes Surg. 2010 Nov;20(11):1530-5. PMID 20803098.

4. Yang JG, Wang CC, Huang J, et al. [Laparoscopic Roux-en-Y gastric bypass surgery for treatment of type 2 diabetes mellitus]. Nan Fang Yi Ke Da Xue Xue Bao. 2010 Jun;30(6):1373-5. PMID 20584680.

Reject Other

1. Moore HS, C. Hooper, L. Cruickshank, K. Vyas, A. Johnstone, P. Ashton, V. Kopelman, P. Dietary advice for treatment of type 2 diabetes mellitus in adults. Cochrane Database Syst Rev. 2004(3):CD004097. PMID 15266517.

2. Qin LK, Mirjam Corpeleijn, Eva Stolk, Ronald. Does physical activity modify the risk of obesity for type 2 diabetes: a review of epidemiological data. European Journal of Epidemiology. 2010;25(1):5-12.

3. Van de Laar FAL, P. L. Akkermans, R. P. Van de Lisdonk, E. H. De Grauw, W. J. Alpha-glucosidase inhibitors for people with impaired glucose tolerance or impaired fasting blood glucose. Cochrane Database Syst Rev. 2006(4):CD005061. PMID 17054235.